NURSES
TAKING
THE LEAD

Personal Qualities of
Effective Leadership

NURSES TAKING THE LEAD

Personal Qualities of Effective Leadership

Fay L. Bower, RN, DNSc, FAAN

Nurse Consultant
Clayton, California

W.B. Saunders Company
A Division of Harcourt Brace & Company
Philadelphia London Toronto Sydney

W.B. SAUNDERS COMPANY
A Division of Harcourt Brace & Company

The Curtis Center
Independence Square West
Philadelphia, Pennsylvania 19106

Library of Congress Cataloging-in-Publication Data

Nurses taking the lead: personal qualities of effective leadership / [edited by] Fay L. Bower.—1st ed.

p.   cm.

ISBN 0–7216–8169–7

1. Nursing services—Administration.   2. Leadership.   I. Bower, Fay Louise.
[DNLM: 1. Nursing.   2. Leadership Nurses' Instruction.   WY 16N97338
2000]

RT89.N635 2000   362.1′73′068—dc21

DNLM/DLC   99-31083

NURSES TAKING THE LEAD:
PERSONAL QUALITIES OF EFFECTIVE LEADERSHIP   ISBN 0–7216–8169–7

Printed in the United States of America

Last digit is the print number: 9   8   7   6   5   4   3   2   1

This book is dedicated to David, Carol, Dennis, and Tom,
my four children.

They are now adults with their own children,
but it is being their mother throughout the years
that has given me my best understanding
of what it means to "take the lead."

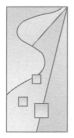

Contributors

Linda Arnold, RN, MSN
Psychiatric Clinical Nurse Specialist
President, Linda Arnold Motivates
Consultant and Professional Speaker
Brunswick, Maine

Fay L. Bower, RN, DNSc, FAAN
Nurse Consultant
Clayton, California

Gregory L. Crow, RN, MSN, EdD
Professor, Department of Nursing
Director, Nursing Leadership and
    Case Management Program
Sonoma State University
Rohnert Park, California
Senior Consultant, Tim Porter-
    O'Grady Associates
Atlanta, Georgia

Nancy Dickenson-Hazard, RN, MSN, FAAN
Executive Officer
Sigma Theta Tau International
Indianapolis, Indiana

Laura R. Mahlmeister, RN, PhD
President, Mahlmeister & Associates
Staff Nurse, The Birth Center at San
    Francisco General Hospital
San Francisco, California

Cynthia S. McCullough, RN, MSN
Senior Consultant, HDR, Inc.
Omaha, Nebraska

Terry W. Miller, RN, PhD
Dean and Professor of Nursing
School of Nursing
Pacific Lutheran University
Tacoma, Washington
Professor Emeritus
San Jose State University
San Jose, California

Daniel J. Pesut, RN, PhD, FAAN
Professor and Department Chair
Department of Environments for
    Health
Indiana University School of Nursing
Indianapolis, Indiana

Carol M. Rehtmeyer, RN, PhD
President, WellCom Group, Inc.
Omaha, Nebraska

Jane A. Root, PhD
Manager of Education and Training
Trustee Leadership Development
Curriculum Consultant
National Institute for Managed Care
    Education
Indianapolis, Indiana

Kathleen Rose-Grippa, RN, PhD
Professor and Director, School of
  Nursing
Ohio University
Athens, Ohio

Debra A. Sanders, RN, MAM
Director, HDR Consulting
HDR, Inc.
Omaha, Nebraska

Robinetta Wheeler, RN, PhD
Staff Nurse
Palo Alto Veterans' Health Care
  Systems
University of California, San
  Francisco–Stanford Health Care
Palo Alto, California

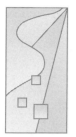

About the Authors

Linda Arnold, RN, MSN
Linda Arnold is a nurse entrepreneur with over 25 years of experience in nursing. She holds a bachelor's degree from Columbia University in New York and an MSN from the University of California, San Francisco. Before venturing forward as a nurse entrepreneur as president of Linda Arnold Motivates, she was a nurse administrator in a large community hospital. She also is a motivational speaker addressing topics such as transition, stress management, limit setting, and caretaking. She has also published a series of articles on the subject of co-dependency.

Fay L. Bower, RN, DNSc, FAAN
Fay L. Bower is an independent consultant with 40 years of experience in nursing. She earned a bachelor's degree from San Jose State College and master's and doctoral degrees from the University of California, San Francisco. She currently is a consultant to nursing and higher education and serves as an expert witness in malpractice health care cases. Her career has included a variety of positions. She was a faculty member, chair, coordinator of a graduate program, Dean, Vice President of Academic Affairs, and Director of Institutional Research and Planning before becoming the President of Clarkson College in Nebraska. Her professional activities include many positions with the National League for Nursing and the presidency of Sigma Theta Tau International during 1993–95. She has written many journal articles and books about a variety of issues in nursing. Her first book introduced the nursing process in the '70s. Her research has focused on nursing education and has been published in a variety of peer-reviewed journals.

Gregory L. Crow, RN, MSN, EdD
Gregory L. Crow has over 20 years of experience in nursing in a variety of roles and settings. He earned a bachelor's degree and a master's degree from the University of California, San Francisco, and a doctorate in education from the University of San Francisco. He has had a variety of administrative and leadership positions as Clinical Supervisor, Director of Nursing, and Assistant Hospital Administrator for Patient Care Services. Currently he is Professor and Director of the Nursing Leadership and Case Management Programs at Sonoma State University. He also directs an off-campus graduate program with Kaiser Permanente of California. He is an expert in organizational and systems development, creating motivational work environments, transformational change, and whole systems shared governance and is a senior consultant with Tim Porter-O'Grady and Associates.

Nancy Dickenson-Hazard, RN, MSN, FAAN

Nancy Dickenson-Hazard earned a bachelor's degree from the University of Kentucky and her master's degree from the University of Virginia. Currently she is the Executive Officer of Sigma Theta Tau International, the only honorary society in nursing and the second largest voluntary organization in nursing. She is a pediatric nurse practitioner with 12 years of experience as executive director of the National Certification Board of Pediatric Nurse Practitioners. She has served on numerous nursing editorial boards and is the author of many articles in peer-reviewed professional journals and nursing texts. She recently completed institute education in trustee leadership development.

Laura R. Mahlmeister, RN, PhD

Laura R. Mahlmeister is a nurse entrepreneur who received her bachelor's degree in nursing from Wayne State University and her master's and doctoral degrees from the University of California, San Francisco. Currently she is the president and co-founder of Mahlmeister & Associates, a national firm providing health care redesign and risk management consultative services and continuing education for health care professionals. She also has a part-time position as a labor and delivery nurse at San Francisco General Hospital, and serves as an expert witness in perinatal malpractice cases. She is co-author of *Maternal and Neonatal Nursing*, published by JB Lippincott, and is completing a textbook on legal issues in perinatal nursing. She co-authored two editions of *Comprehensive Maternity Nursing*, published by JB Lippincott, which won the 1990 AJN Book of the Year Award.

Cynthia S. McCullough, RN, MSN

Cynthia S. McCullough earned a bachelor's degree from Slippery Rock University and a master's degree in nursing from Clarkson College. She has over 16 years of experience in hospitals as a staff nurse and manager, including clinical manager of a nationally recognized transplant center, medical surgical units, outpatient clinics, and home care. She also has experience in patient-focused care, clinical and operations re-engineering, and self-directed work teams. Currently she is employed as a consultant with HDR in Omaha, Nebraska, which is a hospital designer and builder with services for the re-engineering of hospital staffing and care delivery systems.

Terry W. Miller, RN, PhD

Terry W. Miller earned two bachelor's degrees, one in nursing and another in zoology and chemistry, from the University of Oklahoma and his master's and doctoral degrees from the University of Texas, Austin. He currently is the Dean and Professor of Nursing at Pacific Lutheran University and prior to that held the positions of Associate Dean of the College of Applied Sciences and Arts and Professor at San Jose State University. He is also the only nurse to serve as chair of a baccalaureate level Department of Aviation. He and his wife, who is also a nurse, have a consulting firm, Miller-Randolph Associates, which provides services to health care agencies interested in risk management and program planning. He has frequently served as an expert witness and has done case analysis regarding policy failure and professional negligence.

Daniel J. Pesut, RN, PhD, FAAN

Daniel J. Pesut received his bachelor's degree from the University of Illinois, De Kalb, his master's degree from the University of Texas Health Science Center, San Antonio, and his doctoral degree from the University of Michigan. He has had many years of experience as a nurse clinician, educator, and researcher. Currently he is Professor and Department Chair of the Department of Environments for Health at Indiana University School of Nursing in Indianapolis, Indiana. Before that he was Associate Dean for Administrative Affairs in the College of Nursing at the University of South Carolina. He is a recognized master teacher, writes a monthly article on Futures for the *Journal of Professional Nursing,* and has an impressive list of publications in psychiatric nursing and critical thinking. His latest contribution is the publication of a book entitled *Clinical Reasoning: Art and Science.*

Carol M. Rehtmeyer, RN, PhD

Carol M. Rehtmeyer is a nurse entrepreneur. She has had many years of experience as a nurse clinician, educator, and researcher. After receiving a bachelor of science in nursing from Creighton University, Carol worked in a hospital and then returned to school to obtain a master of science in nursing from the University of Nebraska Medical Center, Omaha, and a PhD from the University of Nebraska, Lincoln. She held a faculty position and served as an academic dean. Following these experiences she was in sales and research positions. She also ran a home health care business and was Vice President and Chief Operating Officer for a 200-member physician group. Carol's latest venture is the successful launching of a telehealth business, WellCom Group, Inc.

Jane A. Root, PhD

Jane A. Root earned a bachelor of arts in speech and English, a master of arts in radio-television, and a doctorate in education. She is Manager of Education and Training at Trustee Leadership Development (TLD), a national leadership education program funded by Lilly Endowment. She is also a curriculum consultant for the National Institute for Managed Care Education. Prior to joining TLD, Jane worked for 23 years in hospital education and training.

Kathleen Rose-Grippa, RN, PhD

Kathleen Rose-Grippa has been active in nursing for 30 years. She received her bachelor's degree from the University of Kansas and her master's degree from the University of California, San Francisco. Her doctoral degree was earned from Stanford University. Her initial faculty position was at San Jose State University, where she taught critical care and psychiatric nursing. She joined the School of Nursing at Ohio University in 1987 and has been the director and professor since 1988. The program of nursing is an RN to BSN and serves the nurses of southeastern Ohio using distance education strategies.

Debra A. Sanders, RN, MAM

Debra A. Sanders earned a bachelor of science and master's in administrative management from Bellevue College (now University) in Bellevue, Nebraska. Currently she is employed as Director of Consulting at HDR, a national architectural firm that builds hospitals and other kinds of health care facilities. She has more than 20 years of nursing experience as both a clinician and a manager. Prior to joining HDR, she was a director, managing multiple product lines and locations in a large health care system in Omaha, Nebraska. She was instrumental in planning and implementing the Patient Focused Care delivery model for that system, which was one of the first locations in the nation to do so.

Robinetta Wheeler, RN, PhD

Robinetta Wheeler received a bachelor of science in nursing from New York University, her master of science in nursing from San Jose State University, and a PhD in sociology from the University of California, San Francisco. Her experiences include clinical, management, education, research, and entrepreneur assignments. In addition to working as a faculty member at San Jose State University, she worked with the University of Phoenix, San Jose campus. She has had considerable experience with community-based public/patient education programs focused on behavioral change. She is currently employed at UCSF-Stanford Health Care and the Palo Alto Veterans' Health Care Systems.

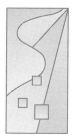

Preface

There is probably nothing more discussed or written about than leadership, for it is a particularly popular subject now, especially with the massive changes in the health care systems in the United States. This book is about leadership, but not the kind of leadership you usually read about. Many texts, popular publications, and presentations suggest that you can assume leadership roles if you have certain personal characteristics (the "great man" theory), can exert a particular style of leadership (autocratic, participatory, or laissez faire), know how to motivate others, or have a position of authority with the concomitant responsibility. This text presents a different perspective by pointing out that anyone can be a leader and that leadership occurs at many levels. Anyone can learn to take the lead using the twelve principles explained in this text; there are no special educational requirements. However, there are definite attitudes and important skills that allow one to be a leader.

Throughout the '90s there has been an incredible shift in the health care system from transactional-based medicine (fee-for-service) to aligned-lives health care (managed care). Hospitals, third-party payers, and physicians have entered into agreements on a per member per month (PMPM) basis whereby the cost of care is prepaid for a defined population. When changes of this magnitude take place, there is a rush to get into the action and thus a need for someone to "take the lead." Those who are quick enough to get to the table first with an attractive proposition are those who stage the changes. In the current arena of health care, physicians moved quickly to form associative businesses; hospitals were quick to entice physician groups to contract with them; and insurance companies were quick to package proposals no one could refuse. But where was nursing?

Pesut (1997) has said that nurses too often take a "wait and see" attitude and that "for too long nursing has been associated with the past or the here and now" (p. 107). He urges nurses to adopt a future-think perspective. That is what this book is about: taking the lead using futurist thinking. It is about ways that nurses at every level, in every kind of job, and in every type of practice can step forward and forge the way. It is about the kind of skills nurses need to develop so that they can take the lead, and it is about the attitudes that nurses need to cultivate that will put them in the forefront of change.

It is not too late for nurses at all levels to get into the act and to shift from being here-and-now doers to future-thinkers and shakers of the system. Each chapter of this book presents a different leadership principle and an example of how the principle allowed a nurse leader to take the lead. Nurses at different levels in a wide variety of jobs and positions were asked to share their experiences with change and to describe how the principle they write about helped them make that change.

No other collection of experiences like those found in this book is available; thus, this book is an excellent resource for nurses everywhere: for those in positions of leadership and for those wanting to be leaders, for those looking for something to "challenge them," and for those who feel "devalued" by the system. Hospital nurses, occupational nurses, home care nurses, community nurses, school nurses, entrepreneurial nurses, nurses attending college, and students preparing to be nurses will find this book a powerful asset for their careers no matter what they want to accomplish. It will be especially useful to student nurses who are developing skills for future use because they will need skills to fit the changes that have altered health care delivery, such as patient-focused care using self-directed work teams. Further, since more care is provided outside of the acute care agency, the nurse's ability to "take the lead" is more important now than ever before. New knowledge and expanded responsibilities and the ability to function with few resources and to make critical decisions demand that nurses have a new repertoire of leadership skills.

I am pleased to present this collection of future-thinkers and their contributions to system change, for I truly believe they have taken "the lead" and are excellent models for nurses everywhere. This book should help others to do the same.

FAY L. BOWER

Pesut, D. (1997). Facilitating futures thinking. *Nursing Outlook,* 45(4), 155.

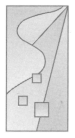

Acknowledgments

No author succeeds in completing a book all alone, even when there are no contributors. This book, however, would never have become a reality if it had not been for the wonderful nurses who contributed their stories about how they had "taken the lead." To them I am most grateful, for I know how hard it was to write about some of their experiences.

I also want to thank Mae Timmons for being the kind of friend every author needs. Her frankness and constructive criticism, while at times hard to accept, gave the book clarity, readability, and authenticity.

To all the nurses, administrators, and friends who I have been lucky enough to know and work with and who may recognize themselves in my stories, I also owe a huge thank-you. Their part in my professional career helped me learn to use the 12 principles outlined in this book and gave me the courage to share them with others.

Thanks also go to my husband, who is always there providing support, critique, and encouragement. Once again he urged me to pursue an idea, sustain the effort when I was tired and wished I hadn't begun, and complete what I believed needed to be published: stories about living heroes in nursing.

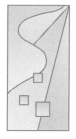

Contents

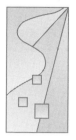

Chapter 1

Setting the Stage: An Introduction to the Principles

Fay L. Bower

Taking the lead . . . is leadership at a fundamental level. It is being aware of who you are, not being afraid to rock the boat, and being ready and willing to take a risk. Being at the lead is often not comfortable, but it is an exciting way to function. Taking the lead is not a new idea, for people have provided leadership throughout history. Some have been religious leaders, some have been politicians, and some have been military men.

Probably one of the most influential persons who has taken the lead was a nurse, Florence Nightingale. Like other leaders, she had a mission (in her case, a calling), the timing was right, change was needed, and she had the skills to take the lead. She was intelligent, resourceful, strong willed, and not willing to take "no" as an answer to her requests. Thus, she is seen as a visionary, a risk taker, and a proactive self-directed individual who devoted her life to the improvement of health care at a time when health care reform was needed. This occurred in the late 1850s (Lewinson, 1996).

Many other nurses have stepped forward to take the lead. Some have made it into history, such as Margaret Sanger, who was the founder of Planned Parenthood, and Lillian Wald, who was the founder of public health nursing. They were ordinary nurses doing what they believed was important at a time when there was a need for change. Many of these women devoted their lives to the mission they had adopted. Some even went to jail for the cause they believed in. However, many leaders in nursing have gone unnoticed even though they used the same skills as these great leaders. They went unnoticed not because their contributions were unimportant but because the changes they initiated occurred at every level and at a time when change was happening everywhere. Regardless of the kind of change or the level of its occurrence, the same leadership characteristics were present and are demonstrated by those who share their experiences in this book.

It has been said that there is leadership potential in every person. The mission of this book is to highlight the attitudes and skills of a leader so that more leaders can emerge. Leadership can be developed using the 12 principles outlined in this book:

1. Knowing self
2. Looking forward: being and becoming a futurist
3. Seeing the big picture (having a vision)
4. Building self-directed work teams
5. Taking a risk
6. Recognizing the right time for action
7. Seeing change as an opportunity
8. Being proactive, not reactive
9. Communicating effectively
10. Mentoring others
11. Letting go and taking on
12. Keeping informed

Every nurse must develop the attitudes, the motivation, and the skills to be a leader at any level. Attitudes, motivation, and skills are not birthrights, nor are they necessarily gained via education, although having an education helps. These leadership attributes can be acquired by anyone interested in their attainment. Because nurses are licensed to care for and protect the public, it is essential that these skills be possessed by every nurse and that every nurse act and take the lead.

The popular literature is full of information about the importance of leadership and how each individual must develop leadership skills. Clearly, leadership is defined differently today because what we face in this decade and what we will face in the next decade are different from what was previously experienced. In the 1950s, 1960s, 1970s, and 1980s, most nurses looked to others to provide "the way." Now it is the responsibility of every nurse to assume "the lead." In fact, there are those who suggest that leadership is a shared responsibility. The 12 principles support that position while making it clear that leadership occurs at many levels and at various times. One is not a leader all of the time, but a leader knows when the time is right to take the lead.

KNOWING SELF

Knowing who you are, state Prestwood and Schumann (1997), is the beginning of the journey to becoming a leader:

> We must understand what we know and what we don't know about ourselves. We must assess our resistance to—and tolerance for—change, our fears, our preferences, and our skills and abilities (p. 68).

Essentially, leaders must be aware of their strengths, their weaknesses, and the obstacles that keep them from exercising their ability to lead. They must be able to let go of personal agendas, become a member of the team, and use their abilities to help the team achieve their desired outcomes. Too often, nurses with valid and desirable goals fail to accomplish them because the goals are not those of the group. Personal awareness helps the individual know whether to lead, to follow, or to get out of the way. The kind of leadership that works in today's environment is to know which choice to take.

There are many ways to learn about one's self. Self-inspection is one way, and feedback from others is another. Frequent feedback on performance from colleagues, those in other departments, subordinates, supervisors, customers, and suppliers is one way of getting to know one's self. Getting ahead just because colleagues think the performance is great is not enough; getting ahead occurs when peers, the boss, or subordinates give good marks. And the more this happens, the more the workplace is democratized because everybody is working together to improve overall performance.

Leaders must know what others think about them if they expect to get respect and followership. Chapter 2 provides an account of how one nurse learned more about himself and how he used this knowledge to improve his leadership skills. Although an awareness of self seems easy to acquire, this nurse's story highlights the lengths to which he went to learn more about himself and how that affected his ability to lead and get others to follow. So that others can do the same, the author presents a model of self-knowledge that can easily be replicated.

LOOKING FORWARD: BEING AND BECOMING A FUTURIST

In the Industrial Age, we learned how to analyze data, to isolate the problem, and to determine a course of action without knowing whether the outcome would be what we imagined or hoped for. In the age of managed care, we must look beyond the situation and determine how we would *like* things to be. This strategy is known as *establishing the preferred future*. Instead of waiting for the future to reveal itself, we create the future we want. Knowing what is wanted today for tomorrow allows nurses to develop strategies that create that tomorrow.

According to Hancock and Bezold (1994), futures can be considered in four ways: as possible, plausible, probable, or preferred futures. *Possible futures* are what *may happen*. They encompass everything we can possibly imagine, no matter how unlikely. Possible futures include those dramatic and seemingly implausible changes that occur very swiftly. The recent health care changes might be considered a possible prediction; who could have known that the entire health care system would change so dramatically and so quickly? Such a change suggests we should consider all possibilities when making decisions.

Most planning efforts do well to focus on dealing with more *plausible futures*, which are what *could happen*. They represent a smaller scope of possibilities that seem to make sense given what we know today. For instance, it is being predicted that in the future, informatics will control most of life's operations and that we will depend more and more on the World Wide Web and the Internet for our information. This seems plausible as we watch the growth and expansion of informatics today; trends are progressing very rapidly. Preparing for that kind of future is our task today.

Probable futures are what *will likely happen* and are based on an examination of the present situation and an appraisal of likely trends and future developments. They are an extension of the present. An example of what will "likely" happen is the plight of Social Security. With the knowledge that the "baby boomers" will place a huge demand on the Social Security trust fund in the not-too-distant future, it is predicted that the fund will be bankrupt unless something is done today to guarantee its availability in the future. However, there are those who predict the fund will not be bankrupt if loans taken against the fund are paid today. How likely bankruptcy is to occur depends on what is done today, and such a prediction helps us do what is necessary while there is time.

The *preferred future* is what *we want* to happen and is sometimes called *prescriptive futurism*. Preferred futures are hard to define because we usually let the present get in our way; however, setting out a preferred future allows us to work for a goal and to pave the way for what should be rather than what might be or could be. For nursing, this would mean that nurses must determine the role they want to play in health care delivery and the obstacles and facilitators involved in reaching that goal and then plan for ways to make the goal a reality. Futures thinking is not new. Futurists have been helping people use strategies that create the future in many aspects of life, but few nurses have used futures thinking (Pesut, 1997). In Chapter 3, the author lays out a model for futuristic thinking and shares his experiences as a futurist. His review of the literature is particularly helpful, and his personal stories clearly illustrate how futures thinking provided him with one of the skills so necessary for taking the lead in today's managed care environment.

SEEING THE BIG PICTURE

An important principle of leadership that often is neglected and leads to unsuccessful outcomes is the inability to see the entire parameters of a situation—that is, to see the forest as well as the trees. It has been said that everything is connected to everything else, and once this is understood, it is easy to expand one's vision. It is essential for nurses to "live in the situation" long enough to see the endless possibilities available to them and how the issue of concern affects and is affected by other aspects of the total situation. For instance, a concern about the number of staff per patient in an acute care facility may mean there is a need to look beyond the question. The shift length, staffing mix, third-party reimbursement criteria, or type of delivery system used (or all of these aspects of care) may affect the patient-to-staff ratio. Simply changing the number of staff per patient may not be the only or the best way to improve the quality of care. Sometimes an action fixes the immediate concern but does not, in the long run, correct the real issue or, even worse, it creates other problems.

Because nurses have not always been included in decisions affecting patient care, there is a tendency for them to look for quick fixes. Leaders can see beyond quick fixes; they are much more system focused. This means that nurse leaders must see the big picture. They must be able to think about the whole, knowing that everything affects something else, and to ask the right questions. Posing several perspectives in the search for actions that benefit the most while reaching the proposed goals is the most desired way to see the whole. In many ways, seeing the whole picture and looking forward are related.

In Chapter 4, the author presents a framework for seeing the big picture that includes three elements: paying attention, using networks, and connecting what is learned with what is known. It also includes the experiences of the author and how she used seeing the big picture to provide leadership.

BUILDING SELF-DIRECTED WORK TEAMS

During the early 1990s, there was a move by innovative acute care institutions to direct more of the time of the health care workers to the patient and to despecialize their work skills. Decentralized services, cross-training, and self-directed work teams were initiated. Although some of these changes were included in the reengineering efforts of many hospitals during health care reform, what was learned about groups of people and how they could direct themselves helped improve patient care by using a new pattern of shared leadership.

There were many who believed this shift from hierarchical leadership to shared leadership would only create chaos. Few believed that a group could govern itself without an identified leader; however, although some groups did find it hard to function in such a different manner, self-directed groups did work, and they did demonstrate that a shared effort is not so new or innovative after all. Prestwood and Schumann (1997) likened this shared leadership to "barn-raising" efforts. Like the pioneers who came together to help someone build a barn using their talents and to form teams to accomplish specific tasks, self-directed health care worker teams place emphasis on teamwork through a shared purpose and the use of each team member's energy, skills, and abilities. Community is formed, and the members of the team see themselves working as a whole to accomplish a shared goal.

The skills used by self-directed team members are important for the team's success, but they are also useful to other groups. The ability to trust, to seek consensus, to lead while following, to serve while being served, to support while being supported, and to keep faith in the group's ability to reach its goals are clearly skills that help groups of people function more effectively (Jackman and Waggoner, 1996).

From another perspective, successful self-directed teams share attitudes. They believe that honesty, appreciation, and respect are essential and that listening is an important attribute. Humphries (1996) also believes that these values and attributes are important for all leaders to possess.

In Chapter 5, two nurse authors provide the theoretical backdrop for the newest team approach in health care. They also tell an important story of how they led a group of nurses in a large hospital into a self-directed work team format. The good and the difficult are explained, and what nurses in other institutions must do if they take the lead into a self-directed adventure is described.

TAKING A RISK

We live in a world of uncertainty and often feel victimized by forces beyond our control. Steven Covey (1997) points out, however, that "you have to remember to create your own future" (p. 5). This often means taking a risk.

Many see taking a risk as scary and something they would never do, or they see everything as a risk and therefore avoid doing anything.

According to DeBecker (1997), Americans evaluate risk in odd ways:

> There are Americans who would not visit Egypt for fear of being killed there, so they stay home where the risk of murder is 20 times greater. Though smoking kills more people in an afternoon than lightning does in a year, there are those who calm their fear of lightning during a storm by smoking a cigarette (p. 4).

Clearly, there are many risks in stepping forward, particularly if the position taken is an unpopular one. Like the worry about lightning in a storm, however, many of the worries nurses have about taking the lead are nothing more than unwarranted fears. Unlike real fear, unwarranted fear is rarely logical. In the new world of managed care, worrying about whether a preferred futures proposal will be accepted when all of the proposals presented are beyond the usual is illogical. Nurses hold back when they often have very good ideas. Interestingly, nurses often do not take the lead because they are afraid of looking inappropriate or foolish or feel they will be mistaken, when logic later often indicates they were on the right track. As DeBecker (1997) states:

> Unwarranted fear has assumed a power over us that it holds over no other creature on Earth. It need not be so (p. 4).

Taking a risk means the unwarranted fear that keeps nurses from taking the lead must be removed. Mark Twain once said, "I have had a great many troubles, but most of them never happened." Like Twain, nurses need to take reasonable precautions but should not let their worries and fears direct their actions. For women, risk often is the deterrent to action, and because most nurses are women, the tendency to avoid risk is prevalent. The author of Chapter 6 addresses this issue in much greater depth. The story of a nurse who took a huge risk and succeeded underscores the importance of risk taking. This nurse was able to become a leader in the new world of entrepreneurs, which set the stage for the development of a new role for nurses as business owners who provide a variety of care options.

RECOGNIZING THE RIGHT TIME FOR ACTION

Taking action often depends on whether the time is right for what needs to be accomplished. Many failures for change have occurred because the time for action was not right—that is, the forces against change outnumbered those in favor of change. Using force field analysis (Lewin, 1951), it is possible to analyze each situation to determine whether the forces in favor of change are worth the risk to move forward with the change. For instance, the move in 1978 for the "entry to practice" to begin with the baccalaureate degree was premature. There was not enough support from community colleges, the Council of Associate Degree Nurses of the National League for Nursing, and many other large and influential groups to ensure that the proposal would be implemented. The time was not right because the necessary support was not there. Support for that move is quite different now because the passage of time has created a very different set of circumstances.

There are times when change occurs without support—the timing was right even though the apparent support was not there. A good example of this is the recent health care system reform. In this case, the force for the change—high cost—was so impelling that regardless of how many other forces resisted the change, it still occurred. Thus, the force for change can be one of either magnitude or intensity. It is essential for the person interested in making change to determine whether the time is right for the change by assessing the magnitude of support or the apparent intensity of the need for the change.

There are other ways to assess readiness for change. Keeping the big picture in mind and looking forward can help one predict change. Using probable futures prediction, knowing what is happening, and projecting forward those events can also help one recognize when the time is right for change intervention. Essentially, a key dimension to the recognition of the best time for action is keeping in touch with events, especially because everything is related to everything else. Health care reform did not occur in isolation of other events. It occurred when other entities were also changing and when cost was an issue for Congress in Washington. Health care reform is happening everywhere in the world, which underscores the effect cost has around the globe. In Chapter 7, the author provides an account of how a nurse was able to use timing to take the lead. She describes a variety of experiences during her career to demonstrate how important the timing of an action can be.

SEEING CHANGE AS AN OPPORTUNITY

Because change is inevitable and occurs all of the time, nurses must learn to view change as an opportunity. Covey (1997) believes the "only way to navigate the upheavals that are bound to happen is to act as if you were in business for yourself. Make sure you know your value to the organization, and never expect the organization to support you" (p. 4). He continues, "too many people have become institutionally dependent, blaming others, looking for someone else to take responsibility" (p. 4). He suggests that nurses become career entrepreneurs when following these three steps:

1. Look objectively at your skills, and figure out what is missing.
2. Find a way to improve your skills and learn new ones. If the company does not offer training, find courses at local colleges or perhaps attend seminars in your field.
3. Know your industry. Attend conferences, join associations, and maintain a network of colleagues outside and inside your company. The idea is not to enhance your visibility so you can climb the corporate ladder but to expand your knowledge so you can grow more effective (p. 5).

Opportunity is available when change occurs if the individual is ready. Nurses must see that change is not an invitation for their demise but instead a call to opportunity. It has been said that problems are opportunities in work clothes;

this means nurses must see change as an opportunity to do some important work.

Many nurses have been doing exciting things since there have been massive changes in the health care system. It is all a matter of perspective! Those who viewed those changes as opportunities have made huge career advances; those who viewed the changes as a threat have missed the opportunities. In Chapter 8, a nurse entrepreneur gives an account of her adventure and how she made the loss of a job an opportunity for an entirely new kind of career in health care.

BEING PROACTIVE, NOT REACTIVE

Being proactive is a lot like preventive medicine—it is better to prevent a problem and to be prepared for change than to wait for something to happen and then to resist or complain about it. In the first instance, control of the situation is in the hands of those who look forward and take action to shape the future. In the second instance, the individual has given control to someone else and is reacting to what occurs. Being reactive is to disempower oneself.

Most writers with an expertise in leadership would agree that it is important for leaders to take control, particularly of themselves. Those who take control of themselves are usually ready for change because they have done something to address the change before it arrived. For example, Covey (1997) states that to be indispensable in the workplace, it is necessary to make sure the job fits, behave like an entrepreneur, seek feedback, move beyond mentors, think teams, take risks, be a problem solver, and balance life. Essentially, he is saying that the individual must take control of himself or herself. These actions are proactive and place the responsibility for what happens squarely with the individual.

Leaders in the traditional sense have always been urged to take control, but in this new world of competition and change, all workers at all levels must take control and be proactive. Reaction to change robs the individual of the right to make choices. Proactive decision-makers reach beyond their usual areas. Nurses in patient-focused care environments have learned how to take radiographs and electrocardiograms and to draw blood. They also have assumed responsibility for the patient's environment by keeping it clean and orderly. They took the lead when it was offered and realized that being proactive was a better position to be in than standing back and reacting to the proposed changes made by others. The author of Chapter 9 focuses on how proactive behavior helped her take the lead. She shares experiences in her career at various times and experiences in her personal life. A model for contextual decision-making is presented in a way to demonstrate proactive decision-making.

COMMUNICATING EFFECTIVELY

Communication is a vital skill for leaders; in fact, ineffective communication often is the reason most individuals who want to be leaders are *not* effective leaders. Being an effective communicator means being a good listener, validating what is heard, and seeking clarification.

Because communication is a two-way system, being a good listener is an essential aspect of being a good communicator. Telling or talking at colleagues and subordinates is not sufficient; listening to what others have to say conveys that their message is important.

There are many barriers to good listening. Raudsepp (1990) believes that most people develop poor listening habits because they allow their mind to wander while someone is talking to them or they are thinking about their reply before the person has finished talking. He offers seven listening skills:

1. Take time to listen.
2. Teach self to concentrate.
3. Do not interrupt.
4. Listen to what is being said, not how it is being said.
5. Suspend judgment.
6. Listen between the lines.
7. Listen with the eyes.

Dr. Shirley Chater (Sponselli, 1997), a nurse and the former Commissioner of the Social Security Administration, points out that "it's as important to listen so that you know what's going on in the other person's mind as it is to try to be persuasive" (p. 24).

Another way to be an effective communicator is to make sure that the message received is the message that was intended. This step in being an effective communicator includes understanding the communication; words, gestures, body position, and one's experiences are part of understanding what has been said. Often, this process of understanding is called *decoding* the message that was sent.

The more experiences the sender and the receiver have in common, the more likely the intended message will be communicated. When leaders have different experiences than those with whom they are communicating, there is a likelihood that there will be miscommunication. To avoid miscommunication as a result of the sender's and the receiver's having different experiences, decoding is necessary. Decoding is the analysis of the verbal and nonverbal messages with the intent of ensuring that they are *congruent*. If someone says they are fine yet there is a facial grimace or sadness in the tone of the voice, then the verbal and nonverbal messages are not congruent. This noncongruence creates a *mixed message* that the receiver of the messages must validate—that is, the receiver must determine which message the sender wants to convey.

One way to validate the message to make sure that there is a shared understanding of the communication is to clarify the message. Simply asking "did you say . . . ?" or "do I understand you correctly when you say . . . ?" helps the receiver of a message determine whether the message that was sent is the message that was received.

Other barriers to effective communication include physical distance, noise, stress, expectations, and language differences. In Chapter 10, the authors share their experiences with effective communication in a large organization and the ways in which barriers to communication can be removed so organizational communication is effective. A framework that includes the characteristics of effective communication, how the culture of an organization effects communication, and the importance of feedback is also presented, with examples on how the framework can be used to improve one's personal and organizational communication skills.

MENTORING OTHERS

Mentoring is a common aspect of every leader's career, both as the person being mentored and as the mentor to others. Having a mentor has been linked with achieving faster promotion and higher pay, greater knowledge of both the technical and organizational aspects of business, and higher levels of productivity and performance of both mentors and those being mentored (Clawson, 1979; Dalton et al., 1987; Jowers and Herr, 1990; Lunding et al., 1978; Queralt, 1989; Roche, 1979).

Most mentoring follows the tutelage model. A person with an established career selects a novice to do a specific task because it is believed the individual has a special talent. The mentor may construct additional tasks that naturally arise from the responsibilities assigned. The protégé experiences a "watch" time for proving merit. This phase doesn't last long because most mentors are reasonably good judges of character and talent (Moore, 1982). Once the mentor is satisfied with the protégé's performance, the relationship moves into another phase. The mentor and protégé work closely together, which moves the protégé into the inner circle, where new skills are learned and new relationships are formed.

An important aspect of the protégé/mentor experience is the impact on the mentor and the organization. Protégés get things done. They learn and develop while they work for the mentor, thus gaining experience while helping the mentor meet his or her goals for the organization (Bower, 1993).

Mentorships take many forms and allow different aspects of personal and professional development to be accomplished. Some mentorships are formal arrangements; others are very informal. Some are planned, yet many simply happen. Some mentors are close acquaintances of their protégés, but many mentors are nothing more than models of excellence. Mentorships can help protégés learn about ways to succeed, ways to dress according to the position, ways to maneuver the political scene, and ways to meet the "right" people. The author of Chapter 11 tells how mentoring facilitated her leadership career and how she provided mentoring to others as they advanced their careers. The advantages and barriers to good mentorships are discussed, and the ways to be a good mentor are highlighted.

LETTING GO AND TAKING ON

"Letting go" can occur at least two ways. You can "let go" of an idea, a plan, or an action and move to something else, or you can "let go" by *delegating* an action to someone else. Leaders do both! Letting go is important when change is occurring and when what we do is no longer working. For many nurses, letting go is difficult because it tends to feel like failure. Too often, nurses hang on to thinking that if they just work harder and longer, things will get better. However, if working harder and longer does not work and the stress from the effort is making the situation worse, then it is time to let go. It is amazing how many nurses fail to see the signs and symptoms of stress and to connect it with the time, energy, and stamina it takes to hang on to something that isn't working, is never going to work, and should be allowed to die.

To drop an idea or a plan, it is important to know when to do it and why dropping an idea or action is the right thing to do. Some ideas are premature given the situation, and some ideas should be dropped because they are just not right for the time and situation. An assessment regarding "timing" and whether the idea is appropriate should occur shortly after the idea is generated.

Letting go of an idea, a plan, or an action does not always mean that it is inappropriate or suggested at the wrong time; it could also mean that someone else should carry it to completion. Frequently, leaders delegate to others. Although an action can be delegated to someone else, the responsibility for that action may still remain with the delegator. In nursing, there are many opportunities to delegate. Many of the changes initiated during the implementation of managed care have increased the use of unlicensed assistive personnel who are assigned tasks by nurses. To delegate appropriately, there are several principles of delegation that must be followed:

1. A task is delegated, but not the responsibility for satisfactory completion of the task.
2. The person assigned the task must have the skills to accomplish it.
3. There must be adequate time for the delegate to satisfactorily complete the task.
4. Evaluation of the quality of the performance of the delegate must be done to determine whether the task was completed properly and efficiently.
5. More than one person may be assigned to complete a task.
6. Communication between delegator and delegate or delegates must be established and maintained by the delegator.
7. Directions regarding who, what, where, when, why, and how must be clearly stated by the delegator.
8. Evaluation of the delegated task is the responsibility of the delegator and those who were assigned the task.

Delegation of tasks is a helpful way to improve the use of time and to develop the commitment of others. Nurses who desire greater challenges generally become more committed and satisfied when they are given opportunities to pursue significant tasks. A lack of delegation can stifle initiative.

There are many barriers to delegation. For instance, delegation can be stifled when the leader believes the following:

1. No one else can do the task.
2. She or he can do it better.
3. There is no time to tell anyone else how to do the task.
4. She or he cannot trust or have confidence in anyone else to do the task.
5. She or he will lose power if the task is given to someone else.
6. The task is too risky for someone else to do it.
7. There is no way to follow up on the delegation.
8. Delegation creates competition.

The use of delegation takes different forms depending on whether nursing care is organized in a team format, as primary nursing, as case management, or in self-directed work groups. The author of Chapter 12 provides the reader with a framework for letting go and describes how the psychological transition can be made during a change.

"Taking on" is a different concept and occurs in a variety of situations. Obviously, "taking on" can occur because someone has delegated a task, but more often, it occurs when an action is needed and someone steps forward to initiate it. Several personal qualities are needed to initiate action when it is needed: confidence, knowledge, the ability to take risk, and trust in others. Fear of failure simply must not get in the way. There is extensive research that indicates that persons who have a need to achieve can accept responsibility, expect feedback, and handle risk (Robbins, 1990). These are the kind of people who "take on" the responsibility and the tasks when there is a need for action. These issues are discussed in length in Chapter 12.

KEEPING INFORMED

Keeping informed is an important principle for taking the lead; it includes knowing what is happening so actions that are taken are not out of sync with the rest of the world's events. Many opportunities could be missed if the leader does not know what is happening in current affairs. There are many changes, and if one wants to assume a leadership position, keeping informed is vital.

Keeping informed is different from looking into the future or seeing the big picture. It is having an everyday awareness of what is happening in health care and in society in general. As Covey says, "everything affects everything else," so it is important to know what is happening in every arena possible. If Bill Gates makes a decision, there will be an impact on most aspects of the business world; undoubtedly, one of those businesses will be health care, and if health care changes, so will nursing—everything does affect everything else. Thus, nurses must read newspapers, watch television, and keep up with current literature in which events are reported and analyzed.

Some years ago, there was a threat to nurses when the American Medical Association decided to prepare "care providers." It was proposed that care providers be used to substitute for nurses, at a considerably lower cost. If nursing leaders had not been listening and keeping track of events, they would not have been prepared to mount the effort they did to stop that initiative. It took a lot of effort, but because the American Nurses Association and other organizations were alert, the preparation of care givers did not even get started. At that time, there was a nursing shortage, and the cost of recruiting foreign nurses was becoming a problem.

There was an earlier incident when a television program was launched called "The Nightingales" that portrayed nurses as flighty, loose women. A nurse took the lead to have that program removed from television, and it was because she was alert and keeping informed that she was able to stop the program. She mobilized nursing personnel through a massive letter-writing campaign that stopped a noted television producer from airing that program. Leaders must be informed.

In this age of informatics, keeping informed means the nurse must have computer skills and know how to "surf the net." Technology has made it easy to read newspapers from all over the world while sitting in an office or at home. It is also possible to communicate with people all over the world through the Internet. The author of Chapter 13 tells how the use of the Internet helped him with the activities of his professional life. He also provides a wonderful quick lesson in the language of informatics and in how to use the Internet for a variety of purposes.

SUMMARY

This chapter introduced the principles that are discussed in detail in this book. Although the principles are not new, they are presented in a way that any nurse at any level can use. The reader must keep in mind that anyone can be a leader if the will and the desire to do so are nourished. All of the nurses who tell their stories in this book are leaders and used the principle about which they wrote. Their stories are validation that the principles work, regardless of the position of the nurse. Each nurse did what he or she did at the right time, although he or she did not necessarily do the "right thing." They were taking the lead, and the circumstances were not always favorable.

It is also important to understand that these 12 principles do not operate in isolation from one another; they often function together. For instance, when the nurse is seeing the big picture, it may also be appropriate to look forward. And when the nurse is communicating, there will be a need to be informed so the communication is not out of date. Taking a risk will involve letting go and seeing the big picture; there is almost no incidence when these principles are not used together.

Taking the lead is being influential and thus means the nurse must not only be aware of opportunities and be skillful in the use of these as principles but also see himself or herself as capable of initiating change. It is not enough to have the skill to make change if there is no expectation that it is possible. The stories in this book are real; ordinary people took the lead and made changes not only in themselves but also in others and in the environment.

REFERENCES

Bower, F. (1993). Women and mentoring. In P. T. Mitchell (Ed.). *Cracking the wall: Women in higher education administration* (pp. 90–97). Washington, DC: CUPA.

Clawson, J. G. (1979). *Superior-subordinate relationships in management development.* Unpublished doctoral dissertation, Harvard University.

Covey, S. (1997, August 29–31). How to succeed in today's workplace. *USA Weekend*, pp. 4–5.

Dalton, G.W., Thompson, P. H., & Price, R. L. (1987). The four stages of professional careers—A new look at performance by professionals. *Organizational Dynamics, 6*(1), 19–42.

DeBecker, G. (1997, August 22–24). Conquering what scares us. *USA Weekend*, p. 4.

Hancock, T., & Bezold, C. (1994). Possible futures, preferable futures. *Healthcare Forum Journal, 2*, 23–29.

Humphries, A. C. (1996). What employees expect from managers. *The Pryor Report Management Newsletter, 12*(3a), 8.

Jackman, M., & Waggoner, S. (1996). Key players have definable traits. *The Pryor Report Management Newsletter, 12*(3a), 11.

Jowers, L., & Herr, K. (1990). A review of the literature on mentor-protégé relationships. *NLN Productions, 15*, 49–77.

Lewin, K. (1951). *Field theory in social science.* New York: Harper.

Lewinson, S. B. (1996). *Taking charge: Nursing, suffrage, and feminism in America 1873–1920.* New York: NLN Press.

Lunding, G. I., Clements, X., & Perkins, D. S. (1978). Everyone who makes it has a mentor. *Harvard Business Review, 56*, 89–101.

Moore, K. M. (1982). The role of mentors in developing leaders for academe. *Educational Record, 63*, 22–28.

Pesut, D. (1997). Future think. *Nursing Outlook, 45*(3), 107.

Prestwood, C. L., & Schumann, P. A. (1997, January–February). Seven new principles of leadership. *The Futurist,* p. 68.

Queralt, M. (1989). *The role of mentor in career development of university faculty members and academic administrators.* Unpublished doctoral dissertation, University of Miami.

Raudsepp, E. (1990). 7 ways to cure communications breakdown. *Nursing 90, 20*(4), 132–142.

Robbins, S. (1990). *Organizational theory: Structure, design, and application.* Englewood Clifts, N.J.: Prentice Hall.

Roche, G. R. (1979). Much ado about mentors. *Harvard Business Review, 57*, 14–28.

Sponselli, C. (1997, August 4). Chater trades top government post for academic life. *NURSEweek,* p. 24.

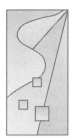

Chapter 2

Knowing Self

Gregory L. Crow

Have you ever wondered why some people are good leaders and others are not? Has it ever occurred to you that one of the reasons some individuals are good leaders is that they know what they know and have a strong sense of who they are? Research suggests that *knowing self* is a very important aspect of being an effective leader.

This chapter is about how leadership development is enhanced by knowing self. Primarily, this chapter contains models and theories about knowing self and is supported by real stories about a nurse with an emerging career for whom knowing self advanced his career into leadership positions.

Many things in this chapter will stimulate your thinking about a career and about how becoming a leader is much more than obtaining an academic degree; rather, it is the interrelationship among education, experience, and knowing self that shapes people, nurses, and leaders. These subjects and others are laid out as a framework for knowing self and its relationship to taking the lead.

At the outset, I think it is important to tell you that I am grateful that my life experiences led to nursing. I am not saying that I have loved all there is about nursing, because I have not. And I surely will not as my career continues to develop. There have been occasions when I was so sick of nursing and nurses that I thought of leaving the profession, but leaving never surfaced as a viable action. There is one overarching reason I did not leave; I felt it is my obligation to leave nursing in a better condition than I found it. To date, I have made some important inroads to that goal, but I am not finished. There is still much to learn and do, and I intend to do it!

If life is to have meaning, the extent to which you know yourself is the most important work you will ever do. And because life is a process of emergence and becoming, it is a journey, not a destination. If there is a destination, it must be that moment when you know all you can about yourself, and I am certain there is a sense of peace at that moment.

For me, the thing that brings the most peace in life is knowing self. Peace, in turn, brings richness to life and allows us to live and die with grace. Knowing self is the first and most important step in the process of pursuing dreams and goals. One key element is to be secure enough in yourself to allow others to influence who you are and where you are going. Please note it is influence, not control. If you are insecure in who you are, odds are that you will not be open to love, caring, and the help of others (De Beauport, 1996).

Knowing self is much like Maslow's highest need in his hierarchy of needs—self-actualization. Just like self-actualization, complete self-knowledge is also fleeting. You have it and it goes away as new challenges interact with each developmental stage; however, once you have experienced the feeling of self-actualization and realize that it is not permanent but rather discontinuous, it becomes that experience to be sought over and over again. At that point, all your thoughts and actions are focused on gaining more and more self-knowledge because nothing is more fulfilling.

All aspects of our life (physical, social, intellectual, emotional, and spiritual) are connected. If one area is neglected, the others suffer. Seeking balance among work, love, and play is an important aspect of living a healthy life. If there is an imbalance in one or more areas, the other areas help regain the balance.

With all the pressures and priorities in our lives, how does one get these aspects of life in balance? To start with, honesty with self is essential; that means doing the work necessary to garner the skills, knowledge, and abilities to develop in a positive way. Time must be provided for meditation and thinking about what is really important. Striving for the big picture is also important. And it is absolutely essential to understand the "I" in relation to the world in which we live.

Have you ever noticed how easy it is to get stuck, locked into one level of achievement—a sort of cul-de-sac way of thinking and behaving? The same things happen and the same results occur; nothing seems to ever change. You wake up one morning and ask, "How did I get here?" "What happened to my dream?" Things just get so comfortable that no one questions what is happening and why one's dreams did not materialize.

It is also easy to get stuck when not living up to your capabilities; in fact, it is easy to get to a place where you lose confidence and as a result your competencies eventually fade. In time you find yourself out of sync with what the world is demanding—you may even feel obsolete. I cannot imagine a more horrifying moment than to observe my own obsolescence.

Getting stuck can also occur by forgetting that life is a process of continual striving and challenge, of pushing farther than was thought possible. Sometimes it's the gentle, or not so gentle, nudge that moves one into action. Nudges often come in different forms, such as getting passed over for a promotion, failing a course in school, having to deal with children who are acting out, or having a significant relationship fall apart. These nudges are the signal to reexamine priorities. They are telling us, in the strongest voice that the universe has, to "wake up."

CONCEPTS

Concept of Self

The self, according to De Beauport (1996), embraces all our conscious and unconscious self-knowledge. The goal of the process of knowing self is to merge the known with the unknown. This merging is what creates you, that unique person unlike anyone else in the world. To know self is to embrace all there is about yourself—the good and the flawed, the conscious and unconscious.

Achieving success and being a productive leader is not easy, but if you can understand who you are and where you want to go, if you can believe in the possibilities (as well as manage the struggles) of your life, and if you believe you deserve to achieve your goals, you will most likely achieve them. Believing that you deserve and can achieve self-knowledge is of prime importance in your career.

Not everyone will take the journey to knowing self because the work—and it is hard work—can at times feel overwhelming and painful, as well as joyous. I believe that the primary reason many people will not take this journey is because it is a journey of accountability. The image in the mirror is the one at whom you must point the finger; the reflection is the one to hold accountable.

We are all born and exist in a world that simultaneously loves and challenges us. The trick is not to let the challenges alone determine the outcome or to shun the challenge. Wishing the challenge to go away or negatively responding to it could mean missing an embedded meaning and a lesson to be learned. The trick is to know how to respond to challenges so the most is gained from the experience.

Failing to create a balance between the impact of the two forces of love and challenge on the human spirit is what creates misery. Surely, you have worked with people who never seem happy no matter what happens to them. They have a chronic life of misery and victimization. They want the world to respond to their misery with sympathy. As long as they are stuck in the victim-sympathy cycle, they never have to take accountability for their lives. If they were to win the $10 million lottery and were congratulated for it, they would hang their heads down and say, "But I really needed $12 million." These people talk in terms of "if only," "had that been different," or "if he or she had not blocked me." A victim's words, actions, and deeds are about his or her never-ending potential, a potential that is never actualized.

Concept of Leader

Leaders actualize. They, too, have "if only" thoughts; however, the "if only" is the call to positive action on a continuous life journey. They deeply understand, as Victor Frankl (1984) described in *Man's Search for Meaning,* that the purpose or meaning in life can be independent of circumstance and that the ability to live productive, meaningful lives lies in response to adversity, not in the adversity itself. In other words, circumstance does not define the person.

The informed and fully integrated person who knows self has the skills and knowledge necessary for a leadership role; however, the fully integrated and informed person does not seek leadership positions for the power that he or she may achieve, because power is not the goal. True leaders do not seek to take what others have in order to be more powerful. They understand that their power comes from within; if it is taken from someone else, it will be available only temporarily because some day it will be taken away. Throughout my career, I have witnessed this cycle of power-taking and the great damage it has done to individuals and to nursing as a profession. As long as we continue to wrestle power from each other, nursing will never be powerful.

The word *leader* in the context of this discussion does not describe a nurse manager or chief nurse executive. It is used in a more generic sense. Every nurse, whether at the bedside; employed at a hospital, clinic, or community setting; or as an educator, researcher, or private practitioner, has the potential to be a leader. Leadership is not defined by role; it is defined by actions. Nor is this discussion meant to be a recipe for knowing self or becoming a leader. It is meant to be a description of one journey and the lessons that can be drawn from reading about it.

THEORETICAL MODEL FOR KNOWING SELF

Every person is born with an innate drive to grow and develop and to understand self within the context of his or her life. Growth and development are guided and affected by many things that in and of themselves help one know self, such as

- Inspiration and motivation
- The environment
- Behavior patterns
- Systems thinking
- Change management

There is, however, a sixth factor, called the "X" factor, used when describing a system's wholeness. When defining a system as a whole, it is said that it is greater than the sum of its parts. But what is the factor that makes a system greater than the sum of its parts? That factor is meaning, the meaning we derive from both our professional and our personal lives that makes us more than the sum of our parts (Fig. 2–1).

Humans have long used symbols to convey information because they are expedient and allow thoughts and feelings to be conveyed simply. The model in Figure 2–1 is derived from the experience of 21 years as a nurse and 47 years as an emerging and developing person. This model emerged as I sat down to write this chapter about knowing myself and the role that self-knowledge played in how I developed as a leader. This model is meant to be flexible and continuous, not static. If I were asked to do the same project in 5 years, the model, the elements within it, and their interrelationships would probably be different.

As background to understanding the theoretical model about knowing self, I must tell a story about how I got into nursing. My nursing career began in September 1974, when I entered Samuel Merritt Hospital School of Nursing in Oakland, California, after my discharge from the military. I was drafted—the only lottery I ever won—into the Air Force during the Vietnamese War and was fortunate enough to be assigned (you had no choice then) to be a medic. While in the Air Force, I worked in the areas of medical-surgical, emergency, and—my favorite—labor, delivery, and postpartum. I also was appointed to various leadership positions. In 1974, I was granted an 8-month early discharge because the war was winding down. I entered nursing school and graduated June 1977. I took the state board examinations 1 year early and worked as an on-call nurse in a psychiatric unit until graduation.

When my basic nursing education was completed, jobs were hard to come by because the anesthesiologists were on strike and hospital admissions were

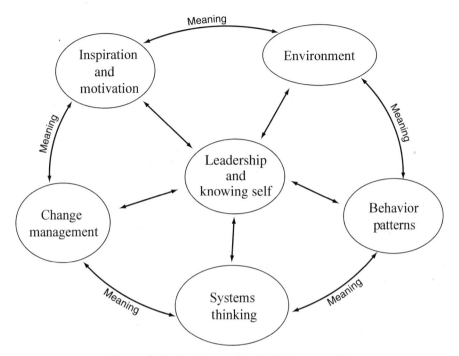

Figure 2-1. The theoretical model for knowing self.

down drastically. Undaunted, two friends and I fanned out over the entire San Francisco Bay area in search of not one, but three jobs.

My two colleagues and I were hired into the critical care unit of a 240-bed community hospital, full time, on the night shift. We took the jobs and the shift with great enthusiasm because we were the first new graduates to be hired into critical care at this hospital. In addition to critical care, I worked as shift supervisor, educator, and recruiter at this same hospital during my tenure there.

In 1980, while at the community hospital, another friend mentioned a 3-year program at the University of California, San Francisco (UCSF), that offered a bachelor of science and a master of science degree. We applied and were accepted. I had numerous prerequisites to complete, so I went to on-call status and attended two community colleges and two state universities over the next year to meet the entrance requirements.

While at UCSF and during my administrative residency, I was hired as the assistant administrator of patient care services at the hospital that was the host site for my diploma program. I stayed there for 4 years. While there, a friend in the education department thought it might be nice to return to school for a doctorate. We submitted our applications and were accepted to attend the University of San Francisco (USF) School of Education. I resigned from my nurse administrator position and, while in school, taught full-time for the School of Nursing at the same university.

After completing my doctorate, there were no full-time tenure-track teaching positions at USF, or anywhere else in the San Francisco Bay area. As luck would have it, one of the members of my dissertation committee worked for Kaiser Permanente Regional Headquarters in Oakland, California. Kaiser was recruiting for a nurse to produce live television programs on management and leadership development for the Northern California region. I interviewed for the position and was hired. I held this position for 1.5 years.

When the position at Kaiser was nearing its end, a full-time tenure-track position became available at Sonoma State University, Department of Nursing. I applied, was hired, and am teaching there today. In addition to teaching, I am a senior consultant with Tim Porter-O'Grady and Associates, Atlanta, Georgia. I primarily consult in the areas of leadership and management development and implementation of whole systems shared governance.

The discussion that follows will unfold in a linear fashion, beginning with the role that inspiration and motivation have played in helping me know myself during my professional life, and will end with a discussion about managing change. Before I start, I offer a word of caution—life is anything but linear. Although inspiration and motivation have played significant roles in my life, at times they were not the most important factors in my developing role as a leader. The elements of this model play off one another and sometimes collide. Which one happens to be most powerful at any given time has a lot to do with circumstance. This means that you can start with any section you choose and still hear the whole story.

Inspiration and Motivation

Inspiration and motivation have played a significant role in how I have gained and used knowledge about myself to actualize my leadership potential. *Inspiration* is a means to enlighten or illuminate (American Heritage Dictionary, 1994) an aspect of life and can serve as a stimulus that motivates one to take action (Covey, 1989). This momentum to take action is created deep inside by inspiration that helps develop new behaviors, knowledge, and abilities, as well as expand existing ones.

The experience of being inspired and motivated, whether initiated by a person, event, or thing, increasingly causes that fulfilled feeling. When one is inspired, a biochemical change occurs in the body. It occurs countless times over a life span. It might happen when viewing a painting that moves us, watching an athlete in the Special Olympics cross the finish line with pride and determination, or seeing joy in the eyes of a newborn's parents when they first see or touch their infant.

Motivation musters the will to act. What is desired that can be acquired becomes a reinforcer to motivation. The interplay among inspiration, motivation, and reward is circular and never-ending (Fig. 2–2). The more motivated you become, the more you will want to accomplish. The reward, to be truly meaningful, must not be easily accomplished. Things that first appear just out of reach or require significant effort often are the most motivating and rewarding.

To realize the "I can" stage of the inspiration/motivation/reward cycle (IMRC) is what De Beauport (1996) states is the call to action to make significant contributions to the world. Covey (1989) agrees with De Beauport when he

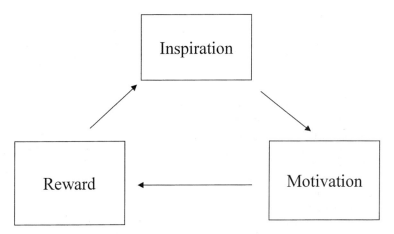

Figure 2–2. The inspiration-motivation-reward cycle.

remarks that the highest level of human motivation is derived from a sense of personal contribution. The intrinsic nature of meaningful personal contributions to the world is more rewarding than public acknowledgment.

Wheatly (1992), in *Leadership and the New Science,* comments that motivational theorists are shifting their attention from the power of external rewards to the power of intrinsic rewards. Intrinsic rewards appear to have the greatest positive force. Block (1993), De Beauport (1996), Peck (1987), Wheatley (1992), and Wilber (1998) state in various ways that commitment to communities (world), dignity in one's own and others' lives, and love in every aspect of one's life are the strongest initiators of the IMRC.

Knowledge about what inspires and motivates self is of prime importance in personal leadership development and in assisting others in their own journey. The connection between knowing self and the IMRC is to find some correspondence between the known (conscious) and the unknown (unconscious) elements of life that drive individuals to action. When you divorce yourself from who you are and separate what you do from what initiates the IMRC, you also remove the meaning of your behavior. If you are always aware of the initial conditions that stimulate the IMRC, then you can call it forward at any time or place.

For leaders, the ability to connect what inspires and motivates colleagues to a call to action is a vital skill. An inspiring and motivating work environment calls people to positive action and not to the petty distractions that so often monopolize the collective energy of people. An environment that inspires people is one in which acceptable behavior patterns are based on open and honest communication. The idea is to create an environment in which people make a choice to behave positively.

The best way to facilitate, coach, and develop new behavior patterns in people is to first change your behavior. It is also true that you cannot directly make a person change his or her behavior on a permanent basis. You might achieve short-term changes by using threats or coercion, but if you want a behavior to change in another person, you must first understand what behavior in you is facilitating or encouraging that person's behavior.

Environment

Inspiring and motivating work environments in which patterns of behavior are focused on growth and proactivity are more likely to weather the storms of change and the ambiguity the entire health care industry is experiencing. Often, the systems we work in do not tap into the intrinsic nature of nursing practice that could initiate the IMRC. Environments characterized by a lack of trust, confusion, top-down control, and rigid rules of work demotivate staff.

In work environments where the strongest force is negative behavior patterns, change will leave the system, and most of the people in it, shaken. Staff and managers may collectively have a sense of low self-worth. Staff who are wounded emotionally and do not believe in themselves deliver little of their potential to their work (Brisken, 1996). They, and hence the system, enter a type of "doom loop" and begin to experience a state in which no matter how Herculean the effort, nothing will ever change for the better. The collective consciousness and behaviors of the system slip farther and farther from its preferred present, let alone its preferred future.

An environment is much more than a physical location. It is a place alive with people, events, symbols, and behaviors that are organized and even controlled toward some purpose. The environment is an integral part of knowing self. If you do not consciously know "where" you are, under what conditions you are "there," and the path you took to get "there," you can never know who you are.

The level of influence and empowerment made available to everyone is a key factor in creating a positive environment. Some important questions to ask yourself while assessing whether your present or new setting is inspiring and motivating are

- Can I grow and develop here?
- Do people engage in inspiring and motivating endeavors?
- Would I choose this environment again or recommend it as a place to work to my best friend?

Nurses are in a state of constant communication and interaction with their work environments, and they both are changed by and change these environments. Wheatley (1992) states that through these exchanges of communication, information is rearranged into new combinations that provide valuable feedback.

Feedback can inform us about the level of meaning that the environment places on our presence and contribution to the success of the system. For instance, organizations that provide a nonmeaningful service in a meaningful way are better appreciated than are organizations that provide a meaningful service in a nonmeaningful way. An example of providing a meaningful service in a nonmeaningful way would be to treat patients like a number, body part, or disease. Many patients and families experience this treatment when interacting with their health care institutions. Some institutions function like cattle drives.

Patients seek help for their health problems that are meaningful to them and then find themselves being herded from one place to another. They exit the system unappreciated and feeling used.

Negative environments insist that people surrender themselves to the cause. In this process of surrender, the price to be paid often is a process of insidious disengagement from what was valued and its meaning. This process of disengagement eventually robs the individual and the system of energy, creativity, and, eventually, meaning. Emerson (1856) suggests that this type of environment has an aversion to openness, self-reliance, and creativity.

Openness, self-reliance, and creativity especially threaten the status quo of top-down command and control practice environments. The people who create or inherit and accept the negative environment will simultaneously despise it and go to unbelievable lengths to hold it unchangeable. They might hate it and tell you so by their words and deeds, yet they prefer it because the routines and rituals are known and predictable. Even negative routines and rituals can bring comfort when facing the unknown; there is more comfort in fighting a known enemy than an unknown enemy.

In his book *The Marriage of Sense and Soul,* Wilber (1998) states that environments are places that are representative of a collective cognitive imperative where the individual is expected to come into line and not to rise above the referent group. DePree (1989) agrees with Wilber when he states that a company will not become more than the majority of staff think it can be or want it to be. If leaders cannot inspire and motivate the masses, then the environment can never become more than it is.

To rise above a stagnant and uninspiring environment is to provide a reason to change. This reason can be that spark of motivation that begins the struggle toward a preferred future rather than one filled with loss, hopelessness, and despair. However, this change is not easy and often takes a Herculean effort. To identify the negative aspects of a culture or to suggest change is to challenge all that is consciously and unconsciously held sacred. This challenge is often met with overwhelming force, sometimes out of proportion to the threat.

These toxic environments are plagued with a sense of hopelessness, victimization, and despair. Staff often see themselves as victims and see management as the victimizer. Neither the victim nor the victimizer accepts accountability for the toxic environment because the other "they" is the problem. The problem with "they" thinking is that there is no "they". This negative line of reasoning is turned around one person at a time. With each person accepting accountability for his or her actions and doing the best possible, there will be a difference. This process begins the personal, professional, and system improvements as everyone asks in what ways activities can be improved, quality can be increased, and resources can be managed more effectively.

The leader sets the tone of the environment. Anyone who consistently strives to squelch any challenge to the status quo will one day find himself or herself a part of a system that appears to be void of soul, ambition, thinking, creativity, and motivation. Everyone becomes what Whyte (1995) describes as "tar babies"—those who are stuck to the past in such a way as to prevent growth. In fact, actions to sustain status quo at times can be so purposeful as to say with words and deeds that "We do not intend to change; you cannot make us change!" There is only one way through this experience: to acknowledge the fear that change creates and to change anyway. Holding onto fear and being stuck to it like a tar baby only increases attachment to the past and weakens our ambition for a brighter future.

How can a leader turn this negative environment into a positive one? A system of shared accountability, such as shared governance, is a powerful alternative. Organizations that implement a shared accountability leadership structure have an opportunity to bring management and staff to the table in an effort to improve the practice environment and to better serve the patient. To be certain, there are tangibles that the environment and the practitioners gain from the practice of shared accountability. Often, in a shared accountability environment, there is a better chance to improve customer satisfaction and profitability; however, these factors, important as they may be, are the artifacts of the change, not the change itself.

The process of knowing and self-transformation can reawaken in us the incredible feelings of exhilaration we felt when nursing and the profession meant much to us. As staff and management shed the yoke of "they" as the problem, an opportunity is created to reattach our collective selves to the meaning of our work as nurses and healers. We can emerge from the transformation with the invaluable knowledge that by asking critical questions that challenge us to be better people and nurses, we can create a better system of health care. The old, yet ever-present, environment of "we at the top think," "you at the bottom do," and "you at the bottom do what we at the top think you should do" is simply inadequate to encourage such a transformation.

When the meaning of care to humanity as defined by the environment and the staff is misplaced, the work of the nurse becomes meaningless to the nurse and the patient. For example, when the nurse comes to work, gets an assignment, and immediately sets about the linear routines and rituals of what should occur hour by hour, or body part by body part, the very essence or meaning of caring is lost. The caring touch of the hand, the compassion of the voice, and the hope conveyed in the eyes become misplaced because the job is seen as a specific service area, on a specific shift, with the same patients day in and day out. The meaning of one of the most important roles any human can play has become disconnected from the person providing it.

Placing meaning back into care is accomplished through shared accountability, not control. The control and command structures of the old nursing matriarchy may have, at one time, served a purpose; however, when a nurse feels accountable for the practice, there is no need for control. Doing the right thing, instead of doing things right, is its own reward. Accountability serves to constantly connect and affirm the meaning in our lives, both professional and personal.

Environments that turn the practice of nursing back to the practitioners at the point of service consistently attract nurses who desire a career instead of a series of jobs. Nurses are attracted to these centers of excellence because they want to be accountable. The administrators of these centers of excellence also clearly understand that it is through shared power and influence that inspirational and motivational professional practice environments are born and nurtured. Additionally, these administrators and practitioners know that knowing self, regarding their behavior patterns, is paramount in this transition from hierarchy to share accountability. Shared accountability calls for—indeed, demands—a very different set of behavior patterns.

Behavior Patterns

De Beauport (1996) points out that "patterns" are the most basic way we organize our world because they are used over and over again. Thus, our parents' behavior patterns pertaining to what is communicated and how it is done and the way patterns of sound mean one thing but not another are learned in our infantile preverbal state.

Patterns of behavior are developed in the individual in relation to family, neighborhood, faith, city, state, and nation and are shared, good and bad, with organizations and professions. The patterns of behavior learned in childhood and passed on from parents and immediate family become so tightly woven into the fabric of one's life that they are often used in unconscious ways. Often it is the unconscious patterns of behavior that can cause the greatest grief in one's personal and professional lives. A significant part of the journey to change behavior patterns is to know all you can about self and the conditions and rewards under which your behavior patterns were developed.

These childhood patterns of behavior were, for the most part, not acquired by choice; they were learned because they were your parents' way. Additionally, it was expected you would learn them and, more importantly, execute them exactly as they were taught. Your parents chose where you would live, with whom you would associate, your place of worship, and your school. Patterns of behavior are usually not challenged until you are exposed to someone outside the immediate circle of family and friends.

There is an insidious and long process of gaining more and more control over identifying which patterns of behavior to choose and which to reject. In addition, parents and family, schools, peer groups, communities, and places of worship all have a very strong impact on behavior. When these patterns of behavior are challenged, there often is shock when someone asks, "Why did you do that?" Too often, the response is, "I don't know; I just do it that way."

Being unaware of your patterns of behavior, and what stimulates them, can often leave a person confused when a smell, event, taste, attitude, or symbol triggers a strong response. Often, these ancient patterns of behavior are called to the surface when an individual is placed back into an old situation, such as a family reunion or visit to a family member. After about 15 minutes, the old patterns of behavior and relating are called back to the surface and, oddly, get the same response they did 20 years ago.

These events, smells, people, attitudes, and symbols are mechanisms that trigger the event; they are not the event. These triggers are sometimes referred to as "buttons." Covey (1989) states that these triggering events can elicit unthinking and robotic behavior. He believes this robotic behavior occurs because time was not taken between the trigger and the action to understand the meaning of the triggering event and to understand that there is time to consider a more fruitful way of behaving.

This time gap between trigger and action is available to make a decision to respond differently. This different action is one that is a considered action, not an unconscious, automatic, long-established trigger-action cycle. With practice and a great deal of power, the cycle can be controlled; however, to exercise control over the trigger-action cycle, one must go through a process that leads to a conscious understanding of the meaning behind the trigger. When the following questions can be answered in a truthful manner, different behavior patterns that are based on new knowledge of self can be chosen.

- What meaning is attached to that trigger that makes me act in that way?
- What behavior patterns would lead to a better outcome, and where and from whom can I learn them?

Given the right motivation, any pattern of behavior can be changed. To be permanent and meaningful, however, the motivation for change has to come from within. External motivators can be short-lived, or worse, they produce behavior that is merely imitative. To be lasting and effective, changed behavior patterns must be integrated into a person's everyday activities.

Patterns of behavior can support success as well as failure. As with our parents and family, mentors can teach appropriate behavior patterns. Mentors play a special and often profound role in facilitating new ways of behaving. Mentors are important and powerful people with whom we associate on some level inside or outside our environments. A mentor does not have to be present, or even alive, to inspire and motivate or to facilitate new patterns of behavior. Important strengths of a mentor are the ability to use feedback and introspection to gain knowledge of self.

Most of us learn new patterns of behavior by imitation. Emerson (1856) posited that there is a limit to the effectiveness of imitation. He goes on to state that although imitation of positive behaviors in life can be helpful, it is not enough. If imitation is used continually, the imitator is a captive of the person he or she imitates. If the one being imitated does not grow and develop, neither does the imitator. At some point, everyone must set his or her own course and increasingly rely on his or her own abilities. This is not to say that you should not seek out the help of others, but an assessment of a mentor's boundaries is important. This is why having more than one mentor is important. First, identify what you feel you need to learn, then target a mentor to assist you. Understand that there will come a point when that mentor may not have the capacity to facilitate your further growth.

Systems Thinking

Ludwig Von Bertalanffy is recognized as the founder of general systems theory (GST) in the 1940s. His genius was to recognize that there is a framework of concepts that are equally applicable to different fields of study (Flood and Carson, 1998). Von Bertalanffy discovered a sameness in how the elements of all systems interrelate. GST has been applied with great success to the social, organizational, behavioral, political, biological, and physical sciences. The basic elements of a system described by Von Bertalanffy are

1. Environment
2. Input

3. Transformation process
4. Output
5. Feedback (positive and negative) (Laszlo, 1996)

Much of the theory development in nursing has relied heavily on GST, which led to the holistic approach of nursing to illness and wellness. The body is viewed as a whole, consisting of interconnecting and mutually dependent parts that interact with each other and its environment for the purpose of homeostasis. With this in mind, it is clear that nurses have an excellent grounding in GST and its application to the body. GST and systems thinking can also be applied to organizations. Organizations are also composed of interconnecting and mutually dependent parts that interact to sustain themselves within their environment.

Wilber (1998) describes the interrelationship of mutually dependent parts as nested holons. A nurse's shift of work is a holon or subunit of a service, which in turn is a subunit of the organization, which is a subunit of a health care system. The subunits nest together to create a whole. So when we think of a system, or a unit of service, it is the quality and quantity of the connections with other units of service that allow the system to operate successfully. Because the elements of a system are interdependent, a change in one part of the system leads to a change in another (Laszlo, 1996).

Systems thinking, or the process of thinking in wholes, is the expression of the science of GST, and when used properly, it can lead to enormous improvements in the way care is provided and organizations are led. Flood and Carson (1998) define systems thinking as "the use of a framework of thought that helps us deal with complex things in a holistic way" (p. 8). Systems thinking is an invaluable tool when used by a system to decide on short- and long-term strategies, identify market opportunities, and make process and structural changes in the system.

During the past two decades, the volume of discussion has increased regarding systems thinking in health care and particularly in leadership. A leader's ability to think in wholes, or to see the big picture, is paramount in leading an organization through change. Leaders see how all the parts of the system currently interrelate and what changes need to occur so the interrelations are strengthened to accommodate changes in the external and internal environments.

The literature is replete with models that guide the user in explaining, predicting, and controlling phenomena in the workplace. A model of the use of systems thinking to diagnose system problems developed by Nadler and colleagues (1982) is a very helpful one. They expanded the transformational process to include the interaction among the person, his or her work, and the informal and formal organizational system arrangements that either facilitate or impede effectiveness. Their thesis is that all four of these elements of the transformation process must work in concert or productivity at the personal, unit, and system levels will decrease.

After years of discussing the absence or presence of accountability in the practice of nursing, a colleague and I began developing a systems model that might help explain why staff and managers either chose or rejected accountability. We also wanted to stop the process that occurs in many organizations of holding staff and managers accountable for achieving productivity levels that could not be reached given the broken system or their level of education. The System, Education, Accountability (SEA) model emerged (Fig. 2–3).

The basic premise of the SEA model (Crow and Debourgh, 1992) is that staff and managers are more likely to choose accountability if they work in a functional system and are properly educated to do what the system requires of them. When productivity at the individual, group, or system level declines, the first question asked is: "Is the system and its infrastructure elements operational, and are they arranged in such a way as to have the capability to meet environmental demands?" The questions, although important to ask and answer, should be asked and answered in the right forum. The correct question asked in the wrong setting will lead to an ineffective answer. It is at the point of service that an organization spends its money, and to exclude the point-of-service staff from identifying system changes is to miss an opportunity for a more complete and lasting strategy.

Frequently, I have discovered that senior executives both ask and answer this question in isolation. They often do not seek the input from either midlevel managers or staff. This is where a system of shared accountability could help improve the quality of questions and answers. Typically, in hierarchical systems, the response to decreasing productivity is to put increased pressure on the managers and staff. The result is increased stress at all levels of the organization, quite often causing further erosion of productivity.

When the system and its infrastructure elements are changed with the full participation of point-of-service staff, it is time to provide education that is specifically targeted at those skills, knowledge, and abilities demanded by the changes. If the leader and staff are confident that the system is functional and everyone has been educated to meet the demands of the environment, then it is safe to assume that acceptance or rejection of accountability is a choice.

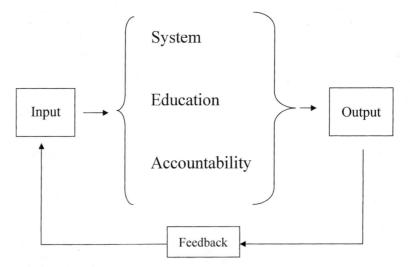

Figure 2–3. The System, Education, Accountability model. (From Crow, G. L., & DeBourgh, G. A. [1992]. SEA: A Model for System Assessment. *NurseWeek, 9* [11], 4–5.)

It has been shown that the vast majority of staff and managers become effective leaders when the system is functional and they clearly understand the expectations. When the above process has been satisfactorily completed, there is confidence that the system is operational, everyone has been educated to the new standards, and some still do not accept accountability, then it might be time to free their future.

Managing Change

I once heard a speaker say, "The only person who likes change is a baby in a wet diaper." After the laughter stopped, I realized the impact of that statement. Many in health care have believed that the future would be much like the past. Nothing could be farther from the truth. Our recent health care past, 1950–1983, was quite simple compared with today's complexities. Many patients entered the health care system, they were treated, a bill was sent to a third party, and they paid it. What could be simpler? The problem with that simple system was that it was fraught with spiraling costs. More hospitals were built than were needed, and they were filled with costly and sophisticated technology and many people. Then reality hit. No longer could we afford the health care system we invented—hence the change from fee-for-service to prospective payment. The entire paradigm has changed. It is no longer a matter of getting more business (customers), but instead the concerns are how to provide care in the shortest amount of time, ensuring high quality, and using the least amount of resources. For many, this journey to more cost-effective health care has left them with jobs that are devoid of meaning.

The response to this change was to attempt to decrease the patient's hospital length of stay (LOS) and get more patients into the system. No one understood that the LOS could be decreased and the cost would still be more than was allocated for a specified outcome. When this did not fix all the problems, much of the care was diverted to outpatient and home care units because the "cash cow" of outpatient and home care had not yet been gored. This did not work either because this migration to outpatient and home care services still required the same amount of resources. The only thing that had changed was the location; that only delayed the inevitable. Eventually, it became evident that a critical examination of the structure and process of care was needed. This process required exquisite leadership skills and could not be accomplished with the old command and control strategies of the past.

Analysis revealed there was a need to change the fundamental way in which the system operated—that is, how to define disease, how to provide care, and how to do both better using fewer resources. It began with an examination of what would truly make a difference in the areas of finance, quality, and customer satisfaction. Many organizations began this examination in earnest, yet they often left one of the most important stakeholders out of the discussion—nursing. Decisions about care were made from a financial (microlevel) perspective. A more effective process would have been to involve the system of care (macrolevel). For many organizations, the increased focus on financial management was not the silver bullet but instead a bullet that proved to be fatal.

Many, if not most, of the financial decisions made about resource allocation in health care organizations were made by senior executives and then handed to middle managers to implement, unchanged, at the unit level. This did not work because the managers and their staff at the point of service had no input into the plan; it was not theirs, and often it was not connected to a larger plan that made sense. It was typical top-down command and control management.

As the point-of-service staff became more and more alienated from management and the organization, the dialogue became louder and more personal on both sides. I remember hearing a familiar chorus from management and staff. The managers would complain that the staff did not care about the financial stability of the hospital, and the staff would complain just as bitterly that management only cared about money. While all this fighting was going on, the organization slipped further and further into significant debt. I describe this as organizational ventricular fibrillation. There is a lot of action, but none of it is directed toward survival. For those who couldn't, or chose not to, face the future, this whole process was a welcomed diversion that allowed them to concentrate on the present and to ignore the future. This was a fatal error. You cannot prepare for the future while expending enormous energy guarding the past. Clearly this behavior pattern needed to change, but how could it change?

A model of change that is familiar is Lewin's three-step change process of unfreezing, moving, and refreezing (Robbins, 1993). Of late I have come to the conclusion that if Lewin was doing his research in today's age of the knowledge worker, rapid technology invention and implementation, and a global economy, his model might actually be unfreeze, move, and slush. The idea of freezing anything in today's fast-paced world, although appealing, is antithetical to what the environments are demanding. The idea that all structures, processes, and products are changeable is relatively new in health care. Today the only realities that can be counted on are

- Eventually and eventuality seem to arrive faster today.
- What we know will no longer be.
- The next way of being will someday run into its boundaries and will need to change again.
- It is a rapid and never-ending process of ending and beginning.

Unrelenting change produces a very common side effect. Many people become hopeless and take up the role of victim; these roles are accepted out of fear and anxiety. What emerges is an organization with staff and managers who feel they have very little influence and power over their future. In fact, they are so wrapped up and controlled by the problems of the day that they are not capable of speaking of, let alone planning for, their future. And as they feel less and less powerful and influential, their commitment to the profession, organization, and each other suffers.

When organizations are rapidly changing, people often feel busier than ever, yet productivity tends to decrease. As they get busier and busier, burnout occurs because it takes enormous amounts of effort to get anything accomplished. This is where the meaning in what nurses do is misplaced or forgotten altogether. This loss of meaning does not occur easily or quickly; it is an insidious process that can sometimes take years and is an artifact of our estranged interaction with the system, its purpose, and our colleagues.

CONCLUSION

Becoming a leader is every nurse's responsibility. All nurses are accountable for the present condition of the profession and, more importantly, its future direction. Health care has never been more complex and, like all evolving systems, will become more complex over time. To truly shepherd nursing into the next century in prime condition to meet the challenges of the next century, all nurses must ask themselves: "What am I doing this moment to improve nursing and myself?" There is no time for petty squabbles. The future is not located in the past or the present; it is exactly where it should be—out there. The pioneers of this great profession were faced with challenges that troubled them, as the challenges of today trouble us. They managed to advance the profession, improve the public's health, establish schools of higher learning, conduct research, and plan for the future. And for many of those courageous pioneers, those challenges were effectively met before they lawfully had the right to vote to change health care at any level of operation. We cannot do less than they when we have more resources, are better educated, and are of sufficient numbers to insist that our lawmakers listen. I believe that the profession of nursing could be strengthened by all nurses' striving for self-knowledge, using it to positively affect their work environments and the health care system at large. If we do this, nursing will emerge in the 21st century as the major force in building a system of health care that more effectively serves this nation and the world.

USING THE KNOWING SELF MODEL TO DEVELOP LEADERSHIP SKILLS: ONE NURSE'S STORY

My stories are like many nurse leaders and unlike most nurse leaders. As an educator, consultant, and clinical specialist, I have had many nursing experiences that I will share as a way to concretize the discussion so far. These stories have occurred at various times in my career and are offered not as *the* way to know self but as the way that worked for me. It is my hope that my stories will alert others about how they, too, can learn more about themselves and their skills as nurses and leaders.

Inspiration and Motivation

The key to using the IMRC is to let what inspires and motivates you, staff, and managers become fully conscious. To know what moves you to positive action is paramount to leadership. I recall a major problem with a practice environment that lacked both inspiration and motivation. I had just been hired as a nursing administrator when the organization was entering a period of significant and rapid change, as they converted from traditional fee-for-service to prospective payment. The patient care services group was experiencing great difficulty in inspiring and motivating staff. The change from fee-for-service to prospective payment involved a different set of skills, abilities, and knowledge. Without understanding the new way, staff and managers were unable to participate in processes that would place the institution in better condition to survive and thrive.

I remember my visit with the staff. I noticed their postures were not straight, their energy appeared low, and, most importantly, they were focusing on what they felt they could no longer do for the patient instead of examining the new possibilities for their practice. I also learned that productivity had declined significantly. And then it hit me; the staff was reflecting back to me what they saw in their leaders. Although the staff may have used different terms and behaviors to describe it, the outcome was the same. They, as well as the managers, were actualizing little of their potential. Rather than just telling them there was hope after prospective payment, I had to tell myself to "role model the new way and coach them." My challenge was to create an inspirational and motivational practice environment with (not for) the managers. The managers could not lead the creation of an environment that inspires and motivates their staff if they were not personally inspired and motivated by their practice. This realization was my call to action.

If I expected the managers and staff to practice in an environment that inspires and motivates, then I was accountable to begin with myself. The question became, "What can serve to inspire me within this rapidly changing health care environment to want to do more with fewer resources and to do it better?" The answer came to me almost immediately, which often occurs when the correct question is asked. The managers and the staff were only part of the problem.

Wheatley (1992) and DePree (1989) have said that when you see a negative pattern in the staff, look for the origins of that behavior in management. I accepted that thought and did a self-assessment in an attempt to discover what role I was playing in crafting an environment that lacked inspiration and motivation. For many, there was no reward worth the effort at the end of the IMRC. I needed an immediate and long-term solution.

That afternoon the director of education came to me with the tape of a speaker whom she had heard at a recent conference. The speaker eloquently outlined how to create a positive and motivating workplace in a rapidly changing health care environment. The problem, as I saw it, was that we were ignorant of how to prosper in the new environment and that our collective ignorance was leading us toward failure. The only cure for ignorance is education, so with the help of the managers, staff, and the education department, we planned and implemented a management and leadership development program that focused on thriving in an age of prospective payment.

Knowledge and mastery over the new way inspired us with know-how and served to motivate because we now had tools that would help. The answer (tool) was not to "do this" so much as it was to understand the new way and know that there were proactive steps (behavior patterns) to take. As it turned out, the garnering of knowledge helped everyone, and I began working on a model that might help explain why staff and managers are often reluctant to accept accountability for outcomes. My conversations with managers and staff continuously brought me back to three elements of a system that affect every-one's ability and desire to be accountable:

- The system in which you work
- The educational preparation you have for the job
- Your acceptance of accountability for the outcome

I observed that these were the three primary elements that affect the work of managers and staff. After this experience, my colleague and I cast the concepts into a systems framework and developed the System, Education, Accountability (SEA) model (Crow and DeBorough, 1992) (see Fig. 2–3).

During this experience, I learned that all too often mangers are accused of not wanting to be accountable. My task then was to change that kind of thinking pattern because many times the problem is not the lack of desire to be accountable but whether the staff and managers work in a functioning system with an infrastructure that supports their roles. Additionally, I found that both the staff and management must be educationally prepared to function in a new environment. My conclusion was that if the system was functional and every-body was prepared to enact their roles, then most would desire to be account-able.

As a result, I set about creating an environment in which inspiration and motivation played a pivotal role in facilitating the development of informed behavior patterns to deal with rapid change. We all learned that the process of re-creating our practice and ourselves had meaning. Creating a work environ-ment that inspires staff to bring their whole self to the practice and the self-knowledge that is derived from that experience created shared meaning about our purpose as nurses.

The Environment

In my role as a consultant, I sometimes find myself in toxic settings where managers and staff do not trust each other. When I find myself in these settings, I try to get managers and staff to identify the forces that brought them to their present situation and the forces that are keeping them in place. Acknowledging how the past is influencing the present and preventing the future is the first step in moving toward a preferred future. I also believe that a thorough accounting of the present state can be accomplished only on a solid foundation of knowledge about self.

I try to help managers and staff understand the following:

1. The process of forgiveness—granting and receiving it—is a primary step in letting go of the past, which frees people to work toward the future.
2. Embedded beliefs, values, and behavior patterns carry tremendous power.
3. You cannot change the environment using old rules because those rules are a part of the problem.
4. Change should be guided by where the organization and its staff need to go, *not* by where it has been.
5. By acknowledging the "good old days" (which were old, but not so good),

one makes a conscious effort to reconstruct the path to the present and to define what should be changed and what needs to be deconstructed and thus begins the process of constructing the future.

Behavior Patterns

Changing behavior is often a part of my work as an educator and a consultant. I begin the pursuit of behavior pattern change by focusing on myself. I use a four-step process that involves knowledge about myself to develop my leadership behavior patterns. The first step is to decide what behavior pattern or patterns must change; I decide this by scanning all the environments with which I have been in contact to determine what made other people successful. Studying what made others successful in their environment helps me contextualize the behavior. Understanding successful behavior patterns in relation to where and under what conditions they occur helps me incorporate specific behavior patterns for specific situations. I have learned there must be a close fit between behavior patterns and the environment.

Second, from those I respect, I simultaneously seek specific feedback about what I can improve. I have discovered that selecting specific colleagues to provide pinpoint feedback on how I can improve is enormously helpful. Their honesty and candor are very important

Third, I limit the list of changes I will undertake to no more than three at a time. When the list of changes to be made is lengthy, the energy needed to accomplish them is diluted so there may not be sufficient energy to accomplish much. By paying close attention to a few issues one is more likely to bring about change.

Fourth, the behavior pattern or patterns that I want to change have to lead to a competitive advantage. The work it takes to change behavior must be goal directed and rewarding. Changing behaviors to those that can give a competitive edge not only adds to your talents but also can advance your career.

Leaders who want to assist others in changing their behavior patterns must not overlook a critical part of the process. To have a lasting impact, the strategies and structures of systems that trigger and reinforce the old behavior patterns must also be changed. Leaders must do this constantly in an effort to align behavior patterns with the demands of the internal and external environments.

Changes in behavior patterns that will make shared accountability successful are numerous for staff and managers. As a consultant, I follow a few basic steps. First, I help the staff and managers identify the behavior patterns that are keeping them locked into place. An important question to ask is "How is this behavior pattern rewarded by colleagues, the system structure, or environment?" I then ask them to specifically identify who encourages the behavior pattern. Often the person or persons who encourage the behavior pattern are the most powerful leader or leaders, formal or informal.

Second, I encourage an honest and thorough examination of how the current system structure, environment, and people are facilitating negative behaviors. In traditional hierarchical systems, rigid structures often encourage learned helplessness and rob everybody of the opportunity for accountability; however, changing the structure is never sufficient. Structure can help in changing behavior patterns, but the norms around what behaviors are acceptable must also be analyzed. Changing the structure without a close examination of the behavioral norms of the culture will result in only cosmetic change. The process of deconstructing the old norms is paramount in building a future. Deconstructing the old way allows everyone the opportunity to identify the limitations of the present behavior patterns, as well as the behaviors patterns that will help everyone move into the future (Crow, 1997).

The process of deconstructing the past and the present is very difficult and at times very threatening. It is a threatening process because of the deeply (although not always consciously) held behavior patterns that are symbols of the culture. The culture of an environment is most evident at the point of service (Crow, 1996a, 1997). Before a strategy to change behavior patterns is planned, an assessment of point of service activities should be accomplished. As leaders identify behavior patterns that are keeping the organization locked in the old way, they can simultaneously build a support system that will facilitate change at the point of service.

Third, I recommend changing the performance appraisal criteria because the performance appraisal process can be a powerful tool in shaping behavior patterns. It can serve as a check-and-balance function for everyone. The new performance appraisal criteria should reflect skills that will, when implemented, place the organization in alignment with its environment. The essential question regarding new behavior patterns covered in the performance appraisal should be "How is what you are doing consistent with current expectations?"

I also recommend that staff and management have the same performance appraisal criteria. The new appraisal system should specifically target professional behavior patterns that will support staff and management accountability for patient care quality and resource management. Shared accountability becomes the arena where management and staff begin the process of identifying what behavior patterns are most likely to propel the organization along the path to their preferred future.

Systems Thinking

System thinking abilities have helped me immeasurably throughout my career at the bedside as a clinician and as an administrator, consultant, and educator. While at the bedside, the major issue that affected my work was staffing. I wanted the staffing that I thought I needed to care for the patients in the manner that felt comfortable to me—end of discussion! I held this view for 4 years; then I took an on-call shift supervisory position. That is when I realized that my unit was only one of many subunits demanding resources within the organization. I had been aware that the coronary care unit was connected to the rest of the hospital, but this was a superficial understanding. After all, I was working in critical care, and we should have all the resources necessary to do our work.

The balancing act of resource allocation is done in the hope that resources can be allocated to the subunits in such a manner as to keep any subunit from collapsing. The balancing act was not well understood by me because of my narrow perspective on the issue. I viewed the hospital and its pool of resources from the perspective of my unit; this was not systems thinking. Clearly, I should have viewed the subunit (microview) from the perspective of the whole system (macroview). I wish I had learned this earlier.

At a another point of my life, the SEA model helped me in my role as educator. When students are not "getting it," I do not immediately jump to the conclusion that they do not want to "get it" or that they are not putting enough effort into studying. I ask myself whether the course is organized in such a way as to lead to learning. I look at it as a total system. This begins with the close examination of the course and the learning methodologies. I rely on student feedback to tweak the course during the semester. I might adjust the course for everyone or let specific students approach the learning in a way that they feel comfortable as long as the outcomes are met.

After the course has been adjusted, I look to the educational elements. The question becomes, "Do the students possess the requisite knowledge, skills, and abilities to master this body of knowledge?" If I find that several students do not have the requisite skills to master the content of the course, I feed that information back to the curriculum committee. This feedback becomes valuable information to ensure that the curriculum is interconnected and sequential. It also can inform a subunit (my class) or the school if the course is interconnected (part of a whole) and in sync with other courses.

Managing Change

In my work as a consultant in the implementation of whole systems shared governance, I never assume that all the executives, managers, or staff have a clear understanding of how their systems work. It is rare for dietary personnel to understand the challenges facing environmental services, and vice versa. What I do find is that most think they know what nursing does. When there is dialogue about how all the subunits operate and the demands they face, people are always surprised by what they learn, especially about nursing.

Before any implementation strategies are designed, the implementation team (or whoever is in charge of the change) must first understand the organization, the interrelationships of each subunit, and how that organization must be continuously in alignment with its environment. This holistic view, in conjunction with the environmental assessment, is the most vital step in placing the organization in the best possible position to build a sustainable future. Again, the SEA model is helpful.

After the implementation team has a clear understanding of the organization and its environment, the team must consider how to transform themselves from where they are to where they want to be. This is a powerful and sometimes anxiety-producing process of deconstructing old ways, based on knowledge, and constructing new ways.

Today's volatile environment of health care demands that an organization be able to rapidly respond and adjust its strategies. This means the organization must be as flat (without hierarchical decision-making) as possible so it can be more flexible (Crow, 1997); however, the structures in place to support the hierarchy will not go without a struggle. There is usually a tremendous amount of education necessary that clearly outlines the strategy for shared accountability, as well as the rationale for it, before any change can be initiated. This ability of the organization to sustain itself within its environment, even though it is changing, follows Darwin's theory (i.e., the environment dictates the quality and quantity of the organization's outputs). If the organization cannot provide these specific outputs, the environment will have little or no need for the organization (Crow, 1996a, 1996b).

SUMMARY

Clearly knowing what you know and being able to use it effectively are important aspects of effective leadership. Knowing how to inspire and motivate people and to understand the impact the environment can have on those people and their thinking are essential characteristics of those who want to take the lead during times of rapid change. Knowing how to focus on the system as a whole makes management of change a lot easier. My stories are testimony that the knowledge of self model presented in this chapter helped me as a nurse, an educator, and a consultant make change in my own life and the lives of others. It is my hope that others will try it and have the same kind of success.

REFERENCES

American Heritage Dictionary. (1994). New York: Dell Publishing.

Block, P. (1993). *Stewardship: Choosing service or self-interest.* New York: Berret and Koehler.

Brisken, A. (1996). *The stirring of soul in the marketplace.* San Francisco: Jossey-Bass.

Covey, S. R. (1989). *The seven habits of highly effective people: Powerful lessons in personal change.* New York: Fireside.

Crow, G. L. (1996a). Developing a change management strategy. *Journal of Nursing Administration, 26*(2), 17–18.

Crow, G. L. (1996b). Shared governance in the world of chaos, change and evolution. *The Journal of Shared Governance, 2*(3), 13–18.

Crow, G. L. (1997, Winter). After the merger: The dilemma of the best leadership approach for nursing. *Nursing Administration Quarterly, 21*(2), 13–16.

Crow, G. L., & DeBourgh, G. A. (1992). SEA: A model for system assessment. *NURSEWeek, 9*(11), 4–5.

De Beauport, E. (1996). *The faces of mind.* Wheaton, Ill.: Quest Books.

DePree, M. (1989). *Leadership is an art.* New York: Dell.

Emerson, R. W. (1856). *Essays.* New York: Little Leather Library Corporation.

Flood, R. L., & Carson, E. R. (1998). *Dealing with complexity: An introduction to the theory and application of systems science.* New York: Plenum Press.

Frankl, V. E. (1984). *Man's search for meaning: An introduction of logotherapy.* New York: Simon and Schuster.

Laszlo, E. (1996). *The systems view of the world: A holistic vision for our time.* Cresskill, N.J.: Hampton Press.

Nadler, D. A., Tushman, M. L., & Hatvany, N. G. (1982). *Managing organizations: A systems approach.* Boston: Little, Brown.

Peck, M. S. (1987). *The different drum: Community making and peace.* New York: Simon and Schuster.

Robbins, S. P. (1993). *Organizational behavior: Concepts, controversies, and applications.* Englewood Cliffs, N.J.: Prentice Hall.

Wheatley, M. J. (1992). *Leadership and the new science: Learning about Organization from an orderly universe.* New York: Berret and Koehler.

Whyte, D. (1995). *The heart aroused: Poetry and the preservation of the soul in corporate America.* New York: Currency.

Wilber, K. (1998). *The marriage of sense and soul: Integrating science and religion.* New York: Random House.

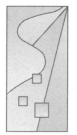

Chapter 3

Looking Forward: Being and Becoming a Futurist

Daniel J. Pesut

I was at a futures conference. Suddenly I realized I was the only nurse in the room. Everyone else was in insurance, health education, or pharmaceutical research. The speaker was talking about a new kind of health worker—a health coach. A health coach would work with individuals, families, or groups. The mode and method of communication and interaction would be via 24-hour telecognitive communication networks. Through the use of in-home computer workstations and interactive educational software, this coach would assist people with the development and maintenance of healthy lifestyles. Health coaching efforts would be organized around diet, exercise, nutritional counseling, and preventive health practices. Hospitals, insurance companies, corporations, and community agencies, as well as private citizens, would employ health coaches. Health coaches would be people who would capitalize on the values of wellness and lifestyle change for healthy living. There was a great deal of excitement in the room about this health coach prediction.

I raised my hand at this meeting and commented to the group, "Such a health care provider already exists—registered nurses are health coaches! What you describe is already happening. Haven't you experienced the skilled care of a nurse practitioner or clinical nurse specialist?" The futurist who was leading the session, a female pharmacist, looked at me and said, "Who are they? What do they do? How would I know where to find one? Are these people knowledge-able about clinical information systems and instructional simulations? Will they be able to navigate the health information infrastructure? Do these people understand the nature and consequences of combined genetic and pharmaceutical use? We are talking about a very different kind of health practitioner here."

Few nurses were present at the meeting to give voice to nursing's contributions. I was shocked that this group did not value, see, or understand the role of nursing in the future. Many of the people attending the meeting were influential advisors and consultants to companies and organizations that would shape the future. They were clueless about the role the nursing profession could play in a preferred health future. Since that time, my quest has been to learn more about futures studies and to encourage my colleagues to do the same.

To create a preferred future for nursing, we need nurse leaders with foresight. We need nurses who are lifetime learners, attuned to emerging trends. We need resilient, curious, creative, and courageous nurses. We need clinical scholars who act on values that support their visions. We need individuals who commit time, energy, and talents to looking ahead and who are willing to be and become futurists. Clearly, to be an effective leader, one needs to learn about and appreciate the role of futures studies in the development of effective leadership.

This chapter is about futures and leadership. The first section contains a presentation of the strategies for being and becoming a futurist that includes a "pledge" to future generations developed by Allan Tough. The second section is concerned with how I use these strategies and how I demonstrate taking the lead in an area of immense importance to nursing.

VISIONARY LEADERSHIP AND FUTURES THINKING

A 1991 Healthcare Forum Leadership Gap study identified five priority leadership needs for 21st century heath care organizations (Bezold and Mayer, 1996):

1. Visionary leadership in terms of risks and opportunities
2. Systems thinking—an understanding of the complex problems and interrelationships and a different view of the health care system
3. A shared vision of what to create in a health care system
4. A redefinition of health that focuses on healing, changing lifestyle, and the holistic interplay of mind/body/spirit
5. Social missions that weld health care organization goals, objectives, and actions with community service coupled with a never-satisfied attitude that supports continuous quality improvement

Visionary leadership is the first priority on this list. One of the keys to effective leadership is the vision factor—looking ahead and being a futurist. *Visioning* is looking ahead and anticipating the future. It is clear to me that being an effective leader involves futures thinking. Dr. Jay Conger is the executive director of the Leadership Institute at the University of Southern California. He studied the strengths and weaknesses of leadership development programs during a 2-year period. He interviewed more than 150 participants in these leadership development programs to gain knowledge of and to identify the necessary components of an ideal leadership course (Conger, 1996). He concludes that effective leadership training programs should address three major areas:

- Shaping strategic vision
- Aligning the organization
- Mobilizing the troops

Embedded in each of these areas are skill sets necessary for effective leadership.

Visionary leaders and leadership development programs should develop a futures orientation, challenge the status quo, and provide leadership development participants with tools and techniques that help them master future industry trends and demographics. Additionally, leaders must learn how to conceptualize strategic initiatives into a vision, which means they need to communicate a strategic vision, be role models, and develop a leadership philosophy and value set and persuasion skills to help leaders manage organizational change and set direction in decentralized organizations. Finally, leadership development programs should help leaders develop skills that mobilize the troops. Such a skill set involves trust building, empowerment skills, inspirational speaking skills, and the ability to master human resource systems and build effective teams. The most important skill of leaders is shaping strategic vision, and this requires developing a futures orientation.

Strategies for Being and Becoming a Futurist

Effective leadership is the process of creating and aligning vision, outcomes, and actions with ethics, energy, and resources in a network of relationships. The creation and alignment of vision and outcomes require leaders who are looking ahead and are futures oriented; being and becoming futurists would require

- Attention to time and the time spirits that influence individual and organizational behavior
- Learning about the future
- Appreciation and understanding of people's reactions to learning about the future
- Active monitoring of trends and industry forecasts
- Discernment of the consequences of trends
- Influence over change through the use and application of emotional intelligence
- Creation of vision-based scenarios
- Stimulation of strategic conversations about espoused visions

These eight strategies shape effective leadership. The following is a brief discussion of each of these strategies and their relationship to being and becoming an effective leader.

■ Attention to Time and Time Spirits That Influence Individual and Organizational Behavior

Being a futurist involves understanding the nature of time and its influence in leadership initiatives. A leader's success requires an understanding of time. How does time influence your current leadership style? Are you focused in the here-and-now or in the future? Images of time influence action and planning. There are many types of time that leaders must attend to, such as clock time, emotional time, mental time, quality time and compressed time, seasonal time, developmental time, and planning time.

There is no future without attention to the effects of time and the time profiles or imprints of individuals and organizations with whom leaders work.

Leaders pay attention to people's time profiles. A *time profile* is an assessment of the time frame or preferences of those with whom we interact. For example, if you had to classify the time profiles of people with whom you work, how would you go about it? For sure, you know individuals or groups of people who are always talking about the "good old days." Do you know anyone who is thinking so far into the future that they have no sense of current events? The words and language people use give clues about their time profiles. For example, people who look ahead often use words and phrases that have a future tense like "anticipate" and "expect." People who have time profiles and preferences for the past often use the past to filter their thinking. They are more likely to use words like "regret" or to invoke traditions as a way to solve problems or make decisions. Time profiles leave time prints. *Time prints* influence the degree to which people perceive they can plan and influence the future. The time profile for an effective leader is future based. Attention to time and time shifting is a personal leadership resource that helps create and reproduce competence.

The skill of reflective time shifting (Rechtschaffen, 1996) enables leaders to run future scenarios and alternative courses of action in their heads. Individual and strategic organizational planning efforts are often hampered because individuals or groups in the organization lack look-ahead time-shifting skills. Time shifting requires mental imagination skills. *Reflective time shifting* is the ability to analyze thoughts, feelings, and beliefs associated with experiences in a specific moment of time. The skill of time shifting allows leaders to visit past personal experiences and reframe experiences through hindsight. Time shifting supports changes in perceptions. Time shifting enables leaders to imagine stepping inside someone else's shoes. Choices in leading, managing, feeling, and behaving are byproducts of a leader's skill in reflective time shifting. In addition to time profiles, effective leaders are aware of the effects of time spirits on organizational change.

Arthur Mindell (1992) observes that time spirits are evident when there are tensions among past experiences, present opinions, and future aspirations. Time spirits can be memory fragments of some past happening that influence current and future practice or the development of tensions among competing group ideologies. Attention to the time spirits of organizations is an important aspect of effective leadership. Effective leaders understand and honor other people's time spirits and realize that to lead effectively, they must anticipate the future and look ahead. Effective leaders have their eyes on the future and make investments in learning about future trends, research methods, strategies, and studies that bear on their thinking and leading. Leaders use what they learn about the future to craft visions and scenarios about possible and preferable futures. In summary, effective leadership involves curiosity and commitment to the future while attending to issues in the present, because the values and heritage of the past are respected.

■ Learning About the Future

Not all nurses or leaders must be health care futurists, but we need a critical mass of future-sensitive leaders to shape thinking and create the future. Consider the pace of cultural change. Medical knowledge is doubling every 8 years, and 85% of the information in the National Institutes of Health computers is upgraded every 5 years (Cetron, 1994). Genetic engineering will do $100 billion worth of business by 2000. Newborn babies may be be artificially endowed with particular disease immunities. The ethical issues raised by technologies such as organ transplantation, the use of artificial organs, genetic engineering, and DNA mapping will cause growing public debate and opportunities for nurses. The physical fitness and personal health movement will remain strong—a market for nurses as health coaches. Breakthroughs in aging research will provide longer life spans of vigorous good health. What are the consequences for nursing? How many nurse leaders have investigated the consequences and implications of future health care projections? Foresight is a human attribute that allows us to weigh the pros and cons, to evaluate different courses of action, and to invest in possible futures (Slaughter, 1995). As a profession, we must engage in futures thinking (Pesut, 1997a, 1998b). *Futures thinking* presupposes learning about the future and using information from futures studies to inform and guide leadership initiatives.

Effective leaders who are capable of looking ahead are likely to hold some of the following beliefs and assumptions that provide a foundation for futures studies (Bell, 1997):

- New beliefs foster renewal and creation.
- The consequences of action always lie in the future.
- There are no facts about the future.
- The future is not totally predetermined.
- The future is uncertain and represents freedom, power, and hope.
- Leaders have a need to know the future and how the past and present produce future effects.
- Futures thinking is essential for human action.
- To a greater or lesser degree, future outcomes are influenced by individual and collective action.
- To act effectively in the world, humans need to estimate consequences of a given action and to guard against unintended and unanticipated consequences.
- The interdependence of people in the world necessitates a holistic perspective and a transdisciplinary approach for the organization of knowledge for decision-making and social action.
- A preferable future is one that you would like to have happen.

Given the universal nature of many of these assumptions and beliefs, it is interesting that there are different schools of futurist thought. The purpose of futures studies is not to predict the future but rather to envision desirable futures and avoid or to prevent catastrophic ones. Wendell Bell (1997) outlines several tasks related to futures studies:

1. Studying possible futures
2. Studying probable futures
3. Studying images of the future
4. Studying the knowledge foundation of futures studies
5. Studying the ethical foundation of futures studies
6. Interpreting the past and orienting the present
7. Integrating knowledge and values for designing social action

8. Increasing democratic participation for imaging and designing the future
9. Communicating and advocating particular images of the future

Each of these tasks has a leadership "spin." Each has professional consequences. Effective leadership requires individuals who can invent and project preferred futures.

There is a difference between assessing the likely future and creating a preferred future (Bezold and Hancock, 1996). However, Howard Didsbury (1994) suggests that futures thinking can be classified into the following six schools of thought:

- Scientific optimism
- Technological pessimism
- Omniscience
- The sustainable society school of thinking
- Transformationists
- Global community

Which perspective fits with your values and beliefs? Scientific optimists advocate that tomorrow will be like today but better. Scientific optimists believe solutions to the serious problems confronting humanity will be found through the application of scientific insight and technological innovation. In contrast, technological pessimists warn that our high-tech civilization is doomed. The pessimists warn that continued technological growth leads to dehumanization, depletion of resources, and doom. If you are concerned about privacy and the threat to individuals posed by a high-tech society where data banks are capable of checking up on people, then you may be member of the omniscience futurists camp. Futurists who advocate a sustainable society believe balanced growth or a steady-state economy is the key to a preferable future. Members of this school of thought advocate technological use tempered by wisdom and foresight with a special emphasis on attention to environmental science. Politics is the currency in a sustainable society. Transformationists are futurists who debate issues associated with value shifts. These people monitor value shifts and changes. An example is the shift in values from a postindustrialist age to new age consciousness. Futurists in this school suggest a spiritual transformation is needed to shape a preferred future. Finally, some believe a cooperative global community is a path to futures thinking. Given the interrelatedness of all peoples and the increase in technology and communication, this school of thought proposes that humankind must cooperate on a global scale or perish. Cooperation among national communities is the goal of members who adhere to this school of thought.

Given the fact that there are so many schools of futurist thinking, it is important to consider people's reactions to learning about the future. Learning about the future has consequences. Effective leaders appreciate the range and depth of people's responses to anticipated or unanticipated futures developments. Consideration of the intellectual, emotional, and existential byproducts of future developments is a challenging task for effective leaders.

- ■ Appreciation and Understanding of People's Reactions to Learning About the Future

Dr. Martha Rogers (1997a), a Canadian nurse scholar, has conducted research about learners' reactions to the study of the future. Based on her research, she identified three patterns of response to learning about the future. She eloquently describes these responses as patterns of the mind, patterns of the heart, and patterns of the soul. It takes a keen mind to understand futures issues. Such issues generate strong feelings; the feelings generated relate to existential issues of meaning, purpose, and soul.

Learning about the future means thinking about the long-term future and the generations to come. Thinking so far ahead challenges the status quo and projects one beyond present-day realities into uncertain future possibilities. Uncertain future possibilities generate a variety of feeling states (Rogers, 1997a). Anticipation and learning about the future evoke feelings that range from depression to elation, anger to acceptance, anxiety, happiness, sadness, and fear. Grief and hopelessness, as well as courage and hope, are emotions evoked by futures thinking. Attention to feelings is about patterns and responses of the heart, says Rogers (1997a).

A third pattern Rogers (1997a) uncovered in her research was unexpected but makes sense; her research revealed that learning about the future seems to affect people at the level of the soul. A consideration of the future somehow taps existential issues of meaning and being, values about the purpose of life, and an individual's responsibility toward justice and care, social action, and legacy. Looking ahead as a futurist requires that leaders understand the mind, heart, and soul consequences of looking ahead.

- ■ Active Monitoring of Trends and Industry Forecasts and Discernment of the Consequences of Trends

Shaping the preferred future requires a pattern of mind. Effective leaders who have their eyes on the future are always asking and answering the following sets of questions (Liff, 1998; Nanus, 1992):

- Is my view of the world out of date?
- Do I spend 20% of my time staying up to date?
- Am I ready for the next industry revolution?
- How do I prepare myself to get on the competitive leading edge of change?
- How do I prepare myself for scanning the environment for trends that have a consequence for my profession and my organization?
- What major changes can be expected in the needs and wants served by my organization in the future?
- What changes can be expected in the economic, social, political, and technological environments in the future?

As a leader, once these questions are answered, one is in a good position to shape the future. Often, we do not go far enough with our thinking about current trends and their nursing care consequences. Trends are the raw ingredients the mind uses to create and craft visions.

In his book *Visionary Leadership,* Bert Nanus (1992) suggests the following clues provide evidence about the presence or absence of a vision in an organization. If there is evidence of confusion about a purpose or there are disagreements among key people about clients, services, technologies, opportunities, and threat issues, the vision factor may be deficient. If people in the organization complain about insufficient challenge or say they are not having fun anymore—if they are pessimistic about the future or cynical about the present, then vision may be lacking. If there is a decline in organizational pride or individuals work only for their paycheck without a real sense of commitment or belonging, then vision is unclear. If people avoid risks and abide by narrow job descriptions and are unwilling to accept ownership for new projects or resist change, then organizational vision is not compelling. If there is an absence of a shared sense of progress or momentum or future aspiration, then the vision factor needs attention. If there is a hyperactive rumor mill and people have to find out through the grapevine what is in store for them or the organization, then the vision factor is not operative. These signs and symptoms suggest the direction for an organization is not being communicated well. The vision factor is deficient. Either the vision is not understood, or the vision is no longer there.

Nanus (1992) offers the following as ingredients of vision or the "look-ahead" factor:

> Vision is composed of one part foresight, one part insight, plenty of imagination and judgment, and often a healthy dose of chutzpah. It occurs to a well informed open mind, a mind prepared by a lifetime of learning and experience, one sharply attuned to emerging trends and developments in the world outside the organization. Creativity certainly plays an important part, but it is creativity deeply rooted in the reality of the organization and its possibilities (p. 34).

Foresight, insight, imagination, judgment, chutzpah, creativity, and attention to emerging trends within and outside of the organization, although abstract terms, give us clues about the elements of the looking-forward factor. Looking-forward leaders are value driven, attend to the future, are proactive and creative, and seize opportunities with a passion and commitment.

The look-ahead factor supports the development of mental models of the future to which people can aspire. Visions unify beliefs, values, actions, and identities. Visions are created on several levels: personal, professional, and organizational. Effective leaders have personal visions for themselves. These visions serve as the blueprint for their personal and professional aspirations. A personal vision statement helps one set priorities, make decisions, and guide actions. Visions are ideas that shape thought and action with a future in mind. For visions to succeed, people must believe the future can be influenced. Unfortunately, such beliefs are seldom reinforced in large institutions where present-centered and crisis mentality are combined with nonsystemic thinking to limit both the existence and breadth of vision (Rejeski, 1993).

To have vision, one needs to contrast the present reality with a desired future, using one's values as a guide. It is the essential tension between the present and a desired future that creates the energy, commitment, and momentum for change. Effective leaders play an important part in this process.

To shape the preferred future of nursing, we need nurses who are skilled in futures thinking methods. Future-casting, according to Kurtzman (1984), is the art and science of charting a way into the future to test alternative futures before they occur. Examples of future-casting methods are environmental scanning, trend analysis, polling, the Delphi technique, scenario development, technology assessment, cross-impact analysis, simulations, value-shift assessment, and gaming (Jarratt et al., 1994; Morrison et al., 1983). Once trends are identified, scenarios about the future can be created. The missing ingredient in most conversations about preferred futures for nursing is the fact that scenarios associated with visionary leadership are underdeveloped. For example, how will nurses react when major chronic diseases can be identified in utero and gene replacement therapy is initiated so the disease no longer occurs? What are the consequences for nursing if people live to be 115 to 120 years old and are in good health? How will nurses interface with 24-hour health education and advances in telecognitive learning and telehealth and telemedicine?

Visions stimulate the creation of scenarios or stories about the future. Are health care organizations and people currently prepared to work and function with these projected trends? Although the intellectual challenge of developments is exciting, the challenges have emotional counterweights. Feelings about the future are directly related to the degree of one's emotional intelligence.

■ Influence Over Change Through the Use and Application of Emotional Intelligence

In their book *Executive EQ: Emotional Intelligence in Leadership and Organizations,* Cooper and Sawaf (1997) write

> Emotional intelligence emerges . . . from the workings of the human heart. EQ is not about sales tricks or how to work a room. And its not about putting a good face on things or the psychology of control, exploitation or manipulation. The work of emotion may be simply defined as applying 'movement' either metaphorically or literally to core feelings. It is emotional intelligence that motivates us to pursue our unique potential and purpose, and activates our innermost values and aspirations, transforming them from things to think about to what we live. Emotional intelligence is the ability to sense, understand, and effectively apply the power and acumen of emotions as a source of human energy, information, connection and influence (p. xx).

To shape the preferred future of nursing, we must develop and use our emotional intelligence. We must pay attention to matters of the heart. The use of emotional intelligence enables us to direct our feelings and creative intuition from present experience to past experience and then to future experience. Time shifting enables us to choose new opportunities, based on an awareness of past experiences and lessons learned. People who develop time-shifting skills are more flexible and adaptable to circumstances. They innovate. They get stuck less often. They flow.

■ Creation of Vision-Based Scenarios

Visions without scenarios are empty (Cooper and Sawaf, 1997). By definition, a *scenario* is an outline of a natural or expected course of events. Scenarios enhance understanding of the present and past in light of future trends and developments. Scenarios provide clues about indicators to track and how decisions relate to organizational procedures. Scenarios help reframe decisions based on learning. People in an organization "test" choices and decisions in the context of a scenario. Creating and sharing stories about the future helps shape perceptions and mental models about what is possible and desirable in light of what is known, expected, and envisioned. Scenario discussions foster commitment to visions and provide paths for action. Scenarios are projections of a potential future. Scenarios help structure meaning.

Other purposes of scenarios are to augment understanding. They promote an understanding of the present and past in light of future trends and developments. Scenarios identify appropriate indicators to track, link specific decisions to organizational procedures, and help reframe decisions based on learning. Scenarios challenge the mindsets of individuals in an organization by developing plausible alternative story lines that require reflection (Van Der Heijden, 1996). Scenarios set the stage for strategic conversations that are vital to organizational development. Scenarios foster learning and help people explore the issues of mind, heart, and soul as well as the range of choices and corresponding results of decisions made in the context of a scenario (Van Der Heijden, 1996). Strategic conversations in an organization require leaders to motivate and mobilize the civic and self-leadership (Anderson and Prussia, 1997; Reed, 1996) inherent in individuals in the organization. Strategic conversation energized around civic and self-leadership lead to organizational learning. Through the application and use of scenarios (Fahey and Randall, 1998) and a consideration of the third- and fourth-order consequences of proposed visions and by creating scenarios that stimulate strategic conversations about the future role of nursing, leaders help align organizations and mobilize the troops.

Nurse leaders who participate in scenario-based discussions with each other and with those in the organization in which they work are more likely to be effective leaders than are those who do not participate in this scenario development process. For example, in 1992 Bezold crafted four scenarios of healthcare:

- High technology-continued growth
- Hard times—focused innovation
- Global business
- The new social contract

Each evolved from forces, plot lines, and end states that were plausible. These scenarios served as the backdrop for a variety of analyses. In 1998, we see elements of each of the health scenarios playing themselves out. Unfortunately, the nursing perspective in regard to these scenarios was and remains underdeveloped. It is time to update these scenarios. The more nurses are skilled in scenario development and are involved in the strategic conversations, the greater their influence in creating and shaping preferred futures.

Another example of the profession's lack of attention to scenario learning is the Belmont Vision. In 1992, C. Everett Koop was a member of an expert panel that developed the Belmont Vision (Bezold and McNerney, 1996). The purpose of the project was to craft a vision for 21st century health care. The Belmont Vision was shaped by considering trends projected to influence health care—specifically, the public-priority setting, cost-effective innovation, better design of financing and deployment of personnel, broader and better-measured therapeutic approaches, reduction in unnecessary complications, and integrated public policy. The Belmont Vision suggested the following criteria to judge health care reform initiatives:

• To what extent do plans broaden definitions of health and health care?
• How clearly do plans delineate the rights and responsibilities associated with the social contract for health care?
• Is universal access to services that improve health a part of the plan?
• How much caring and change are built into health care delivery?
• To what degree does each plan finance care on the basis of public priorities?

The Belmont Vision dealt with specifics for each of these areas. The vision suggested an expanded notion of health with an emphasis on prevention and education. The vision advocated a public/private partnership that would capitalize on the creative talent of the private sector and the social justice factor of the public sector. The Belmont Vision called for the creation of a new health care worker called a *health associate.* This individual would be community based and extend the effectiveness of physicians, nurses, and the health care team. Financing of 21st century health care would be accomplished through an alignment of risk and responsibilities, incentives, economic choices, tort reform, and competition based on quality and service.

If the Belmont Vision were realized, what would the nursing story be? Unfortunately, the consequences of the Belmont Vision for professional nursing are yet to be developed. There are some visions of nursing that require and demand strategic conversation, such as the work of Dr. Martha Rogers. American nurses have much to learn from our Canadian nurse colleagues in the area of strategic conversations with a futures focus.

■ Stimulation of Strategic Conversations About Espoused Visions

Canadian nurse futurist Rogers (1997b) was commissioned to develop five scenarios about Canadian nursing in the year 2020. Rogers suggests, when thinking of scenarios, that the following questions help focus thinking and reacting:

• How plausible does the scenario seem?
• What thoughts does it bring to mind?
• What feelings, if any, does the scenario generate?
• What are the implications for society, health, health care, and nursing?
• If parts of the scenario are desirable, what actions must be taken to increase the chances of the scenario happening?
• If portions are undesirable, what actions should be taken to prevent them from happening?

Consider this set of questions as you read the following scenarios about the future of nursing in Canada. Consider the issues and strategic conversations these scenarios raise for the nursing profession in the United States.

The title of the first 2020 scenario is *Technology Eclipses Care.* In this story, health care and health management are technology driven. Hospitals are high-tech centers. Sensors, monitors, and voice-activated equipment and smart machines monitor and adjust care parameters. Genetic engineering decreases or eliminates disease development. For example, enzymes dissolve organs like the appendix and gallbladder. A cast of health supporters that includes massage therapists, palliative care assistants, elder care assistants, health communication specialists, and child development specialists emerges and supports health initiatives. Nursing disappears. Analysis reveals that the reason for nursing's demise was its definition of the practice as a set of skills and tasks rather than as knowledge-based care (Rogers, 1997b).

The title of the second 2020 scenario is *Control, Manage and Measure*. In this scenario, because of debt, social programs are eliminated. The business of health care is organized around programs of managed care. Health activities are centralized. Genetic fingerprints result in predicted illness patterns. People are given personalized care maps based on genetic analysis. Compliance is monitored via a personal health record, called a "smart card." People who do not follow the care map are required to finance their own health care. Physicians are directors of medical teams and choose whom to hire. Nurses on teams decrease in number because others are less expensive. A small band of nurses who believe in the power of nursing continues to exist.

The title of the third 2020 scenario is *Return to Care*. Social, political, and economic stability leads to "values-based" politics. Health is a value. Resources are shifted from illness care to health care. Some believe nursing can be replaced with more cost-effective workers; however, the panacea of managed care did not realize its promise. In fact, managed care contributed to increases in complications and death and an increase in consumer dissatisfaction. Nursing studies contributed evidence that supported the achievement of health outcomes by nurses. Healing rooms and lay learning centers accelerate healing and maintain health. Collective political action results in nursing education reforms.

In a fourth 2020 scenario, entitled *The Transformation,* society discovers that caring and spiritual development begets better health and a meaningful life. The quest for balance results in an appreciation of diversity, a balance in work and play, and a renewed interest in the concept of community. People conclude that not everything can be measured. The mystery of life is valued. Boundaries among health disciplines blur and are replaced by educational programs for healing and health. Healing competencies are documented on smart cards. The international exchange of ideas contributes to global health.

These stories are excellent examples of how futures methods can be used to create conversation and action toward the development and creation of a preferred future. Creating and sharing stories about what we do not want to see as well as what we do want to see helps shape perceptions and mental models about what is possible and desirable in light of what is known, expected, and preferred. The effect of scenarios and futures-oriented thinking is to stir the souls of people in their organizations.

Paths to Effective Leadership: Stirring Soul in the Workplace

In his book *Stirring Soul in the Work Place,* Alan Briskin (1998) writes, "The soul remains a vital metaphor, particularly during periods of change because it speaks to timeless longings for meaning and purpose" (p. x). Creating the preferred future of nursing requires that we wake up our corporate soul and pay attention to spiritual politics. According to authors Corinne McLaughlin and Gordon Davidson (1994) in their book, *Spiritual Politics: Changing the World from the Inside Out,* the meaning of the word spiritual is far broader than a specific religious connotation. *Spiritual* applies to anything that relates to the expansion of consciousness, that drives an individual or society forward toward some form of development—physical, mental, emotional, and intuitive—that develops greater love, beauty, and understanding. Creating and celebrating a preferred future for nursing requires waking up nursing's corporate soul. The four paths to corporate soul are also the four paths to effective leadership (Klein and Izzo, 1998).

The first of the four paths is the *Path of Self:*

> Soul awakens when people are aware of their own passion, in touch with their core values, and when they actively bring these alive in their daily work. Although this path is primarily about the individual discovery of vocation, leaders are responsible for developing a climate that fosters the kind of self-discovery required to be sure people bring their values and passion into the workplace (p. 23).

Futures thinking involves understanding the path to self. The path of self leads to the path of contribution.

In walking the *Path of Contribution,* people discover the deeper reason for their work, both now and in the future. The value and meaning of people's contributions come alive as they recognize daily efforts to serve worthy goals. When people see the outcomes of their work as valuable, especially when connected to service, soul and commitment are evident and present. Contributions have a past, present, and future tense. Contributions involve craft.

The *Path of Craft* is the development of an intense enjoyment in the moment to moment action of work. Craft focuses on the ongoing process of learning and mastery that turns most mundane tasks into artistic activities. People come alive when they are engaged in activities that call forth their highest level of skill, when they discover unknown capabilities, and when they can take their learning with them into the future.

Finally, people find soul on the *Path of Community* when their connection to others goes deeper than a job description and touches the heart, transcending traditional team efforts. Through the Path of Community, individuals join together to bring out the best in each other and secure a preferable future. Successful futures thinking involves community members who see each other's limits without blaming and who call forth each other's riches without demanding.

As Rogers (1997b) observes:

> Every nurse has the capability to influence the future: to create a positive future for the profession as well as health, and health care of those we serve. To make informed decisions and choices we need to think about the future beyond tomorrow and or the next day. We need to explore the possibilities, both good and bad. We need to use our minds, hearts, and imagination to generate images of the future, use our voice, hands and feet to create our destiny (p. vi).

If the nursing profession is to play a significant role in the future, we must get out our stories and influence the futurists, who influence the strategic planning efforts of businesses and corporations and educational institutions. To have a significant voice in shaping the future, more nurses must extend their influence to people outside the profession of nursing. For nurses to play a role in a transformed health care system, we need individuals who can transcend the present, anticipate the future, and create vision-based scenarios that show how resources are aligned with action to achieve well-defined outcomes. As Nanus (1992) said, we need leaders with "one part foresight, one part insight, plenty of imagination and judgment, and a healthy dose of chutzpah." We need leaders who have open well-informed minds prepared by a lifetime of learning and experience, who are sharply attuned to emerging trends and developments in the world. We need leaders who are creative and deeply rooted in the reality of their discipline and organizations. We need leaders who can translate visions into stories about the future that provide paths of direction and action. As a profession, we need leaders who are looking forward and being futurists. As we learn about the future from futurists, futurists learn about nursing from us. Connection with the futures community enhances effective personal and professional leadership.

Sentiments and values about looking ahead and being a futurist are contained in the thoughts developed by Allen Tough (1993) (Box 3–1). As you read and reflect on the messages contained in this pledge to the future, consider the consequences and implications for the development of qualities related to your effective leadership talents.

BEING A FUTURIST: MY USE OF THE EIGHT STRATEGIES FOR BEING AND BECOMING A FUTURIST

The last section of this chapter focuses on my stories as a futurist as they relate to the eight strategies described in the first half of this chapter. I have had a long-standing interest in futures-oriented issues. Recently I was introduced at a meeting as a nurse futurist. I don't remember exactly when I became a "futurist." I do know that working in leadership positions in several academic and nursing service organizations forced me to consider the future and anticipate the consequences of projected future trends. To some degree, I believe we are all futurists and must pay attention to the role time plays in our professional careers and organizations in which we work.

Paying Attention to Time and Time Spirits

Professional development and leadership require attention and reflection about the role of time and how time spirits influence your personal and professional decision-making. As one pays attention to time, it is important to reflect on the past, present, or future of one's day-to-day thinking. The context in which one works also influences one's sense of time. For example, if you work with people on a day-to-day basis, present realities are the focus. However, as an academic, it is easier for me to spend time thinking about the future because planning for the future is an important part of educational administration.

Box 3–1

A Pledge to Future Generations

Although humanity is far from perfect, it is definitely worthy of my respect, affection, compassion, and nurturance. I am fully aware of the pain, suffering, ignorance, selfishness, and greed in the world, but I do not condemn human civilization nor write it off as hopeless. I believe that a satisfactory future is possible if enough people care about future generations, understand today's options, and make appropriate choices.

For me, it is very important that humanity and other life on our planet continue to evolve in positive directions. Nothing is more important than the continued flourishing of human culture and society over the next few decades and beyond. Because I care deeply about humanity and its future, I do my best to live up to the following principles.

1. I care about the well-being of future generations. Their needs are just as important as those of today. When I am making a major choice in my own life, when I am involved in policy-making or decision-making, I take into account the needs of the next two or three generations. No short-term or narrow goal should be allowed to jeopardize humanity's long-term future. My choices support the principle of equal opportunity for each future generation: We should not cause their opportunities and well-being to be less than ours.

2. I choose paid work or volunteer work that makes a positive contribution to humanity's flourishing. I do my work with conscience—and with respect for the well-being of future generations and our planet.

3. I play my part in halting the deterioration of our environment and I support efforts to achieve a sustainable relationship with our planet. I try particularly hard to avoid actions that might reduce the ozone layer or increase global warming. I understand that people who own and consume more than they really need do even more harm to the environment than the desperate efforts of the poorest one-fifth of the world's population to survive.

4. I understand and support humanity's urgent need to halt population growth in all countries. In my own personal decisions, I am strongly influenced by this. I take highly effective steps to avoid pregnancy except when I have made a careful and thoughtful decision to have a child.

5. Because the institution of war causes so much harm over the years, I speak up against all wars, terrorism, organized violence, and arms manufacturing. Better ways exist for handling conflicts, greed, anger, and the urge for revenge. Because I believe the world's storehouse of weapons should be kept below the level capable of ending civilization as we know it, I support campaigns for a huge reduction in nuclear, biological, and chemical weapons.

6. Through words and actions, I support some of the additional goals and directions that will help human civilization to survive and flourish over the next few decades. Examples of positive goals and directions include the following: the health and well-being of children; understanding and coop-

Box continued on following page

eration among diverse cultures; a deeper understanding of the universe and our place in it; a more profound body of knowledge related to world problems and our future; widespread human rights, civil liberties, and political participation; a designated spokesperson for future generations in all political and military decision-making; experiments with innovative policy-making and governance.

7. I support local organizations, political parties, government policies, and international organizations that foster these six principles. I oppose those that do not take seriously our responsibilities to future generations.

8. When deciding how to spend my money and time, I seek an appropriate balance between my own needs and those of future generations. Instead of choosing luxuries and activities that harm the environment, I focus on my most significant underlying needs, such as relationships, learning, giving, contributing, vigorous health, a spiritual connectedness to nature, and other simple joys of life. I do not use material goods to meet my psychological and social needs.

9. I continue learning about the world's problems in some depth, and about our various potential futures ranging from highly positive to extinction. I face my feelings about these problems and possibilities, and avoid becoming stuck in hopelessness and paralysis. I speak up to counter misinformation and untruths, but I also keep an open mind to new ideas and perspectives.

10. I live in a decade during which some of the most important choices in the history of human civilization will be made. I happily join others in facing the heroic challenge of this decade—to move from our present catastrophic path to a new path that will dramatically improve our prospects for a flourishing future.

Tough, A. (1993). Making a pledge to future generations. *Futures*, 25(1), 90–92.

I believe many nurses operate "in" time and not "through" time. It is easier to focus on the here-and-now. Nurses pride themselves on caring moments, immediacy, intimacy, and being present. People who operate in the present are often content. People who have aspirations are likely to be focused in the future and restless in the present. People who focus on the past live with regret and often are angry and resentful. Psychiatrist Dennis Gersten (1997) suggests that people who have a tendency to worry about the future need to work on issues of faith, trust, and surrender. People who have a tendency to focus on the past need to work on issues of forgiving, letting go of resentment, overcoming blame, and releasing guilt.

When I began to assume leadership positions, my relationship with myself and others and my professional aspirations shifted my orientation to time. Clearly, nurses who think of nursing as a career have a different time perspective than do those who consider nursing a job. My own experience is an example.

Fundamentally, I am a worrier. As a worrier, I try to anticipate events and plan appropriate reactions. I was the firstborn child in my five-person family. I often had responsibility for my younger brother and sister. Being responsible involved worry and anticipation of what the future might bring. Such worry created a hypervigilance that is still with me. In recent years, I have transformed my hypervigilance into a concern about the consequences of future health care developments for the profession.

After I graduated from my baccalaureate degree program, I went into the Army. I was a product of the U.S. Army Student Nurse Program. As a neophyte nurse, I enjoyed working with burn victims and their families. My early years were spent as a staff nurse at the Brooke Army Medical Center at Fort Sam Houston in San Antonio, Texas. As a staff nurse, I was challenged one day at a time. I didn't look much beyond an 8-hour shift or a 2-week schedule. In fact, during tense codes, it was second to second and minute to minute.

For a while, I was content with my knowledge, skills, and abilities as a burn nurse. I particularly enjoyed the evening shift; I was in charge. The tempo of time is different on evening shifts. I could work more closely with patients and their families. I helped people cope. For example, as I watched and learned how burn patients coped with the pain and trauma of multiple dressing changes, surgeries, skin grafting, healing, and rehabilitation through occupational and physical therapy, time shifted me.

I started to worry about the lack of attention to burn patients' psychosocial needs. I reasoned that the acquisition of mental health knowledge would augment my nursing care through time—for example, from the present to the future. I began to think about a future in which I would have advanced practice skills and be able to do more and offer more to patients and their families.

I soon realized that a graduate degree would offer me the skills I needed to be more effective. So, with an image of a preferred future, I enrolled in a graduate program in psychiatric mental health nursing. Returning to school altered my relationship with the here-and-now of my professional aspirations, patients, and military assignment and put me on a fast track to the future. I was lured into the future by the promise of a different set of advanced practice nursing skills that I believed would make me a better nurse.

After completing my master's degree at the University of Texas Health Sciences Center in San Antonio, I developed a psychiatric clinical nurse specialist role at the Army Medical Center. I received the Army Commendation Medal for my efforts. The spirit of future time moved me from day-to-day nursing care to working with families, groups, and staff in an effort to design programs and treatment plans that would serve as models that could be replicated and to extend nursing care influence through time. Reflecting on time in regard to your roles, responsibilities, and aspirations is one of the first steps one can take to look ahead.

Learn About the Future

Depending on the role you play in an organization, your affinity for learning about the future may be great or none at all. Graduate school is an open invitation to learn about the future. Most graduate programs offer courses in professional issues, policies, and politics. Graduate students are encouraged to immerse themselves in the current literature and discern consequences derived from application and testing of knowledge. I enjoyed the opportunities to examine the past, live the present, and shape the future. My years as a doctoral student introduced me to and reinforced for me the importance of futures thinking.

I first became aware of futures thinking and the World Future Society (WFS) in the early 1980s. The WFS is a nonprofit educational and scientific association. The society is independent, nonpartisan, and nonprofit. *The Futurist* is one of the official publications of the WFS; *The Futurist* publishes articles and reports dealing with (1998)

- Significant social and technological trends and informed forecasts about where they may lead
- Methods for using information about future possibilities in decision-making
- Other topics of interest to people seeking greater success in the future of their organizations and themselves

Reading *The Futurist* opened my eyes to the issues and challenges facing the world in a variety of areas: demographics, economics, ecology, lifestyles, technology, health, and finance. I often used *The Futurist* as a starting point for references and resources about emerging future issues. Following up on articles and experts, I was able to track down leads, research, and resources that were useful in my learning. Exploring the futures literature, I discovered the importance of creative thinking in the design of preferred futures. Many futurists systematically use creative thinking strategies to build scenarios and associations between and among trends and consequences. "How," I asked myself, "do some futurists get these ideas? What is the essential dynamic of a futurist's thinking?" The answer seemed to be these people had well-informed minds and a knack for creative thinking.

I set out to learn as much as I could about creative thinking. Eventually, I wrote my dissertation on the topic: *Metacognition: The Self-Regulation of Creative Thought in Nursing*. Because the nursing profession was struggling to develop a scientific base for practice, I reasoned the following: Nursing science needs a scientific base. Science presupposes research. Research presupposes a significant research question. Significant research questions presuppose clinicians who have well-developed critical and creative thinking skills. Creative thinking is essential to science. If one could help nurses develop creative thinking skills, then the development of questions that could be translated into research to inform the future could be posed. After all, isn't that one of the reasons we engage in theory development and testing—to inform the future? Although it seems self-evident now, at the time this was a big insight for me!

My interest in creativity fueled the desire to learn more about the future. Conversely, my interest in the future supported my study of creative thinking. Along my career path, I continue to use what I have learned about creative thinking. My knowledge is especially useful in my teaching role. I continue to write and lecture about the importance of creative thinking for personal and professional excellence. I have always enjoyed teaching; I take special delight when I use a metaphor or story that makes a point, and I see the lightbulb go on and students make discoveries or insights that shift their thinking, doing, and feeling. One of my greatest honors was receiving the Edith Moore Copeland, Sigma Theta Tau, Founders Award for Excellence in Creativity in 1993.

In 1995, I became a Fellow of the American Academy of Nursing. Because I had a growing interest in the future, I approached the editor of *Nursing Outlook*, the official journal of the academy, and offered to contribute a short feature on selected aspects of the future. The feature is called *Future Think* (Pesut, 1997a, 1997b, 1998a, 1998b) and is designed to stimulate thought, reflection about future-oriented trends, and consequences. I enjoy writing these "think pieces" because this is one way for me to challenge myself and others to learn more about the future; remember that people's reactions to the future vary.

Appreciate and Understand People's Reactions to Learning About the Future

Effective leaders understand the range of responses people have in regard to the future. I have come to believe that reactions to the future are fear based or aspiration motivated. Fear-based responses are motivated by the need to protect and defend one's current modes of responding to change. Fear often is derived from a scarcity mentality and a belief that there are insufficient resources to accomplish change. In contrast, aspiration-based responses are rooted in a learn-and-grow paradigm and motivated by an abundance mentality in that there are sufficient resources to get what one wants.

I have worked in organizations in which the predominant style of responding is avoidance or moving away from the future. Often in such organizations, people are invested in protection and defending and operate to minimize threat. Scarcity of resources is often invoked as an obstacle to innovation and change. In these environments, people often focus on problems and engage in blaming, judging, or demanding. They lack the creative thinking to move beyond the problems to obtain useful solutions. Organizations with these dynamics erode spirit because the fear/scarcity/avoiding organization is often too busy defending and protecting itself. In these organizations, the future receives limited attention.

In contrast, I have also worked in organizations that adopt a learn/grow/aspire/abundance orientation. In these organizations, learning and renewal revitalize everyone in the organization. These organizations respond to obstacles with flexibility, resilience, and an eye on the long view. These organizations strive to create the future and reinvent the industries of which they are a part. In these organizations, people more often focus on end results or outcomes and then work backwards in an effort to get what they want. They bring the future into the present.

It is important to consider people's personality types or interpersonal styles as you study reactions to the future. A model that has been especially useful to me is one developed by Robert Dilts (Dilts and Bonissone, 1993). He modeled the creativity strategy of Walt Disney. Dilts considers creative thinking to be a strategy of communication and negotiation among various "parts" called the *dreamer, realist,* and *critic.* Every organization has dreamers, realists, and critics. When one takes the time to discover them one can discover one's own inner dreamer, realist, and critic!

These parts need a manager and broker because each part has a different sense of time and a different intention in the planning process. Dreamers establish new goals and outcomes. In terms of time, dreamers are oriented toward the future and long term. Realists implement new goals and outcomes.

Realists are more action and short-term oriented. Critics in an organization push for the establishment of evidence procedures and evaluate progress toward goals or outcomes. Critics often want to move away from what is proposed because they try to evaluate the long- and short-term consequences of change based on their experiences. Effective leaders know the organizational dynamics and the mix of dreamers, realists, and critics to negotiate the future and anticipate people's reactions to proposed plans or projects. When a project must be done, make sure you have the right mix of dreamers, realists, and critics and someone who can manage their talents. It is important to take into consideration comments from all the dreamers, realists, and critics in an organization and then trust your intuitions. I have also learned never to discount the value and contributions of those who take on the critic role. At the heart of every criticism is a positive intention about an important value or belief that is essential to the success of the proposed project.

Influencing Change Through the Use and Application of Emotional Intelligence

Learning how to use the emotions of people to influence change is important. As a director of the nursing service of a psychiatric hospital, an associate dean in a college of nursing, a faculty member, and a leader in a variety of professional organizations, I have learned the following:

- Everyone has a story to tell.
- Every story has emotions linked to it.
- All stories are true and valuable given the individuals' perceptions.
- Behind every story, there is a positive motivation even if the motivation is not clear at the time.
- Given a different context, the meaning and the emotional intelligence of a story might change.
- It is often more important to attend to the emotional intelligence embedded in the story than the content of the story per se.

Along my career path, I studied a model of human behavior and communication known as neuro-linguistic programming (NLP). Some of the many things I value about this model are the presuppositions on which the model is built. I also value the degree to which emotions as drivers of change are incorporated into the model. I have described elements of the NLP model and how the model can be applied in practice (Pesut, 1989, 1991). Two important building blocks of the model are an outcomes focus and a flexibility that results from reframing the meaning of events depending on the content or context of a given situation. Being flexible and focused on outcomes is important. For example, given health care's shift to primary care, is it possible to blend the competencies of clinical specialists and nurse practitioners? What are the outcomes, meanings, and emotions involved in such an issue?

Many clinical specialists do not want to learn nurse practitioner skills; however, the market supports clinicians with nurse practitioner knowledge. As much as I value my role and identity as an adult psychiatric mental health clinical specialist, the transformation of health care offers greater opportunity for those individuals who have advanced practice nursing knowledge consistent with skills of a primary health care nurse practitioner. In an effort to obtain some data about a blended role, a group of supportive colleagues and I were able to examine the emerging competencies for advanced practice (Williams et al., 1998) and design a curriculum that prepared individuals for both roles.

Moving away from the emotions of "either/or" to one of "both/and" in terms of practitioner-specialist preparation sustained a learn-and-grow dynamic in lieu of a protect-and-defend position. It is too early to tell what the consequences of such curricular evolution will be, but data from the project are likely to be influenced by people's emotional intelligence and their predilections for change. What is clear is that learning/growing and using emotional energy directed toward future aspirations create time and space for innovation. The emotional energy related to protecting and defending may promote comfort but not necessarily safety as the trends and projections transform the health care industry of the future. Consider the importance of monitoring trends and discerning consequences.

Monitoring Trends and Discerning Consequences

Projected future changes in health care are mind boggling. The most significant shift to affect health care will be the shift from a "diagnosis and treat" to a "predict and manage" health care paradigm (Bezold and Mayer, 1996). This shift is especially important as one considers developments in genetics, advanced practice roles, and informatics, as well as community-based care. What, for example, will the nursing care consequences be if chronic diseases can be identified, treated, and genetically altered in utero? How do past trends and future projections relate to each other? What skills will nurses need in the future given the shifts in the health care industry? How can nurses be best prepared to manage change and to reason effectively about patient care scenarios?

With the shift to an outcomes-oriented health care industry, I believe nurses are disadvantaged because of the educational focus on the nursing process, which is a stepwise, sequential problem-solving process. How can we as a profession blend the best of the problem-solving experience with the development of outcomes-based reasoning? My 28 years as a nurse educator are beginning to help me formulate an answer to this question.

I think the answer lies in the development and dissemination of a different model of reasoning. Traditional nursing process has changed over time. I continue to work to develop models of clinical reasoning that have relevance for contemporary nursing practice (Pesut and Herman, 1998). I think I have identified three generations of the nursing process. Taking the long view, it was clear that each generation of the nursing process was influenced by the state of knowledge development and contemporary forces operative during its formation. The first generation (1950–1970) focused on problems and process. The second generation (1970–1990) highlighted diagnosis and reasoning. The outcomes/present state test (OPT) model that Dr. Jo Anne Herman and I developed represents a third-generation nursing process model that emphasizes reflection, outcomes specification, and testing within the context of patient stories. The OPT model provides a structure for clinical reasoning that is consistent with the needs of the future. The OPT model builds on the heritage of the nursing process yet is more responsive and relevant to contemporary and future nursing practice needs. As a profession, I want nurses to develop expertise in clinical reasoning. To do so, I think the profession will benefit from a shift in thinking from problems to outcomes. Putting ideas out in lectures, the classroom, articles, and books is one way to stimulate strategic conversation and dialogue.

I often contrast the use of the nursing process with the OPT model to illustrate differences in the thinking that emerge from each model. For example, if pain is identified as a nursing diagnosis, most nurses talk about "no pain" or "alleviating pain." They are quick to point out pain management nursing interventions. However, in the OPT model, the pain situation is framed differently given a specific client story. One realizes reasoning is not just about pain and pain management but more about the contrasts between pain and comfort and the decisions and actions nurses use to promote comfort. This is a subtle and importance difference for teaching and learning clinical reasoning. In a forthcoming book, I discuss clinical reasoning and the critical and creative thinking strategies that support reasoning. My colleagues and I have tried to "unpack" the thinking used in clinical reasoning. Making these strategies more explicit is likely to help teachers to teach, students to learn, and clinicians to reason better. The model also serves as a structure for teaching clinical supervision and the development of middle-range theories organized around nursing knowledge taxonomies.

My professional vision is that the OPT model of clinical reasoning will become a means for multidisciplinary health care initiatives and provide a structure for accelerating the acquisition of clinical reasoning skills based on future knowledge development activities in nursing and other health care disciplines.

Creating Vision-Based Scenarios

Effective leaders have to do a good job of storytelling to get people in the organization to begin talking about the effects and consequences of espoused visions. Visioning is only one side of the leadership coin; the backside of visioning is scenario development. The work of Rogers (1997a, 1997b) cited in the first half of this chapter is an excellent example of the use and power of scenarios. Her stories about the future of nursing in Canada put different spins on what could happen, might happen, or is likely to happen or what people want to have happen. Scenarios such as these stimulate strategic conversations that excite people to exercise civic leadership in service of a preferred future.

The scenario by Rogers labeled *Technology Eclipses Care* (p. 21) is very plausible. Already, nursing is starting to disappear. In 1998, we see all kinds of nurse substitution taking place. It is also sadly true that nurses are undereducated and underprepared when it comes to genetic advances and biogenic informatics. It won't be long before robots and smart machines are performing many nursing tasks. The reluctance of the profession to embrace nursing knowledge development and classification of diagnoses, interventions, and outcomes leads me to believe that technology may eclipse care unless the nature of nursing is defined, classified, and incorporated into health care delivery information systems and databases that enable nurses to define and track what nursing provides and how nursing care affects the achievement of health outcomes. To think technology could eclipse care generates feelings of surprise and resentment. To think it would never happen is naïve and supports a protect-and-defend mentality that is not conducive to the learning and growing needed to understand the technological developments that are taking place.

A different kind of scenario will have to occur to prevent the *Technology Eclipses Care* scenario. First, nurses will need to develop nursing knowledge activities at all levels so there will be nursing knowledge to support the survival of the discipline. Second, nursing curricula will need to incorporate information about biogenetic and engineering advancements in health care technology. Finally, nurses who are masters in health care technology will need to evaluate, explain, and write about the human-response consequences of technological innovations and discern the nursing care consequences that coevolve with such technology.

Highlighting patient stories, problems, and outcomes supports clinical judgments about technology used in health care contexts and is the responsibility of the profession because nurses are those who will ensure the value of human-sensitive technology versus technology that eclipses care. These expectations are far-reaching and, although plausible, are highly improbably.

Truth be known, it seems we are living the *Control, Manage and Measure* scenario (p. 21) suggested by Rogers. We are moving toward care maps that discount the value and importance of clinical reasoning in day-to-day practice. The smart card is just around the corner, and physicians maintain control of medical teams and make the hiring decisions. Such a scenario breeds feelings of anger, resentment, helplessness, and hopelessness in nurses. The hope or emotional intelligence nested in this scenario is the fact that nursing brings meaning to the control/manage/measure mentality. Nurses are advocates of the meaning in illness and health experiences, and from meaning, people derive resourcefulness. Nurses who collaborate rather than compete for managed care dollars do it because their work means something different than control, manage, and measure. However, this scenario begs for nursing knowledge work in health outcomes research to provide the evidence for our belief and value systems. Such evidence is likely to invite support and inclusion rather then exclusion.

I would like to believe in the *Return to Care* scenario (p. 22), but I believe we are a long way from values-based politics in American health care. I think consumers who have the resources will pay for and get what they want. As a result, in the future, we will continue to struggle with part of the population who "has" and another large part of the population who are vulnerable. The contrast of this condition for the nursing profession will underscore issues and dilemmas of ethics, advocacy, responsibility, and social justice. To return to care, social justice is prerequisite.

As we approach the millennium, I sense a renewed interest in matters of the spirit. People continue to search for balance in their lives. Often, this search is motivated by a desire to serve and contribute to something greater than themselves—a sense of community, or legacy. Effective leaders challenge people to develop spirituality that leads to transformation and a renewed sense of society in which health and caring become part of the social fabric.

As you can see, the scenarios developed by Rogers have elicited many thoughts from me. All of the scenarios are plausible. The forces that will shape nursing in the future are global and far reaching. What and how can nurse leaders contribute to the strategic conversations inspired by these scenarios? The answers lie in recovery of corporate soul and the paths of self, contribution, craft, and community. A community of nurse leaders with global responsibilities are planning scenarios that will influence 21st-century health care.

Global Futures—Thinking

In December 1997, I was elected to a 4-year term on the board of directors of Sigma Theta Tau International Honor Society of Nursing. It is an honor and challenge to serve. President Eleanor Sullivan's theme for the biennium is *Pathways to the Future.* I was invited to participant in the strategic planning for the future of the organization. Taking futures thinking to scale in a global organization is an exciting challenge. Each member of the society was invited to be a member of the "Dream Team." Each was asked to identify values important to preserve in the society's future as well as beliefs they hold dear. Finally, people were asked to suggest what the society needed to hold fast and what the society could give up. Once data are collected, the planning team will have a clear picture of people's values, beliefs, and images of the future. Then, the board of directors can construct scenarios of the future in light of other health care industry trends and Sigma Theta Tau's mission. The scenarios will engage members in strategic conversations about the future aspirations, direction, and mission of the organization. This is another example of the application of futures thinking and planning to organizational development and success.

SUMMARY

To some degree, we are all futurists. Effective leaders look ahead. Being and becoming a futurist involves paying attention to time and time spirits, learning about the future, understanding people's reaction to the future, using emotional intelligence to influence change, monitoring trends and discerning consequences, developing vision-based scenarios, and engaging people in strategic conversations about the scenarios. Looking ahead and being a futurist requires an understanding of the value and contributions of dreamers, realists, and critics in an organization. Finally, being and becoming a futurist is more about learning and growing than about protecting and defending. I hope some of these thoughts and ideas help others consider the relationship of time to their professional aspirations.

REFERENCES

Anderson, J., & Prussia, G. (1997). The self-leadership questionnaire: Preliminary assessment of construct validity. *The Journal of Leadership Studies, 4*(2), 119–144.

Bell, W. (1997). *Foundations of future studies: Volume I: History, purposes, knowledge.* New Brunswick, N.J.: Transaction Publishers.

Bezold, C., & Hancock, T. (1994, March/April). Possible futures, preferable futures. *Health Care Forum*, 23–29.

Bezold, C., & Mayer, E. (Eds.) (1996). *Future care: Responding to the demand for change.* New York: Faulkner and Gray.

Bezold, C., & McNerney, W. (1996). Creating more visionary health care systems: The Belmont vision project. In C. Bezold & E. Mayer (Eds.). *Future care: Responding to the demand for change.* New York: Faulkner and Gray.

Bezold, C. (1992). Five futures. *The Health Care Forum Journal, 35*(3), 29–41.

Briskin, A. (1998). *The stirring of soul in the workplace.* San Francisco: Berrett-Koehler.

Cetron, M. (1994). An American renaissance in the year 2000. Seventy four trends that will affect America's future. *The Futurist, 28*(2), supplement insert.

Conger, J. (1996, Winter). *Can we really train leadership? Strategy and business,* Issue 2. New York: Booz-Allen and Hamilton.

Cooper, R., & Sawaf, A. (1997), *Executive eq: Emotional intelligence in leadership and organizations.* New York: Grossett/Putnam.

Didsbury, H. (1994). *Prep21 course/program guide: A selection of future oriented courses, programs, and instructional resources.* Bethesda, Md.: World Future Society.

Dilts, R., & Bonissone, G. (1993). *Skills for the future: Managing for creativity and innovation.* Cupertino, Calif.: Meta Publications.

Fahey, L., & Randall, R. (Eds.) (1998). *Learning from the future: Competitive foresight scenarios.* New York: John Wiley.

Gersten, D. (1997). *Are you getting enlightened or losing your mind?* New York: Crown Publishing, Three Rivers Press.

Jarratt, J., Coates, J., Mahaffie, J., & Hines, A. (1994). *Managing your future as an association: Thinking about trends and working with their consequences.* Washington, DC: American Society of Association Executives.

Klein, E., & Izzo, J. (1998). *Awakening corporate soul: Four paths to unleash the power of people at work.* New York: Fairwinds Press.

Kurtzman, J. (1984). *Future casting.* Bethesda, Md.: World Future Society.

Liff, A. (1998). Future think: Seven essential questions. *Association Management 50*(1), 39–48.

McLaughlin, C., & Davidson, G. (1994). *Spiritual politics: Changing the world from inside out.* New York: Ballentine.

Mindell, A. (1992). *The leader as martial artist: An introduction to deep democracy: Techniques and stratgies for resolving conflict and creating community.* San Francisco: Harper.

Morrison, J., Renfrew, W., & Boucher, W. (Eds.). (1983). *Applying methods and techniques of futures research.* San Francisco: Jossey-Bass.

Nanus, B. (1992). *Visionary leadership.* San Francisco: Jossey-Bass.

Pesut, D. (1998a). Twenty-first century learning. *Nursing Outlook, 46*(1), 37.

Pesut, D. (1998b). Scenarios: Stories about the future. *Nursing Outlook, 46*(2), 55.

Pesut, D. (1997a). Facilitating futures thinking. *Nursing Outlook, 45*(4), 155.

Pesut, D. (1997b). Connecting with the futures community. *Nursing Outlook, 45*(5), 251.

Pesut, D. (1997c). The future, virtue-ethics, and sigma theta tau. *Reflections, 23*(3), 56–59.

Pesut, D. (1995). Health care reform: From public policy vision to professional personal action. *Nurse Educator, 19*(6), 1–2.

Pesut, D. (1991). The art, science, and technologies of reframing in psychiatric mental health nursing. *Issues in Mental Health Nursing, 12*(1), 9–18.

Pesut, D. (1989). Aim versus blame: Using an outcome specification model. *Journal of Psychosocial Nursing and Mental Health Services, 27*(5), 26–30.

Pesut, D., & Herman, J. (1999). *Clinical reasoning: Art and science of critical and creative thinking.* New York: Delmar.

Pesut, D., & Herman, J. (1998). OPT: Transformation of nursing process for contemporary practice. *Nursing Outlook, 46*(1), 29–36.

Rechtschaffen, S. (1996). *Time shifting.* New York: Bantam Doubleday.

Reed, T. (1996). A new understanding of followers as leaders: Emerging theory of civic leadership. *The Journal of Leadership Studies, 3*(1), 95–104.

Rejeski, D. (1993). Exploring future environmental risks. In C. Cothern & N. Ross (Eds.) *Environmental statistics, assessment.* Ann Arbor: Lewis Publishers.

Rogers, M. (1997a). Learning about the future. *Futures, 29*(8), 763–768.

Rogers, M. (1997b). *Canadian nursing in 2020: Five scenarios.* Ottawa: Canadian Nurses Association.

Slaughter, R. (1995). *The foresight principle: Cultural recovery in the 21st century.* West Port, Conn.: Praeger

The Futurist. (1998). Editorial policy, *32*(3), 2.

Tough, A. (1993). Making a pledge to future generations. *Futures, 25*(1), 90–92.

Van Der Heijden, K. (1996). *Scenarios: The art of strategic conversation.* New York: John Wiley.

Williams, C. Pesut, D., Boyd, M., Russell, S., Morrow, J., & Head, K. (1998). *Journal of the American Psychiatric Nurses Association, 4*(2), 48–56.

SUGGESTED READINGS

Barker, J. (1993). *Paradigms: The business of discovering the future.* New York: Harper Business.

Bargen, D. (1996). Community visioning and leadership. *The Journal of Leadership Studies, 3*(3), 135–162.

Bell, W. (1997). *Foundations of future studies: Volume II: Values, objectivity and the good society.* New Brunswick, N.J.: Transaction Publishers.

Bezold, C., Halperin, J., & Eng, J. (Eds.). (1993). *2020 visions: Health care information standards and technologies.* Rockville, Md.: USPC.

Blancett, S., & Flarey, D. (1995). *Reengineering nursing and health care: The handbook for organizational transformation.* Gaithersburg, MD: Aspen.

Conner, D. (1992). *Managing at the speed of change.* New York: Villard Books.

Cornish, E. (1977). *The study of the future.* Bethesda, Md.: World Future Society.

Dilts, R. (1996). *Visionary leadership.* Capitola, Calif.: Meta Publications.

Dilts, R., Epstein, T., & Dilts R. (1991). *Tools for dreamers: Strategies for creativity and innovation.* Capitola, Calif.: Meta Publications.

Dolence, M., & Norris, D. (1995). *Transforming higher education: A vision for learning in the 21st century.* Ann Arbor: Society for College and University Planning.

Emery, M. (1995). *Intuition workbook: An expert's guide to unlocking the wisdom of our subconscious mind.* Englewood Cliffs, N.J.: Prentice-Hall.

Fairhurst, G., & Sarr, R. (1996). *The art of framing: Managing the language of leadership.* San Francisco: Jossey Bass.

Fisher, J. (1992). *Our medical future.* New York: Simon and Schuster.

Flarey, D. (1995). *Redesigning nursing care delivery: Transforming our future.* Philadelphia: Lippincott.

Hamel, G., & Prahalod, C. (1994). *Competing for the future.* Boston: Harvard Business School Press.

Hesselbein, F., Goldsmith, M., & Beckhard, R. (1996). *The leader of the future: New visions, strategies and practices for the next era.* San Francisco: Jossey Bass.

Hoyle, J. (1995). *Leadership and futuring: Making visions happen.* Thousand Oaks, Calif.: Corwin Press.

Institute for Alternative Futures. 100 North Pitt Street, Suite 235, Alexandria, Virginia 22314-3108. 703-684-5880 (voice) 703-684-0640 (fax), futures@delphi.com (e-mail).

Joseph, E. (1974). What is future time? *The Futurist, 8*(4), 178.

Kaiser, L. (1996). Designer health care for a designer nation: A new paradigm. In C. Bezold & E. Mayer (Eds.). *Future care: Responding to the demand for change* (pp. 189–218). New York: Faulkner and Gray.

Kidder, R. (1996). *How good people make tough choices: Resolving the dilemmas of ethical living.* New York: William Morrow.

Korniewicz, D., & Palmer, M. (1997). The preferable future for nursing. *Nursing Outlook, 45*(3), 108–113.

Kritek, P. (1994). *Negotiating at an uneven table: Developing moral courage in resolving our conflicts.* San Francisco: Jossey Bass.

Loye, D. (1983). *The Sphinx and the rainbow: Brain, mind, and future vision.* Boulder, Colo.: Shambhala.

Malaska, P. (1995). The futures field of research. *Futures Research Quarterly, 11*(1), 79–90.

Marcus, L., Dorn, B., Kritek, P., Miller, V., & Wyatt, J. (1995). *Renegotiating health care: Resolving conflict to build collaboration.* San Francisco: Jossey Bass.

Moore, J. (1995). Synergistic health-care patterns for the future. *Futures Research Quarterly, 11*(1), 47–59.

National Academy of Science (1997). Focusing on quality in a changing health care system. http:www.nas.edu/21st/health/health.html.

Nowicki, C. R. (1996). 21 predictions for the future of hospital staff development. *The Journal of Continuing Education in Nursing, 27*, 259–266.

Schwartz, P. (1991). *The art of the long view.* New York: Doubleday.

Wells, H. (1987, Spring). Wanted professors of foresight. *Futures Research Quarterly*, 89–91.

Wheatley, M. (1994). *Leadership and the new science.* San Francisco: Berett-Koehler.

Woodhouse, M. (1996). *Paradigm wars: World views for a new age.* Berkeley, Calif.: Frog Ltd.

World Future Society. 7910 Woodmont Avenue, Suite 450, Bethesda, Md., 20814. USA Telephone: 301-656-8274, FAX: 301-951-0394.

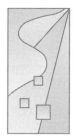

Chapter 4

Seeing the Big Picture

Fay L. Bower

Seeing the big picture is an important aspect of leadership because it allows the leader to place the present situation and the decisions that need to be made into a larger context. Being able to see the big picture is often called *having the true picture* or *having a total perspective*. Regardless of the name, it is the ability to extend the parameters of a situation to their fullest extent. It is looking at how the present situation is connected to or affected by other situations. It is the ability to see beyond the obvious, beyond the current activity, beyond the present.

Being able to see the whole of any situation creates several advantages for the nurse. First, the nurse immediately has more possibilities and opportunities from which to select when decisions need to be made. Each bit of new information about the whole brings with it a variety of options that were not there when things were seen in a more confined way. Second, because seeing the whole is liberating, this expansion of options doesn't restrict or confine decisions to a narrow outcome; however, having a new and expanded vision may also create a feeling of being overwhelmed and can sometimes scare off the timid, so there is a need to weigh all of the new information carefully before acting.

There are other reasons for wanting to see the total picture of a situation. Clearly, knowing all about an issue colors our attitudes about whether there is hope or a reason to respond. We are also much more motivated to act when we understand all of the aspects of an event. Furthermore, we are much more likely to get involved if we are informed than when we are only partially aware of the total picture. The converse is also true; if we know all about the issue, we may decide to step aside and let others carry the burden of resolution.

There is a saying that "everything is related to everything else," and although at first this may seem an exaggeration, it is true. Nothing we face today occurs in isolation, so although problems in health care and nursing may seem unique, over time we have seen that they are not. For instance, changes in the way that health care is delivered is an offshoot of changes in other kinds of service delivery and are the result of a general overall approach to cost containment. And what might seem unique to nursing when viewed in the context of health care delivery turns out not to be so unique. Everywhere and in every kind of business, there are movements to contain cost, to provide quality service, to improve market share, and to do all of these things in a timely manner.

This relationship of events illustrates how important it is to keep in touch with change, and given the many ways that information is circulated and distributed, it is not too difficult to realize what is happening that might have a bearing on the current situation. Reading the newspaper, watching television, and listening to the radio are excellent ways to determine the bigger picture. Increasingly, "surfing the net" has become the popular way to gain a greater view (see Chapter 13 for a review of how to stay informed). Being available for dialogue with others should not be forgotten as another way to see the whole picture.

Probably the most outstanding value of seeing beyond the immediate situation to the bigger picture is that it enhances the chances of solving the real problem. Seeing only the immediate situation often blinds us to the real issue. We may be responding to a problem that has greater implications and thus a greater impact or a greater or better outcome than imagined. What looks like a fairly uncomplicated issue may really be much more complex and involve many more individuals and operations.

There are many reasons why the bigger picture is often not considered. The most common reason is that nurses are not accustomed to looking beyond the immediate stimuli; they have been taught to respond quickly to patient-related problems. The second most common reason is that nurses are usually in a hurry to respond so that they do not look stupid or unconcerned. They also miss seeing the big picture because they do not see the relevance or the connectivity of one incident to another. And frankly, nurses have not had enough experience with being involved in decisions that affect others to know when they have been short-sighted or missed seeing the total picture.

Having the vision of the bigger picture is not difficult; it simply means not being caught up in the immediate circumstances or what is apparent or is expedient. Quite often, nurses miss the bigger picture because their orientation to quick solutions overrides a more expansive approach. Lately, there is much more emphasis on outcomes than on process, and seeing the big picture demands that we give attention to the process of determining the parameters of the situation. Thus, we may not be paying attention to the big picture.

The process of seeing the big picture is not a hard or concealed process; in fact, it is easy to see the entire picture once you understand the elements of the process and how they can be pursued. It is an easy skill to learn and a valuable way to attack most problems. A discussion of the process and one nurse's experiences with it follows.

MODEL FOR SEEING THE BIG PICTURE

The process of seeing the big picture includes three elements: (1) paying attention, (2) using networks, and (3) making connections between what is known and what is learned. It is a process that one person or a group of people can pursue. It can happen quickly, or it can consume a lot of time.

Paying Attention

According to Bob Waterman (Peters and Waterman, 1981), paying attention is all there is. Many writers have written about "paying attention." In some instances, paying attention has included listening to employees (Peters and Austin, 1985; Peters and Waterman, 1981). Attention according to Peters and Austin involves "managing by walking around (MBWA)" (p. 266). There are many, many stories in Peters' books about the ways in which top firms in the United States have stayed that way because the chief executive officers were in touch with their employees and their competitors. They were able to stay on top because they knew what was going on due to personal contact.

This same strategy (i.e., MBWA) is an excellent way to get a view of the big picture. By walking around and staying close to the action, it is possible to get a more comprehensive view and thus obtain a better understanding of the operations and the problems. Looking, listening, and asking are excellent ways to pay attention. It is amazing how much can be learned by placing yourself in the center of the action and by letting others know that you are paying attention to their concerns and desires.

Most people want to be heard, to be included, and to be part of the "action." By paying attention to what they say, by including them, and by inviting them to become part of the activities, several benefits can be realized. There are a variety of perspectives, a cadre of people who can be the eyes and ears for collecting data, and a group who could help solve any problems that arise. Paying attention does more than provide information; it promotes interest, motivation, and team approaches—while providing a fuller understanding of what is happening.

There are some problems to avoid when paying attention. Some people like attention so much that they block out input to you from others. Their needs for inclusion exclude other views, so the wise thing to do is to weigh their contributions and to keep an open mind while screening out information that appears to be self-serving or unrelated.

Quiet people may need special attention because they often have information that the more vocal ones do not have but they are too shy to share that information. Paying attention means making yourself available to all kinds of people and at all levels of the organization and to seek out those who seem knowledgeable but unlikely to share.

A second potential problem when paying attention is reaching a premature conclusion based on a preconceived notion. Paying attention means that one seeks to enlarge a body of knowledge until the full picture is revealed; it is not seeking validation of what is already known. Paying attention means listening for new perspectives and different versions. There may be similarities in what is heard, but hearing the same thing over and over again may mean that you are not listening for a difference or that you have sought people who have the same perspective as yours. Paying attention does not mean that you seek input to justify your own perspective. One good way to avoid this is to keep track of whom you listen to and to broaden your sample so you have the perspective of a wide variety of people.

A third problem is access. Clearly, no one person can be everywhere, so smart nurses involve others in every aspect of the process of seeing the big picture. There are several benefits to this approach. The most obvious benefit of involving others is the development of a group of people who are prepared to solve potential problems or to initiate new actions as a result of the new information. Instead of only one person having the full picture, there are several who have it. There also is the chance that the group will have a vested interest in seeing any problems solved or initiatives developed because of their new awareness. Both Chapter 5 (Building Teams) and Chapter 12 (Letting Go and Taking On) provide discussions on how groups of people working together can see the big picture and thus provide more effective leadership.

A fourth potential problem with paying attention is that some people have difficulty reaching out. Unless the nurse is willing to approach others and to ask questions and listen to other ideas and concerns, getting the full picture is hard. For some nurses, this approach might feel intrusive or uncomfortable. Being open about your motives is helpful because most workers are cooperative when approached if they know what is happening and if they know that you care about their responses. It also helps to let the workers know what you intend to do with the information. Peters and Austin (1985) point out in their book that when Packard of Hewlitt-Packard managed by walking around, he was clear about his need to know and about what he intended to do with the information.

Paying attention can be deliberate or it can be unintentional. If you are in the habit of listening to the radio on your way to work, of reading the morning newspaper before you leave for work, or of watching the 10:00 p.m. news report on television, you know that there is a lot to be learned. These are easy and deliberate ways to keep informed. It also helps to occasionally have lunch with different groups of workers and to listen to their concerns and ideas. Although you may not be seeking information, there always is the possibility that you will learn something you did not know. This is an example of an unintentional way to pay attention.

For a more systematic sampling of ideas, you may want to select certain groups of people to interview. In this case, paying attention is scheduled to seek particular views given the position, age, gender, or ethnicity of the informants. We know that these variables provide different views and thus provide a fuller picture of the world.

More than anything, paying attention is an attitude, which becomes a habit. Because paying attention helps provide the bigger picture, it becomes part of your repertoire of activities to get the big picture, just like reading a patient's chart helps you learn all you can about the patient's condition. It must begin with the belief that it is important to pay attention and to seek methods of broadening the ways to do it.

Using Networks

Like paying attention, *networking* is an important strategy to determine the big picture. Sometimes paying attention means being in the right place at the right time or being able to get information. This is where networks fit in. According to Gruber-May (1997):

> Traditionally seen as a skill set reserved for nurse executives, proficient net-working abilities must now be developed by nurses at all levels. Once a luxury for augmenting one's professional development, networking has become a

required component for successfully managing the rapidly changing health care environment nurses face every day (p. 25).

Networking is a process of creating a select group of individuals who can supply you with information, other contacts, or opportunities so you can get the best vision of what is happening beyond your immediate situation. Originally, networks were for career advancement, and they still are, but networks are now used for a variety of other reasons. Mergers, acquisitions, buyouts, and the formation of health systems have accelerated change in the health care arena. Nurses at all levels are struggling to stay abreast of the latest knowledge and how their situation fits or does not fit with the rest of the health care industry. Networks are a mechanism for staying in touch with trends; they provide a quick way to find out whether the issues being faced are different or like those faced by others.

Networks also help us keep up to date about the latest therapies, products, and interventions. Networks keep us connected so we can make the best decisions. Spitzer-Lehmann (1994) states, "using the collaborative relationships of networking validates data and enhances access to inside information" (p. 132).

To be effective, nurses must understand the networking relationship, be able to identify who will make a good network member, know what to expect of the network, and be comfortable using the network members for meeting personal and professional needs.

Understanding the networking relationship to see the big picture means that the nurse must follow the 11 guidelines for networking etiquette described by Gruber-May (1997):

1. Stay in touch. Do not overuse individuals in your network. Call when you do not need anything. Maintain a balance in the relationship between what you give others and what you request from them. Establish the relationship first; do business second.
2. Members of your network are your allies; do not misuse them.
3. Offer to help others. After you offer to help, follow through. Give of yourself generously and often to the members of your network.
4. Follow up on all referrals. Report back and update the person who provided the referral.
5. Do not ask a favor that will make your network members uncomfortable. Do not put someone in a position to say no.
6. Share information with your network but use good judgment. Sharing critical business information is important but be careful because you do not want to become labeled a gossiper.
7. Technology has made the world a very small place. Do not burn your bridges. Mean-spirited remarks and pettiness will ruin your reputation.
8. Avoid personal or private questions that make a person uncomfortable. Do not question someone in an interrogation manner. Ask open-ended questions, and share in the conversation.
9. Return calls personally and in a timely manner. Do not ignore others, or they may ignore you when you need them.

10. Know when to use a personal touch; send a handwritten thank-you note, flowers, or a small gift.
11. Give credit where credit is due. Put praise in writing. Make sure your appreciation reaches not only the individual but also his or her boss (p. 29).

Developing a network is a process in which two people, and then more, establish a relationship because of mutual interest and trust. The persons in the network trust one another and use that basic trust as a springboard for other activities. Networks usually begin in school or the workplace as a helping relationship. Networks can begin at conferences, workshops, and other professional functions where individuals discover they have something in common. Networks have even been established by persons who have read about someone and called that person to converse. Over time, the relationship matures, and as trust is established, so is the network. Henderson and McGettigan (1994) offer some tips on ways to boost your networking power:

1. Create opportunities to meet others at conferences, conventions, and workshops; on committees; and during other activities. Introduce yourself and start a conversation. Tell others about your interests, experience, and goals; then listen carefully to their replies.
2. Look for information that might be useful to you in the future as well as now. Check printed programs for biographic information on speakers. Ask for someone's business card; later, write a note on it to remind yourself of the person or topic. Have your business card available to exchange with others.
3. Be patient and persistent as you refine your networking skills. Analyze your strategies and notice what works. Think of ways to improve your weak spots.
4. Be prepared to be a resource for others—networking is a reciprocal process, and you may have information someone else wants (p. 71).

Besides trust, networks involve exchanges. These exchanges must provide, over time, benefits for all parties involved. The nurse's credibility within the network depends on how often he or she requests and provides help and information. O'Connor (1982) contends that network members must periodically identify the mutual gains, direct or indirect, for all parties. The exchange must be equivalent, even if reciprocity is delayed.

Identifying members for a network is an ongoing process. Both men and women, people in and out of the nursing, and social as well as professional people make good network members. A broad base of colleagues creates a strong network.

Network members are often selected because of their particular contributions. For instance, a nurse's network while in school would include other students and faculty. As a clinical nurse, the network probably would include clinicians. As the nurse's career advances, so do the careers of the colleagues, so networks often include people from all over the country and in a variety of positions.

Networks should also include people from a variety of organizational levels. Having a network with too many people perceived as higher than you in position or status is not a good idea. Although it is a good idea to have influential people as a part of the network, it is unrealistic to expect that these people will have the time to help that may be needed. Furthermore, a balance of persons from many levels provides information from a variety of perspectives up and down the workforce. Although top executives may have an important perspective, it is often their secretaries who can give the time and information needed, so secretaries are excellent resources and thus good network members. Of course, it is important to treat everybody, regardless of their position, with respect and consideration.

Networks that span a geographical area provide another perspective that can be helpful when the big picture is needed. Trends often begin on the West and East Coasts and move to the center of the country, so if the nurse wants to be proactive, having a picture of what may occur is important. Managed care is a good example of why a network should have geographical representation. Nurses in California felt the impact of managed care long before nurses in other parts of the country did, so having a colleague in California could provide you with a picture of what could happen long before it does.

Age is another variable to consider when establishing a network. Clearly those who have lived longer have a more complete picture of health care and its many changes. Conversely, those who are younger are free of the constraints older nurses may have and can provide a vision free of "how it was done." Both perspectives are important because they provide a more complete view of any situation.

Currentness is another aspect of networking that is important. Knowing whether your informants are up to date on issues and thus are current could mean the difference between getting information that broadens your perspective and puts you in a proactive position and being stuck with data that are out of date and useless. Currentness is essential because health care change is occurring at a speed unknown in the past. This means that you must be cognizant of your informants' activities so you do not embarrass them or compromise your position with them.

According to Sullivan and Decker (1996), networking with the media also is important and may require attending a meeting of a business organization that features a panel of media specialists and taking the time to let them know that you are interested in building a relationship. It could also mean taking a newspaper reporter or a radio or television commentator to lunch and establishing an ongoing relationship regarding certain topics.

Although establishing a network is time-consuming and sometimes not a comfortable activity, Calano and Salzman (1988) state that the process of establishing a network includes

- Forcing yourself to broaden your perspectives
- Exploring various environments for networking and then focusing on those that have the greatest potential for your purpose
- Using your telephone directory, business card files, and correspondence files as a beginning network
- Recognizing one's position of authority on a current topic; nurses who publish and speak have a way of establishing themselves as experts
- Being proactive and seeking new contacts as well as affirming current ones when the opportunity arises (p. 131).

Dienemann (1998) points out that there are professional networks that nurses can join if they do not have a network. In Washington, D.C., the "Nurse in Washington Roundtable" is a regularly scheduled dinner meeting with a congressional or an administration speaker. For those who attend, it does not matter who the speaker is or what is served for dinner; the most important activity is networking with professional colleagues. What better place could a nurse find that would provide the big picture?

The *Nurses' Directory of Capitol Connections* is a networking directory that lists more than 500 nurses in health policy positions in the Washington, D.C., area and in federal agencies nationwide. To contact these nurses involves only a telephone call, or you could invite one of the nurses to lunch and get acquainted. The network is constantly growing. Another way to get started with a network is to join the state nurses' association or a clinical specialty organization. A list of these organizations is available by calling the state licensing board, by using the telephone directory assistance, or by searching on the Internet (see Chapter 13 for information on how to access the Internet). It is not hard to get a view of the big picture when there are so many ways to establish networks.

All hospitals, clinics, and home care agencies are excellent places for the development of networking groups. Networking often begins when nurses talk and plan together on a regular basis. The move to self-directed work groups, total quality improvement, and patient-focused care has provided nurses with the means for developing networks. Even though these relationships start as work groups, they often expand to networking groups (Tiano et al., 1994).

Knowing what to expect from a network is important if the network is to accomplish what the nurse wants. Because networks are links to others, they are reciprocal relationships; this means you can expect to get if you give. Networks are not one-way conduits to information or help; they are two-way links, and you can expect to give information and help just as you hope to get both from others.

Making your expertise known and working on keeping it current are the responsibilities of every member of the network. It is also important to keep the relationships alive so that when information and help are needed, the persons who can help are easy to find and ready for the request. Keeping the network "alive" means frequent contact with the network members, such as several times a year. A simple telephone call or an e-mail to say hello is all it takes. A note saying "how are you?" is another way to keep in touch. When you want something, then it does not look like the only time you make contact is when you have a request.

Resistance from a network member could mean that serious attention has not been paid to the relationship. Generally, networks fail when the situation was not assessed properly or there was misuse of the generosity of the network (Puetz, 1983). If the relationship has been neglected, it will be necessary to reestablish trust. Poor timing of a request or not clearly knowing a colleague's position on a subject when a request is made could threaten the relationship. In both instances, trust could be lost, necessitating the reestablishment of what once was there. Reestablishing trust could take considerable time and is not always possible, so it is best to keep the networks alive and well through frequent and genuine contact.

Besides keeping current in the field and keeping contact with the network, good network members help other members even when there is no request. They are alert to opportunities and their match for network members; they know what the network members need and do and link them to the appropriate opportunities when they arise. Frequent interaction among network members serves a variety of purposes.

Being comfortable with asking for help from the network is often difficult for some nurses, who believe asking for help is a sign of weakness and therefore do not seek advice or help when needed. Others are afraid to ask for help because they think they should have the information or should know how to get it. Nurses need to understand that seeking information from a network is not like asking for help or information from just anyone. Because the network is there to help the members, asking is expected. Requesting information, help, or contacts is appropriate. Networks can make a positive difference for the nurse who is trying to see the big picture, so being shy not only is inappropriate but also may deter the nurse from ever obtaining the needed information from anyone.

The network should not be overworked or considered the only source of information. Frequently, the network is a referral system by which the nurse obtains the information by being referred to someone else. Being shy with the referral will not work, so if shyness is the problem, the nurse must learn to exert initiative.

Sometimes being comfortable in asking the network for help or information means seeing the network as way to do an assessment, like the process used to gather data about a patient. All nurses know how to assess a patient situation. The use of the network is like consulting the health team or like reviewing the patient record, but instead of doing these things to better understand the patient, the goal is to understand the bigger picture, with the network as the source of that understanding. Seen in this context, use of the network should not be difficult, and contacting referrals made through the network should not be uncomfortable.

Networking is a valuable tool for obtaining a broader base of information and, thus, an understanding of what is happening. Instead of everyone's working in isolation, networks provide a bigger picture and, with the use of cyberspace, a view way beyond what one could even imagine. Obtaining information through paying attention and networking is still not sufficient; being able to connect what you know with what you learn is another important skill that ultimately provides the nurse with the bigger picture.

Connectivity: Combining What You Know With What You Learn

Connectivity is the process of putting together, or linking, one phenomenon with another. In the case of seeing the bigger picture, it is the process of gaining new insights or meanings for data that you have when it is linked to data you have just acquired. Connectivity is recognizing the relationships of one set of data with other sets of data. Connectivity is both similar and dissimilar to the use of information discussion in Chapter 13. What is the same is the way in which you analyze information; what is different is how you relate the analyzed data with what you know.

There are three things to consider in the process of relating new information with your current situation: (1) the currentness of the information, (2) the source of the information, and (3) the usefulness of the amalgamation of what is learned with what is known. Although there may be other issues that need to be considered, these three will help the decision-maker determine what to pay attention to.

The *currentness of the information* gained is very important because if the information you have just acquired is out of date, then the conclusion reached may be off the mark and not a view of the current big picture. If the information is old, then the conclusion reached will also be old and therefore useless. Furthermore, if the information is current and connectivity is delayed, then the same outcome can be expected—the big picture is missed.

It is not unusual for information to reach sources late. Things happen very quickly in health care. Some people know right away when an event is to happen because they have been part of the preliminary activities. The rest learn about change after it has been implemented. When change seems imminent, checking with others helps to determine the possible outcome if the source of the information has already experienced the phenomenon. This is why paying attention and using a network help us get the bigger picture. Wouldn't it have been useful to know in advance that ancillary workers would replace registered nurses in the new world of health care? Some nurses who were worried about the changes going on in their environment checked with other areas in the country and saw the trend of replacement start. They saw the bigger picture and began to prepare by looking for employment for themselves outside the hospital. They found out they had much to offer and were prepared for many kinds of positions in and out of nursing. When registered nurses were terminated and replaced by unlicensed personnel in their hospital, they had already moved on. If they had waited, they probably would have been replaced. Having current information helps one make a timely decision.

The *source of the information* probably is the most important aspect of the usefulness of what is learned. The integrity of the information source is critical to the validity of what is learned and whether it can be used. No one wants information that has little relationship to reality or that is heresy. Good information is often hard to find because rumor and gossip travel fast and reach lots of people; this is why the network is so important.

There are a several rules to follow when evaluating the information source:

1. Be aware of the person who wants to tell you a secret about what is happening in health care, because most of what is happening is not a secret.
2. Avoid individuals who tell you they have information that no one else has, because it probably is information that everyone has.
3. Critically analyze any information given to you that has passed through several people, because most information gained this way is distorted.
4. If you are in doubt about the source, check the information just gained with more than one source or check it out with the network members to determine whether the information is valid.

5. Keep informed yourself by reading the newspapers, by listening to the news on the radio and the television, and by reading the most recent professional journals. Avid readers are usually very well informed and are their own best source of information.

The *usefulness of the amalgamation* of what is known with what is learned is the third way to determine whether you are getting the big picture. Usefulness means being able to use the information gained immediately or in the future because it is somehow is related to what is already known. Usefulness also means that the new information provides a perspective not already known. It must also provide a greater and more inclusive perspective. Furthermore, the new information, given that it is accurate and current, is useful if it allows new possibilities and opportunities for action. Last, this union of what is known with what is learned must provide a picture bigger than either piece of knowledge alone and provide options for action.

If what is heard does not fit with what is going on, it obviously is not going to help to provide the big picture. However, if what is learned has a potential connection with what is happening, it should be tucked away for future use. It may be valuable, and time is the best test of whether it will prove to be useful.

New information, while demonstrating connectivity, could create confusion and doubt or even fear, so it should be evaluated carefully. Getting information that has a negative connotation could push the decision-makers to act quickly, whereas waiting might be the better course. The reverse is also true. Getting information that leads to positive outcomes could raise everybody's hopes when waiting might demonstrate a different outcome. The usefulness of the connectivity of what is known with what has been learned should be viewed over time, not just for its use in the present.

This model of seeing the big picture is best understood when it is supported by real events of real people. The remainder of this chapter is about one person's experience with paying attention, using networks, and connecting what is known with what is learned. Several scenarios are presented so the reader can see how one nurse leader used "seeing the big picture" to provide leadership to colleges and to an international nursing organization.

HOW A NURSE LEADER USED THE "SEEING THE BIG PICTURE" MODEL

My career began early, when I was just 17, and has spanned 42 years. Although it started out rather uneventful and with no plan, I was fortunate to have held leadership roles at several levels and was responsible for people, activities, and budgets of considerable size throughout those years. In retrospect, I wish that I had had a plan and that I had the opportunities available to leaders today. More than anything, I wish that I had had the wisdom I have today when as a novice I "took the lead." Although I learned "on the job" and from wonderful mentors, I also wish that I had had the literature available today.

The story I want to tell is not chronological; instead, I want to tell you about several events in my career in which seeing the big picture paid off in both opportunity and wise decision-making. Although I use the model given in this chapter to present these events, I had no idea at the time that I was using a model. In fact, the model presented in this chapter is grounded in my life experiences as a leader.

Being Director of a Curriculum Grant

One of my earliest experiences with seeing the big picture was when I was trying to establish a new way to move forward a department of nursing in a university that had a faculty of persons who had been my instructors; I was now their leader. Although they were proud of me because I was a product of their effort, they were suspicious of my abilities as their leader. The university was the oldest public university in the state, with a history going back to the 1800s. Things were done as they had "always been done," and for me to suggest a new way was dangerous. I was new in the position of associate director of a curriculum project funded by the USPHS, Division of Nursing; although I was admired for my abilities, the faculty often reminded me that they knew what was best.

We needed a new curriculum because what we were doing was very out of date. We had written a grant for funding to review what we were doing, and after the initial phase of the review, it was determined that the curriculum had to be revised. I knew if I mentioned anything about revision, the faculty would object; they believed the review would find no reason for a revision. I decided to pay attention to their concerns so I could get a clear picture of what obstacles I would have. I also decided to check with my network about what was happening in nursing education and curriculum development elsewhere to see whether what I was experiencing was the same or different from the experiences of others.

I spent nearly 6 months listening to faculty members. Sometimes, the discussions occurred in faculty meetings; on other occasions, I initiated the discussion at lunch or at other off-campus times. At the same time, I contacted my advisors from graduate school and persons I knew at the National League for Nursing. I also worked closely with my mentor, who was the director of the project and who had faith in me as a change agent.

Over and over again, I heard the faculty say, "What will the curriculum look like if we change it?" "How can we teach and revise the curriculum?" "Will we have help with a curriculum change?" "What will we do to change the curriculum?" and "What do we do with the old program while we implement a new curriculum, or will we have to offer the old curriculum while we phase in a new one?"

I listened and listened and thanked them for their input. I did not answer their questions because I did not have answers. I did, however, worry that their concerns might be another way to express resistance, but after listening, I realized they were not resisting change but rather telling me they did not know how to change the curriculum. The lesson I learned from this group is that what sounds like one issue often is another. You have to listen carefully. You can listen to others, but you must *hear* what they say. Sometimes, it is what is *not* said that is important. Listening hard and without bias helps you hear the real message. For a long time, I was listening, but it took me longer to hear what was really being said.

One of the other most important things I did was to check with other programs that had also received funding for curriculum evaluation. This action provided me with the big picture and told me whether what they were doing would fit where I was. There were nine programs in the United States in different geographical areas that were funded by the same source and were doing similar things. During the 5 years I worked on that grant, the directors of those projects and I met yearly to exchange ideas and progress and to support one another. They became my networks; even today, if I have a curriculum problem, I call one or more of those people for advice.

There were other lessons I learned from this experience that have helped me at other times in my career. By listening carefully, I learned that the faculty did trust me and that they would have followed me to the ends of the earth because they believed I knew what I was doing. They knew that I was qualified when I told them that I had checked with other programs and other faculty and that there were many programs going through curriculum revision. They knew then that I had the bigger picture and that we were on the right tract. It is important to share with your coworkers what you know so that they also can get the bigger picture. In fact, they were proud to be in the forefront of change, and they knew that was so because I brought them information that they otherwise would not have had.

Being a University Planner

At a different time in my career, I served as the director of strategic planning and institutional research in a private medium-sized Catholic university. I reported to the president and had the responsibility for getting the university ready for a regional accreditation visit. The university's accreditation status had been placed "on warning" because of its apparent lack of planning, and it needed to demonstrate that there was a planning process at the institution that led to the implementation of the university mission. One would think that given these circumstances the university community would be willing and ready to do what was needed, but instead there was a great deal of resistance to anything I proposed. In fact, the campus was in the throes of a political battle about the entire process. Some faculty did not believe in planning; others did not want me to lead the effort. The vice presidents wanted divisional planning, and the deans wanted no one to tell them what to do. The faculty union wanted to control the process, and the faculty was in a dispute about support for the president, but the president was adamant about an institutional approach and told me to go forward with the process.

I began by becoming informed about strategic planning. I sought help from a national organization of strategic planners. I visited other universities and colleges, talked with planners, and read everything I could on the subject before taking the planning position. I met with all of the deans, having been a dean on the campus for 8 years, and tried to get them to help me. I worked hard to build a network that would support me as I proceeded with the task and that would provide me with ways to maneuver through the political battlefield.

I learned a lot about planning and had to take each bit of information I gained and determine whether it would fit (had connectivity) with what I was attempting to do. Some places I visited had a top-down leadership planning process, and others had implemented a bottom-up planning process. In some institutions, planning was done by a small group of administrators. In others, everyone was involved. I saw every conceivable planning process you could imagine in operation. Some were very successful, and others were getting nowhere. The big picture was very variable; that is, there was no one way of doing strategic planning in a university. I learned that planning, although written about as if there was an agreed-on process, occurs in a variety of ways and that those who succeed do so because they have designed a process that fits the institution.

I also learned that seeing the big picture was important because if I had followed what I read, I would have failed. If I had followed what others suggested, I would have failed. It wasn't that I was given bad advice; it was just that I had to determine what would fit in the environment in which I worked, and I would not have known that if I hadn't looked at other places and seen the variety of ways in which planning occurred.

I also learned that it was not the deans whose support I needed but rather the faculty, and once I was able to include them in the process, things improved. The process never did go smoothly and I never did feel totally supported, but I learned that total support often is not given and that one can make change without it. I learned this from seeing the big picture because in many universities and colleges, not everybody supported the planners, but the presidents always did.

The greatest value of this experience was learning that the big pictures can vary and that although the outcomes can look similar, the processes for getting there can be different. I also learned the value of having the right supportive group and how outside networks really do provide more than information, namely, support and help. They validate what you know is right but might be afraid to do.

Being President of Alpha Gamma Chapter

Like many nurses, I went to college after I had worked as a registered nurse for many years. I was the mother of four children, and my husband and I lived in a university city south of San Francisco. I worked nights at the university hospital and went to school during the day. It took me 6 years of part-time course work to get my baccalaureate degree in nursing, and during that time, I was elected president of the Alpha Gamma Chapter of Sigma Theta Tau International (STTI) at the university where I was going to school. I knew nothing about the organization I had been invited to join, but I was honored because only those who have demonstrated scholarship and excellent academic achievement are invited to become members of the only honor society in nursing. I figured I would complete my term and move on to other things. Fortunately, that did not happen, and by learning more about the parent operation (the bigger picture), my professional life was changed.

I thought that I had better learn more about the organization if I was to be a good president, so I asked the faculty sponsor to help me. She suggested that, beyond reading about the society, I go to the regional assembly, which would be held in San Francisco the next spring. Her advice was the best thing I could have received, and it was the beginning of a 34-year involvement that I continue to this day. I paid close attention to her advice, which was to get involved and stay involved. She said I would be able to establish a network throughout the entire nation of nurses who were scholars and who would be there when I needed them. She was right!

I not only learned about the history and purpose of STTI, but over time, I also established a network of colleagues who have served me well over those 34 years. I met faculty, authors, deans, clinicians, and students from all over the United States who were serving, like me, as officers in other chapters. I learned more about how to serve the chapter as its president and how to promote research. I took from those interactions the things that I thought would work at the university because they fit our mission, goals, and environment.

Over the years, I have served with some of these nurses on regional and international committees of STTI, have used them as references, and have been a reference for them. I have authored textbooks with some of them and written chapters with others. I have conducted research with nurses I met through STTI, and I have had the pleasure of being mentored by some of the most outstanding nurses in the United States. I also have a long list of nurses whom I mentor whom I met while working with the honor society.

Clearly, learning more about the total organization helped me to recognize the relationship of the chapter at the university with the parent organization and prompted me to continue on with STTI long after that presidency was completed. Without this big picture, I would not have been able to serve the chapter properly, nor would I have been able to grow and advance as I did. Many, many opportunities became mine because of my involvement. It was easy to make new friends and to establish working relationships with nurses in STTI because they shared the same values and goals that I did.

Being Involved in a National Professional Organization

At another time in my career, I was elected to the Accreditation Review Board of the Council of Baccalaureate and Higher Degree Programs (CBHDP) of the National League for Nursing (NLN). This board reviews and approves nursing programs for accreditation. I served on that committee for 4 years, and during that time, I learned not only about accreditation decisions but also about nursing education in universities and colleges all over the United States.

Each program that was reviewed received a preliminary review by three members of the board; this subcommittee presented their conclusions, based on the accreditation criteria, to the full board. I reviewed public academic medical center nursing programs, liberal arts college nursing programs, large and small private university and college nursing programs, large and small public university and college nursing programs, distant learning nursing programs, and single-purpose college nursing programs. I saw a lot of different kinds of nursing programs and thus learned a lot about the variety of ways nursing curriculums are organized, how policies and procedures differ, and how students function in a variety of learning environments. I got a vision of nursing education far beyond what one could learn by just being a faculty person in one institution.

I also served as a program evaluator for the CBHDP of the NLN. My responsibility in this role was to visit the university or college to validate the self-study prepared by the institution with what was actually going on. If amplification or clarification was necessary, the director or dean of the unit was asked to submit additional materials. I visited many different types of programs in all areas of the country. I visited institutions that had bachelor's or master's programs or both. I visited institutions that were seeking initial accreditation or continuing accreditation for their programs; some were on warning.

In this role, like that of a board of review member, I learned a lot about nursing education; in fact, my vision of the total picture of nursing education was considerably enhanced during those years as I saw what kinds of activities worked, which ones created problems, and which issues changed over time. I remember when the first "second-step" nursing programs came up for review. They are now called RN completion programs, and there are a lot of them. When they first appeared for accreditation, they were denied, and there was a lot of difficulty getting them accredited because they were new and did not fit the usual model. The same thing occurred when generic master's programs were developed and the institutions sought accreditation. Over time, however, change occurred more rapidly and differences became more common, so the accreditation criteria and the ways in which they were applied to programs during review also changed.

Having this overall big picture of nursing education prepared me for the roles I played in nursing education as dean, vice president of academic affairs, and college president. I knew what to expect during accreditation, how to write a good self-study, how to prepare for the program evaluator visit, and what could and should occur during the visit. All of these things were important because they would be expected of us during our accreditation visit. I also knew what the board would be looking for and what the board could and could not do. I was very well prepared.

As president of a health science college in Nebraska, I knew what other professional accreditation agencies would do and expect because all accreditation agencies are accredited themselves by an accreditation group. When my college, which had nursing programs and physical therapy, occupational therapy, and radiology programs, had accreditation visits and the college had its regional accreditation visit, I knew what we had to do and how we had to demonstrate compliance with accreditation criteria regardless of the discipline doing the accreditation. In fact, while I was president of this health science college, we received initial accreditation of the radiology technologist, occupational therapy assistant, physical therapist assistant, and master's in nursing programs and continuing accreditation of the baccalaureate nursing program. We also received initial accreditation of the entire college from North Central Association during my tenure as president. This we did in a 4-year time frame; I know it would not have been possible if I had not known the process.

My involvement with NLN and other national nursing organizations was probably the best way for me to gain the big picture because it put me in a position in which paying attention, building a network, and determining fit of what I know with what I learned could occur at a national level. It allowed me to meet influential nurses and to establish a name for myself as an educator and consultant. This ability to see the educational big picture all began because I submitted my name for consideration as a program evaluator. Once I received that designation, I met nurses from other colleges or universities, and it was these people who nominated me for the board of review. Once on the board, I met nurse deans and directors of nursing programs who viewed me as a competent educator and evaluator, and they, too, nominated me for different positions. As I met more nurse educators, I advanced in positions and my network of colleagues grew. Everything seemed to snowball forward, and it all happened because I was willing to volunteer my time and expertise to the organizations so I could keep informed. I worked very hard, but in retrospect, I believe I gained more than I gave.

Every position and every nurse I met provided me with new opportunities and these new opportunities provided me with new information, so I always felt like I had my fingers on the pulse of change. It was not hard for me to get the big picture–it was only an e-mail away. I loved those years of professional involvement, and to this day, I volunteer my time when needed.

Being a College President

There are many stories I could tell about being a college president, but I am going to limit my accounts to my political activities at the state and national levels and how these activities helped me acquire the big picture. When I arrived in Nebraska, I was the only woman president of a college in that state. I had come from California, where I had been the only woman dean on a private Catholic campus, so I knew what it was like to be a minority. I knew what it was like to forge ahead with colleagues who were polite and respectful but who seemed uncomfortable in my presence until they knew me well. I knew what it was like to be paid less and to be expected to do more. And I knew that I could do what was needed because I had wonderful mentors (many who were men) and was not afraid of the challenge. I also knew that in a state with a population less than that of the county I had just left, I could do much more than I had in the past. So I set out to learn about the state politics and to get to know the governor, the senators, and the congressman of our district. I did this by getting involved with the state and national associations: Nebraska Association of Independent Colleges/Universities (NAICU) and American Association of Independent College/Universities (AAICU). There always were issues affecting education at the state and national levels, so it was easy for me to keep informed by serving on committees and by attending the meetings. I got to know the governor and the senators because legislation affecting education needed input from college presidents. I responded to requests for information and kept these elected officials informed about how proposed legislation would affect a small private college. I attended many political functions so these officials would see me and connect my face with my name.

To get the big picture of the city, I joined the Downtown Rotary Club so I could get to know the businessmen and women of the city. I served on rotary committees and raised money for the rotary; through those activities, I became friends with some of the most influential people in the city. I included my husband in many of these events because this area of the country valued family and I wanted them to know I did also.

While I was chair of the NAICU, I had the opportunity to periodically lunch with the senators and legislators of the state, which had a unicameral organization. At these events, I was able to state my case for private education and to get a view of what was going on in the legislature. These interactions always paid off because I knew what was happening and was likely to occur and whether it would affect the college. When we had decisions at the college that would be affected by state and national policy, we were prepared because I had paid attention to my colleagues (the network) and had determined from what I heard whether it was something that connected to what we did.

I loved those years of political involvement and now know that my political activities helped me to grow, which in return helped the college advance. The college flourished under my leadership because I had built a strong support system in the state and had nourished support at the national level, also. Those in the city were also more aware of who and what we did, so when threats to education occurred, I knew where to turn. This same process of paying attention, building a network, and making the connections of what is learned to what is known can occur at any level.

Being President of the World's Second Largest Nursing Organization

The last event I want to discuss is what it is like to be the president of the second largest nursing organization in the world, and seeing the big picture was an essential aspect of the role. In 1993 I assumed the presidency of STTI, and for 2 years I traveled all over the world to bring the message of scholarship, leadership, and research to nurses. I had a very supportive and talented board, who, with me, made major differences in what the society would do. We began that biennium with a retreat, where we learned what it meant to be trustees and ambassadors of the organization. I had arranged for this experience because I believed we needed to look at the big picture. Until that biennium, the elected governing unit had been a board of governors. I believed we needed to evaluate our role in light of our responsibilities as a board. I also thought we needed to look into the future and to determine where we wanted to be in 5, 10, and 20 years. My years as a strategic planner told me we needed to think proactively and futuristically. We needed to pay attention to what would be needed in the future.

The retreat made a huge difference for all of us. The board members and I not only learned about what it meant to be ambassadors of the organization but also discovered how important it was to be trustees of the organization's assets, which were considerable. We had tangible assets (the center of nursing scholarship building and its furnishings, the endowed scholarships, and our investments) and intangible assets (the money to be earned on our endowments and investments) that the board needed to protect. By looking at these assets now and in the future, we were able to get a much better idea of the whole and our responsibilities.

As a result of the retreat, we began to establish some guidelines for the generation of revenue from other sources and to devise ways to invest our money in a more aggressive manner. We started to think about the future of the organization in a more holistic manner. Some of the ideas we tossed around were quite daring, and even though many of these ideas were discarded, the group had begun to think differently and to see things in a new perspective. This was the outcome I had hoped would occur.

As an outcome of the retreat, we prepared a work plan for the organization and later introduced the concept to the chapters at the regional assemblies. We wanted to share our newest activity with the network of chapters; we asked our chapter members to start to think in bigger ways and to look forward so their units would remain viable and healthy in the future. It was an eye opener for us to see how much our chapter officers grasped the idea and how eager they were to think big and futuristically once they understood how to do it. They took from us what they believed would fit with what they were doing.

During my tenure, there were other ways that seeing the big picture helped us. For instance, whereas we had been a national organization for much of our 73 years, it was important that we remember to do things that fit our more recent international framework. For example, we had to devise a fee schedule that fit countries beyond the Western Hemisphere, change our written materials so they were reflective of our international membership and change the focus of our publication *Reflections* so there were articles of international interest, and broaden the board complement so it had an international profile. These changes are a good example of how knowing more about your mission helps you create the right context for your operations.

There were many other things that were different once we became international, and some of those things were cultural. For instance, I learned that volunteering in Australia means being available to give ideas and to plan on paper but not to do the actual work. In the United States, volunteers do everything, which tends to keep the cost down; when we planned a cosponsored event in Australia, the event cost more because we needed to hire people to do the actual work, which meant that the price for each participant was higher. We had made the mistake of thinking that what we do in the United States would fit into their culture.

Just as knowing the big picture at the national level helped me function more effectively as a college president, so did knowing the big picture at the international level help me function more effectively as president of STTI. I do not think I could have done my job as leader of any entity without that grand perspective.

SUMMARY

Looking back on my career and the ways in which seeing the big picture helped me function highlights the value of involvement. I cannot imagine how one could get the big perspective by sitting at home or staying in the office. Regardless of the level of involvement, being with those who had the information gave me the opportunity to pay attention, to establish networks, and to make connections between what I knew with what I learned.

However, not every activity I pursued paid off. Sometimes I gained nothing new; unfortunately, it was difficult to predict which activity would produce nothing. "Nothing ventured, nothing gained" was my motto because during any one activity, I usually gained more than I thought I would, so it made up for the times that I learned nothing new.

Another lesson to be learned from my experiences is that seeing the big picture requires that you be willing to give a lot of yourself. My involvement with national and international organizations took a lot of my time and often took me away from home and the job. This is one of the reasons I involved my husband in the activities; otherwise, I would not have seen much of him. Together we saw a lot of the world, and he helped me gain that bigger perspective. And while the time away from the job meant I had a lot to do when I returned, what I gained from voluntary professional work actually made my job much easier because I had the information I needed

Some of the activities I pursued to get the big picture were not much fun; some of the activities were tedious, and some were actually unpleasant. Most of them were challenging and invigorating. This kind of diversity made the task of getting the big picture worth any of the time I spent or energy I expended. If I had the opportunity, I would do it all again.

However, there are some negative aspects that the nurse leader must not be afraid of, such as rejection, criticism, fatigue, or alienation. Sometimes during my career, while I was attempting to get the big picture. I was rejected. If I had reacted to the rejection in a negative way, I would not have obtained what I was pursuing. My advice to all nurses and potential leaders is to sustain the effort and not take things too personally. In fact, I used to remind myself that the task at hand was part of my job and not part of my life. I tried to see the rejection as something that would pass, given time. This is when the network helped. I would call my friends and check things out with them to determine whether I was on the right track or should take the rejection seriously.

Fatigue often was my companion, but it was a fatigue of work. I was tired because of long hours and intense work, not because of despair or disillusionment. Paying attention to what is said and not to what you think is said helps. Frequent short vacations and rest periods also helped me keep up the momentum, and the joy of getting the big picture kept my fatigue at a manageable level.

Criticism, I have learned, is a gift and not to be dreaded. Although it sometimes is hard to take, it is through criticism that we grow and get better. I tried to look at criticism as a way of getting better, so I paid close attention to what was said, and of course, it is important to note who is giving the criticism. If friends criticize, you know it is for your improvement. Some people are mean-spirited and criticize viciously. It is important to know the difference so you can judge the value of the remarks; it is important to know whether what you hear is in any way important regarding what you already know.

Alienation does happen when you lead a large group, such as a college or an international organization, and you are seeking the big picture, but it can occur at any level because frequently you are the deciding vote and thus alienated from others. This comes with the territory and should not be feared. It simply means the network is very important and should be used frequently to validate your inclinations.

Having confidence in self also helps the nurse leader obtain the full perspective. Given the fact that there are pressures on most leaders when they attempt to reach out and up, it is essential that they know themselves and can weather any attack. Chapter 2 describes the importance of knowing self and how that principle can help the nurse move beyond the current situation. When rejection, criticism, fatigue, and alienation occur, it is helpful to have confidence in yourself. Confidence building is a skill easily learned and an essential aspect of taking the lead.

Paying attention, networking, and connecting what is known with what is learned form a model that has worked for me when I needed to get the full perspective. It helped me make wise decisions in a variety of positions, and it opened doors for me as a professional. I doubt that any leader at any level is able to provide leadership without the full picture, regardless of the issue. As Pritchett (1994) stated,

> The world rewards only those of us who catch on to what's happening, who invest our energy in finding and seizing the opportunities brought on by change. And change always comes bearing gifts [preface].

REFERENCES

Calano, J., & Salzman, J. (1988). *Career tracking: The 26 success shortcuts to the top.* New York: Simon & Shuster.

Dienemann, J. A. (Ed.) (1998). *Nursing administration: Managing patient care.* Stamford, Conn.: Appleton & Lange, p. 50.

Gruber-May, J. (1997). Networking for nurses in today's turbulent times. *Orthopaedic Nursing, 16*(2), 25–29.

Henderson, F. C., & McGettigan, B. O. (1994). *Managing your career in nursing* (2nd ed.). New York: National League for Nursing Press.

O'Connor, A. B. (1982). Ingredients for successful networking. *Nurse Educator, 7*(6), 40–43.

Peters, T., & Austin, N. (1985). *A passion for excellence.* New York: Random House.

Peters, T., & Waterman, R. (1981). *In search of excellence.* New York: Random House.

Pritchett, P. (1994). *The employee handbook of new work habits for a radically changing world.* Dallas: Pritchett & Associates, Inc.

Puetz, B. (1983). *Networking for nurses.* Rockville, Md.: Aspen.

Spitzer-Lehmann, R. (1994). *Nursing management desk reference: Concepts, skills and strategies* (p. 131). Philadelphia: W.B. Saunders.

Sullivan, E. J., & Decker, P. J. (1992). *Nursing administration: A micro-macro approach for effective nurse executives* (p. 60). Norwalk, Conn.: Appleton & Lange.

Tiano, J. J., Myers, D. C., Broad, G. C., Staley, D. S., & Thomas, J. (1994, March). Mentoring leads to networking. *Career Scope,* p. 73.

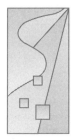

Chapter 5

Building Self-Directed Work Teams

Cynthia S. McCullough
Debra A. Sanders

Teams have been a part of nursing for a long time. Originally, teams consisted of physicians who led nurses and gave them orders. Because of the work of Eleanor Lambertson (1953), teams in nursing changed, with nurses taking the role of team leaders and providing direction for other nurses and for ancillary workers who also provided nursing care. The concept of *team* presented in this chapter is another version of teams that was initiated because hospital administrators wanted a care delivery system that would use workers more efficiently, be less expensive, and increase patient satisfaction. Patient-focused care (PFC) and self-directed work teams (SDWTs) were developed because they had the potential for meeting these criteria at a time when shared governance was popular and in its infancy stage.

A *team* is a group of people working together. It means that more than one person is involved in the care of a patient. Originally, it meant there was a leader with followers and that together they worked out the division of labor. The concept of team presented in this chapter is different. SDWTs have no leaders and no followers. Each member of the team is accountable for the work of the unit and is responsible for certain aspects of patient care. Some activities are unique to an individual, and some activities can be provided by more than one member of the team regardless of the person's preparation or credentials. Cross-training of nurses, x-ray technicians, phlebotomists, and ECG technicians is instituted so a team of individuals can more efficiently meet the needs of patients.

This change in team began in the early 1990s, when several hospitals in the United States formed a consortium to determine a new way to deliver patient care. These hospitals were searching for a way to provide patient care that was consistent with the multilevel changes occurring in health care environments while continuing to meet consumer and provider needs for quality and affordable care. Cost had become a big issue; the hospitals needed to develop a model that would reduce cost, more efficiently use workers, and maintain or increase patient satisfaction. They believed these issues could best be tackled at the system level with the use of SDWTs in a PFC model. The model developed met the following criteria:

- Focus on the patient
- Decentralized services
- Use of a worker skill mix that was more efficient while maintaining or improving patient satisfaction

The service configuration for this PFC model meant that the services had to be close to the patient, so decentralization and renovation were usually needed. To better serve the patient, the radiology department, the laboratory, the pharmacy, and other services were decentralized and moved to the units where the patients were housed. Remodeling in most instances provided the hospital with an opportunity to upscale the facility and at the same time reduce the operational costs due to improved efficiencies and supply utilization. For the first time, the hospital was seen as more than a building. It became a system of health care delivery that provided a continuum of services that were located strategically throughout the system and were specifically organized for the patients. The nurses' station was removed, and the nurse was placed in the room with the patient. The patient's chart, medications, and treatment supplies were also relocated to the patient's room. The goal was to make the organization a place where staff could grow professionally, where they had information and power to get things done, and where incentives to do the work augmented the work. SDWTs were established so this goal could be achieved.

The designers of these systems found that by allowing the staff to practice in milieus of control where they could exercise professional judgment and establish caring, beneficial relationships, job satisfaction increased, turnover was reduced, and the institution's financial condition was ultimately protected (Teschke, 1991).

During the past decade, a number of U.S. hospitals have quietly launched and nurtured SDWTs, which have reduced bureaucracy and increased employee motivation, while at the same time promoting continuous improvement. This chapter describes how a hospital in the Midwest successfully developed and used SDWTs and the roles two nurses played in their development. It addresses the key concepts of SDWTs, how those concepts can be applied to health care, what made this management initiative successful, and the lessons the organization and the nurses learned from the process.

PHILOSOPHICAL, HISTORICAL, AND THEORETICAL ASPECTS OF SELF-DIRECTED WORK TEAMS

Philosophical Aspects

Worker values play an enormous role in the development of SDWTs. According to Izzo and Klein (1998), a 1997 Harris Poll found that 53% of workers were planning to leave their jobs voluntarily in the next 5 years and that more than 80% of North American workers wished they could work for themselves. These figures indicate that workers are mobile and interested in control and self-direction, which are important aspects of SDWTs.

It also seems that workers are looking for different things in the workplace than previously. Although salary is important, being part of the organization in a meaningful way is also very important. For instance, Izzo and Klein (1998) state that workers are looking for the kind of workplace that offers meaning, learning, and community in the midst of change. Peters and Austin (1985) say staff want to work hard, contribute to a satisfying group effort, and get a sense of accomplishment from doing the best job they can.

Izzo and Klein (1998) believe organizations need to create more "soulful workplaces," which they describe as places of compelling intrinsic value in which the energies of workers are engaged and tapped. Several authors (Champy, 1995; Donovan, 1989; Hammer, 1996) suggest that today's workers resist hierarchy and function best in a highly decentralized work environment in which they are empowered to make decisions. Barnum and Mallard (1989) believe that in some respects, knowledgeable workers represent a difficult group. They expect more than wages from their work; they expect to derive a sense of satisfaction and self-esteem from work well done. According to Alderson and McDonnell (1994), workers are looking for corporate cultures that emphasize learning over security and personal responsibility over control. When individuals are truly alive in the workplace, they pour their creativity, energy, and passion into their work.

Traditionally, people have selected careers in health care because of a desire to heal and help. The latest changes in health care based on cost containment often have created a problem because the focus is more on the bottom line than on patient care. According to Morris (1997), the organizations that will survive in the next decade are those that discover how to meet simultaneously the demands of the marketplace and the inner needs of the workplace. Today's workers want community—a sense of contribution, a place to be one's self, and a place to grow professionally. Liedtka and Whitten (1998) believe that decentralized decision-making and flexibility are hallmarks of collaborative processes that increase job and patient satisfaction. Clearly, the values held by workers of today have an impact on how the organization organizes and delivers its services.

Historical Context

Although SDWTs have existed since the 1940s, they are relatively new in the health care setting. Over the years, there have been many organizational patterns for the delivery of care, and these models have at times either functioned independently of each other or been used in mixed forms. In most cases, the number and skill level of staff have dictated the delivery model of nursing care.

According to Marram et al. (1974), the four modalities commonly used for the delivery of nursing care are case method, functional approaches, team nursing, and primary nursing. *Case method* is the oldest form of nursing care delivery, and it is still used today in specialty units, such as intensive care. Case method means that the registered nurse plans and administers care to the patient on a one-to-one basis. Case method is used when the skills of the registered nurse are needed and no other health care worker can provide the care the patient needs; only the registered nurse has the skills that match the acuity level of the patient. This method is not possible in an environment in which the services of nonprofessional personnel are used.

Functional nursing was developed in an effort to provide nursing care in a more efficient manner. By adopting an assembly line approach, workers (registered nurses, licensed practical nurses, and aides) focus their attention on doing tasks. The technical functions of nursing are sorted into levels of complexity and assigned according to the skill level of the caregiver. The nurse aide is given the simplest tasks for a group of patients; the practical nurse is given tasks that demand more training; and the registered nurse is assigned the most complex tasks. The downside of this model is that the identity of the patient is lost because everyone is focusing on "doing things." It is also difficult to coordinate care with this model, so the patient often receives fragmented care.

Team nursing evolved as an answer to a professional care delivery crisis. The nursing shortage caused by World War II left hospitals without registered nurses. To compensate for the shortage of registered nurses, hospitals hired technicians, practical nurses, and aides to provide nursing care. The downside of this move was a reduction in the quality of care because of the inadequate preparation of the ancillary workers and because of an inadequate number of registered nurses to supervise the care provided. Team nursing offered a way to address these problems.

With team nursing, care was provided by a group of nurses, orderlies, aides, and practical nurses under the direction of one registered nurse—the team leader. The team leader was expected to facilitate the team's work by formulating and overseeing the care plan for all patients assigned to the team. The team leader was also expected to know the diagnoses, medications, orders, tests, family problems, and social background of each of the patients cared for by the team. In addition to these duties, the team leader gave and received reports, delivered all of the medications, provided some of the treatments, and planned and delivered in-service training to the team. The downside of this model was the time the team leader spent away from the patient when it was she or he who was responsible for the patient's care.

In the early models of nursing care delivery, hierarchical lines of authority existed; it was therefore easy for nurses to avoid the development of autonomy. With functional and team nursing models, most nurses did not need to assume responsibility. Decision-making responsibilities were easily passed to physicians, administrators, and team leaders. *Primary nursing* was the first attempt to place autonomy in the hands of nurses.

Primary nursing is similar to the case method, except that the registered nurse is responsible for the care provided to the patient over a 24-hour period of time for the length of the patient's hospitalization. Primary nursing is characterized by three qualities: *autonomy, authority,* and *accountability.* The primary nurse assesses the patient, collaborates with the patient and other health care personnel in the development of the care plan, and ensures that the plan is implemented 24 hours a day. The primary nurse delegates nursing care tasks to other nurses through the care plan. Decisions are participatory, involving the patient and the other caregivers most directly involved with the care. Systematic improvements are also promoted with this care delivery model. The downside of this model is that it requires a totally professional staff and thus is expensive. It also is nearly impossible to hire only registered nurses in some areas of the country.

Theoretical Model

As a delivery model, SDWTs challenge the traditional lines of authority and affords caregivers, at all levels, the opportunity to be accountable for their own behavior. Employees are expected to be responsible for creating significant change in the way patient care is delivered and in the cost to the institution for the care delivered. SDWTs are small groups of employees who are responsible for an entire work process. Team members work together to improve the operation, to plan and control their work, and to handle the day-to-day problems. Accountability is the hallmark of SDWTs and the concept that clearly delineates this model from all others.

SDWTs are an innovative approach in the health care setting and are the next step in the evolution of nursing care delivery from primary nursing. Loveridge and Cummings (1996) point out that SDWTs on patient care units are often implemented simultaneously with PFC. In traditional health care organizations, specialization and bureaucratic hierarchies have not supported the use of SDWTs. PFC redesign, however, has caused health care organizations to look at organizational structures that facilitate empowerment within the unit-based multidisciplinary group providing the most patient services. The care of patients is now dependent on the contribution of more than one individual or discipline; thus the team replaces the function of the primary nurse. The literature indicates that member involvement means a sense of commitment to the team, respect for team members, and a growing desire to understand team dynamics. While recognizing their own contributions to the team, they see themselves as part of the whole, striving to reach common goals (Antai-Otong, 1997). The goals of this model are to

1. Achieve high patient, staff, and physician satisfaction
2. Improve patient health care outcomes
3. Decrease the cost of care by increasing resource effectiveness
4. Contribute to staff retention and productivity

The effectiveness of SDWTs is based on the following assumptions:

- Everyone is responsible for fulfilling his or her portion of the care.
- Everyone understands what is expected of him or her.
- Managers relinquish control.
- There are boundaries regarding autonomy.
- Managers are responsible for the environment and culture that determine, in part, the success of the team.

When these assumptions are met, SDWTs can provide a service that no other nursing care delivery model has been able to accomplish.

One of the reasons SDWTs are so useful in a PFC environment is because decisions need to be made by the people who are closest to the patient. Staff need to be able to react quickly to opportunities and problems at the bedside. They need to be able to do what is right for the patient without bureaucracy getting in the way. Because nothing is stable in the health care environment, being able to respond quickly to change is essential. The slow-moving bureaucratic organization cannot compete with the quick response possible by SDWTs. Thus, one of the concepts unique to SDWTs is *quick response.*

Another concept that is unique to SDWTs is *continuous improvement.* Teams of multiskilled workers organized around the delivery of a service can reduce the potential for mistakes and deliver better care and service to the patients. "Working smarter" is achieved with an involved workforce, and teamwork promotes motivation, job satisfaction, and productivity. As the team members examine the team functions, they can self-correct for improvement and thus deliver better service.

The development of a team culture is a process by which there is a conscious transfer of leadership from management to the employees. Orsburn et al. (1990) claim there are five nontraditional characteristics of SDWTs:

1. Specific responsibilities and boundaries for team members are defined by the team.
2. Roles within the team change because teams are structured around an entire process and everyone is equally responsible for the outcomes.
3. Education of the team members focuses on the technical, administrative, and interpersonal skills necessary for people to function within the SDWT.
4. Teams evolve into groups that work with less and less dependence on managers or other leadership.
5. Teams define their own performance measures to identify growth and accomplishments within the teams.

These five characteristics provide a unique set of parameters that define the structure and work of SDWTs.

The development of effective SDWTs is also evolutionary. According to Harper and Harper (1992), as work teams evolve into SDWTs they go through three stages:

1. Turning crisis into opportunity
2. Moving from dependence to interdependence
3. Becoming mature and learning continuously.

Although this process is dependent on the people involved and the organization, it generally takes 2 to 3 years for an SDWT to mature.

Stage 1 of the evolution lasts for approximately 6 months. It is a time of uncertainty for all involved because no one knows quite what to expect. There often is confusion, uncertainty, and frustration throughout this stage; it is usually also filled with excitement and high energy. Much is happening in this stage as the old structure (traditional work) gives way to the new structure. Feeling overwhelmed, frustrated, confused, excited, and energized is perfectly natural. Celebrating small successes and recognizing progress toward the vision are important during this early stage. Rewarding the risk takers with praise and dealing with mistakes (which are inevitable) in a positive and supportive manner are critical.

Stage 2 lasts for 1 year or longer. Harper and Harper (1992) believe that during this stage, team members become united and develop a sense of belonging. The designated team leader is building trust with the team as she or he slowly delegates decision-making to the team to ensure they develop confidence in assuming the task. It is also important to continuously measure cost and quality outcomes and to promptly report them to the group. This allows the team to identify opportunities for process improvements, problem solving, and process redesign. During this stage, the departmental manager transitions to the role of coach and continues to develop the skills necessary for that role.

By the time the SDWT reaches the third stage of development (maturity and continuous learning), most of the training has taken place and team members are comfortable in their new roles. Team members feel ownership of their work and a responsibility for contributing to the achievement of the outcome targets. They believe that each member plays an important role in the team's success and can personally affect the system. Trust, respect, and support among team members have developed. At this stage, tying rewards to productivity (pay for performance, skill-based pay, pay for learning) makes good sense and is an important strategy for pushing teams to achieve higher levels of success.

IMPLEMENTATION OF SELF-DIRECTED WORK TEAMS IN A HOSPITAL IN THE MIDWEST AS EXPERIENCED BY TWO NURSES

Environment for Change

In 1991, SDWTs were introduced into a large Midwest hospital that had a long history of successful operation. It was the first hospital in the state and had an Episcopal church affiliation. Because of the changes occurring in health care delivery throughout the nation and because the hospital needed renovation, in 1989 the board of directors decided to change the care delivery system to a patient-focused model. Individual operating units were developed to bring services closer to the patients in an attempt to broaden the responsibilities of the caregivers. Services were grouped by product lines, and patient floors were renovated to include admissions, dismissals, and medical record services. A satellite pharmacy was added to each floor, and the traditional nurses' station was replaced by a service area within each patient room that included a computer, supplies, the patient's chart, and other equipment normally housed at the nurses' station.

Services offered by the hospital included both inpatient and outpatient on-site locations and several satellite off-site locations. All billing for the off-site locations was centralized at the hospital location.

Before the PFC effort, the hospital used a modified team approach to provide patient care. Two thirds of the staff were licensed practical nurses, and the remaining third were registered nurses. A registered nurse served as the charge nurse and along with a secretary was responsible for processing orders for 50 patients on a daily basis. Charge nurses also made patient and staff assignments and were expected to make rounds with physicians daily. The registered nurse team leader was responsible for the care of 15 to 25 patients and usually directed the activities of three to five licensed practical nurses. A combination of 8- and 12-hour shifts made day-to-day continuity difficult. In this environment, it was common for patients to have contact with 50 staff members or more during their hospital stay. Time from admission to the initiation of orders could be up to 5 hours, a 60-minute turnaround time for STAT medications was common, and information technology support was not an efficient system. Hospital studies showed that nurses were spending twice as much time documenting scheduling and waiting as they did giving direct care. As Berwick (1989) states,

> A test result lost, a specialist who cannot be reached, a missing requisition, a misinterpreted order, duplicate paperwork, a vanished record, a long wait for the CT scan, an unreliable on-call system—these are all familiar examples of waste, rework, complexity, and error in the physician's life . . . for the average physician quality fails when systems fail (p. 53).

This statement is true for any health care worker. Operating systems are the links that hold the institution together and enable the workers to deliver services efficiently. Significant frustration and inefficiencies result when these systems do not appropriately support the way the hospital wants to do business. This hospital was functioning as a failed system, morale was low, and change was needed—it needed something to get excited about.

The primary objective for developing a PFC environment was that the institution recognized it needed change. The staff accepted the move to PFC partly because they knew they could not survive in the current environment, and any change at this point in time was welcomed.

SDWTs are often a method used to reduce layers of corporate bureaucracy; however, at this hospital, those layers had already been removed with the move to PFC, but a clear plan about how the work would be done was lacking. During this "delayering" period, the executive nurse position was eliminated. To complete the decentralization process, the directors and managers of departments were made responsible for the executive nurse's functions.

When jobs are eliminated and processes are not improved, the work does not go away, and it is not long before the jobs are back. We did not want this to happen to us. We believed SDWTs would fit well with the new culture. PFC was being implemented, and the hospital was educating all managers about the continuous quality improvement (CQI) process, so it seemed natural to push forward with the SDWT effort. As leaders of this process, we recognized the opportunity, had the courage to act, and were cognizant of the time it would take. We were planning a delivery model that would function across the continuum of services no matter where they were located in the system.

Preparing for the Implementation of Self-Directed Work Teams

When we began our venture to establish SDWTs, we sought help from the literature as our first step. We found a variety of messages that helped us to get started. Orsburn et al. (1990) state that teams may be organized in a variety of formats, such as natural, systemwide, task force, or cross-functional. They stated that membership could be determined according to whether the individuals depending on each other for success had the experience or skills necessary to work together in an area or had a vested interest and were committed and accountable for outcomes. They also pointed out that teams must establish their own ground rules, actively work to improve their own effectiveness, and determine when and how often to meet.

Donovan (1989) describes the move from a traditional organization to a high performing work team in his article entitled "Employees Who Manage Themselves." He points out that in the traditional organization, the basic building block consists of the individual and a specific task; however, when employees manage themselves, the focus is on the team and its processes.

The literature (Barnum and Mallard, 1989; Booz, Allen, & Hamilton, Inc., 1989; Donovan, 1989; Dumaine, 1993; Swansburg, 1996) clearly shows that in traditional organizations, management plans, controls, and improves. There are narrow job specifications and specialization of work. Each person is focused on his or her job rather than on departmental performance. Information systems are designed for top management and filter down very little information to those who do the work. Accountability is pushed upward. This kind of organization creates several interesting outcomes. A single-skilled job narrows the worker's focus so he or she has no understanding of the overall process and goals. Improvement is always someone else's job, problems are pushed upward, and people often feel powerless.

When traditional organizations are compared with organizations that have instituted SDWTs, there is a different outcome. When teams move to semiautonomous groups, there is "multiskilling" of jobs, an integration of functions, and a whole-job focus. The team begins to assume the responsibility for planning, controlling, and improving. Information is available and used for decision-making, self-correction, and ongoing improvements. As Moffit et al. (1993) point out, a high performing work team is the goal of SDWTs. The team has a clear sense of running a business and assumes full responsibility for setting and achieving business goals. They also emphasize that achieving high performance requires extraordinary effort and commitment.

The literature also indicates that the team is considered the major vehicle or tool for accomplishing the empowerment of employees (Deeprose, 1995). In some instances, employees are prepared to assume this leadership role. In others, training, skill development, and mentoring are essential before the transformation. In general, it has been found that as teams develop, the members gradually accept responsibility for team building and maintenance and perform successfully. Champy (1995) says there are people who argue that cultural change is impossible because values and behaviors are too deeply rooted in people to expect any change. Other authors disagree with this perspective and claim that under the right circumstances and with support, most workers are not only willing to change but also anxious to do so (Davidhizar, 1993).

After this literature review, which took 6 months, we began organizing work groups. We chose to implement SDWTs by organizing around natural work groups. We wanted the teams to be fully connected to the natural work process. Seventeen SDWTs were formed within shift boundaries so members could attend meetings without incurring overtime costs. The discussion that follows includes how the leadership council was formed, how the planning/redesign group was formed and what their responsibilities included, how the boundaries of the team were established, how the role of the manager was changed, and what the training program included and how it was implemented—all based on the characteristics and concepts of SDWTs. What barriers we faced and how we addressed them are also described.

Forming a Leadership Structure

■ The Leadership Council

This council served as the governing body for the department during the development of SDWTs. The council met monthly to review quality improvement reports, facilitate CQI groups, review diagnosis-related group (DRG) reports, monitor the budget, and ensure that resources were available to assist the teams so they could meet their goals. The Leadership Council membership included the medical director, department director, a manager, and representatives from the SDWTs. Supporting the Leadership Council and the SDWTs was a resource team. Membership included a pharmacist, social worker, dietitian, technical specialist, utilization reviewer, and three clinical nurse specialists. Figure 5–1 depicts this organizational structure.

■ The Design Team

We knew a formal structure was needed to plan, guide, and oversee the effort of transitioning to SDWTs, and we knew that the group needed to include both management and staff members. To build ownership across the organization for changes that would correspond with the implementation, representatives from other key stakeholder groups were also included in this planning group. After the completion of the original implementation of PFC in 1991, a design team was formed that included representation from the directors, managers, and staff, as well as hospital representatives from staff development, computer services, human resources, finance, marketing, administration, and a faculty member from a local college. The planning group was charged with the responsibility of devising a sound strategy for converting the present delivery system into an SDWT system. This involved sanctioning the effort, establishing clear goals and objectives, assessing and preparing the organization for change, setting boundaries and guidelines for team activities, and overseeing all phases of the change process from planning to implementation and evaluation.

To perform their roles effectively, the planning group members needed a solid understanding of work teams and what they do, as well as how to go about implementing new kinds of teams in an organization that already had teams. The group spent 6 months reviewing the literature and sharing that information with other team members at a weekly 2-hour session. We discussed books and articles and viewed films about SDWTs. In retrospect, we should have visited other institutions that had SDWTs, but we did not.

Members of the design team were responsible for informing the staff of the progress made by the team, and minutes from every meeting were distributed

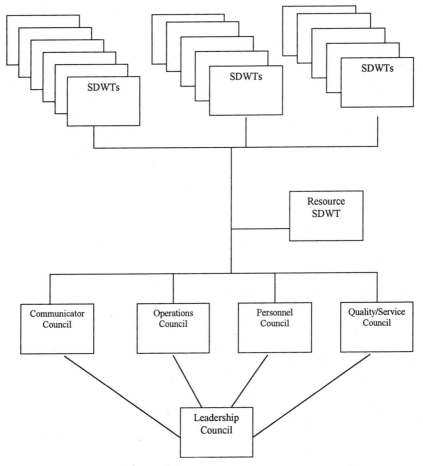

Figure 5-1. Unit organization chart.

to the staff. Furthermore, the design team published a weekly newsletter, which was distributed throughout the organization, and held monthly informational sessions for the staff. We knew that communication was very important.

The first steps the design group took were to develop a mission statement, goals, and a definition of SDWTs. The mission was to "facilitate the creation of SDWTs that would enhance the development of a quality health care environment." The goals were to

- Obtain organizational support for the implementation of SDWTs
- Identify the skills necessary for SDWTs to function
- Develop a transition plan for SDWT implementation

After several weeks of research and discussion, the design team agreed on the following definition for an SDWT: "A SDWT is a small group of employees responsible for an entire work process or segment who work together to improve their operation or product, plan, and control their work, and handle day-to-day problems. They are also involved in organizational issues such as vendor selection, quality, safety, and business planning. Managers now function as coaches and leaders." The design team also suggested that the budget and profit margins be shared and that employees have information about the jobs and tasks of the entire team—not just about a single job or task.

As a result of this definition, the design team was acquiring new skills and demonstrating a commitment to the guidance of a long-term transition to SDWTs. Midmanagers were eager and busy learning new ways to facilitate the process. Employees who were already reaping the rewards of the new PFC environment were eager to master multiple skills and searching for expanded responsibility. All of this was occurring while those in traditional environments in the hospital were watching and expressing skepticism about the success of a transition to SDWTs.

Critical to self-direction is a culture in which executives are willing to support, both verbally and by funding, the plans being formulated by the SDWTs (Orsburn et al., 1990). During this time of change at our hospital, there was strong support from the chief executive officer. He had reviewed and accepted the design team's key concept document and their plan for implementation. And although some senior managers expressed concern about the plans, overall they saw the potential value of expanded employee involvement that would make the organization productive and competitive while producing patient, staff, and physician satisfaction. They agreed the department should proceed with a pilot implementation; however, funds for training were not provided, so a plan was formulated that would fit into our existing budget.

According to Howard (1996), leaders pull others together to collaborate and work as a team. Giving the group a vision, a purpose, and a direction to pursue is the best way to accomplish this task. To educate the employees of this department as it was going through change and to gain input from them into the process, a 3-hour all-employee session was led by the chief operating officer of the organization and the department director. The strategic goals of the organization were presented, as well as the business plan of the department. Findings from the design team literature review were summarized. From these data, the goals and objectives for the teams that were related to the goals and objectives of the organization were developed and shared.

The next task of the design team was to develop a transition plan that was to act as a guide outlining which management duties would be turned over to teams, when that would occur, and when specific skill training would be provided. This plan clearly identified which duties could be transferred immediately and which would require more time because the teams needed to mature. It also included those duties that the employees needed to learn before transfer of the tasks was possible. The design team questioned whether the vendor contracts or the termination of employees should be handled by the SDWTs but decided to revisit these issues after the teams had been functioning successfully for a period of time. Table 5-1 illustrates how the management duties were evaluated for transfer to SDWTs.

The Diamond Concept The design team knew that leadership had to be shared, so they identified four roles necessary for team leadership: communica-

Table 5-1. Transferring Management Duties to Self-Directed Work Teams

Management/Social Duties	Transfer Now	Transfer With Training	Transfer Later	Transfer Perhaps
Scheduling assignments		X		
Timecards			X	
Leading meetings		X		
Hiring		X		
Performance feedback		X		
Customer relations				
Internal/patients	X			
Vendors			X	
Vendor contracts				X
Determining raises			X	
Problem solving/identification	X			
Auditing work/verification		X		
Monitoring quality			X	
Cost containment		X		
Budgeting			X	
Interdepartment communication			X	
Progressive discipline			X	
Guidelines/procedures/protocols			X	
Setting goals/objectives	X			
Responsibility for daily production	X			
Communicate between shifts	X			
Safety/housekeeping		X		
Stocking	X			
Record keeping/documentation			X	
Data maintenance			X	
Manage as own business			X	
Public relations/marketing			X	
Termination				X(?)

tor, operations, personnel, and quality/service roles. These roles were directly tied to the transition plan, which identified the potential responsibilities for each role. The team called this leadership structure "the diamond." Each SDWT had members assigned to these roles.

Communicators played a critical role in the SDWTs. The role was assumed by only one person in each team but was rotated among the team members. Communicators were appointed by the leadership council or selected by the team members using consensus. Whenever possible, team members were involved in the selection of the person who would become the communicator. One of the communicator's major tasks was to balance guiding the group with letting the group assume responsibility. Communicators had to be adept at being leader-members; they had to know when to take the lead, when to let others take the lead, and when to share the lead. When the communicator was also a manager, transition to the communicator role was difficult because the urge to take over was very strong. The person in the communicator role was expected to do the following:

- Enable all members to participate
- Be sensitive to the corporate team culture
- Be interested in solving problems
- Be able to listen attentively (know when to intervene and when to remain quiet)
- Be sensitive to the feelings, opinions, and needs/goals of each team member
- Be able to give constructive feedback
- Understand team dynamics and the process of team development
- Be able to recognize that the role of communicator could inhibit the participation of other members and be able to take steps to prevent that from happening
- Be flexible and secure enough to share the leadership role with other members

Communicators learned a lot about group dynamics. They learned that group members sometimes disagree and that their job was to facilitate resolution of the disagreement before there was widespread discontent. They also learned how to manage discontent and how to avoid "showdowns."

Communicators met monthly with their teams and monthly with the communicator council. A representative of the communicator council was also a member of the leadership council. It was at these meetings that the communicators discussed the problems and shared the successes they were having with the SDWTs.

The persons in the *operations* role were accountable to the team, the operating unit, and the hospital for the financial and operational costs of the department on a day-to-day basis. They were also responsible for increasing the teams' awareness of the fiscal condition of the department. This meant they had to understand the department's fiscal reports, which included the operational statement, cost center detail, the billable supply report, the patient's bill, exception reports and the justifications for variances, and the revenue reports. They were also responsible for auditing patient charges and monitoring team overtime.

The department director, the director of finance, and the unit managers spent a lot of time helping the operations' personnel and the operations council understand the various documents and procedures for which they were responsible. Patient days, productive hours per patient day, cost per patient day, and employee cost per patient day data were graphically portrayed on a monthly report, which was available to the staff at any time. Department-targeted DRG reports were also available on a monthly basis. Operations personnel met with their counterparts from the other SDWTs monthly as a council and had a representative on the leadership council. Again, the leadership council and the director of finance of the hospital were available to the operations personnel so they could work on the problems and concerns they had as they assumed their new roles.

During the implementation of SDWTs, the chief executive officer asked all departments to reduce their operating expenses by 10%. The leadership council worked with the operations personnel from each SDWT to identify opportunities for improved processes that would result in cost savings so reductions in staff would not be necessary. For example, one of the many ideas implemented by the teams that resulted in cost savings without staff reduction was related to supplies. The team evaluated the cost of many supplies, and after 2 months and a review of four products for their effectiveness, cost, and the patient's satisfaction, the team recommended a product be changed. This change saved the department $52,000 annually, had no adverse effect, and provided the teams with the confidence they needed to make further reductions.

The *personnel* role involved the coordination of human resource functions, such as staff scheduling, the orientation of new employees, the coordination of new employee interviews, and helping employees with their time cards. As a beginning, the human resource department provided a session on hiring and firing for the personnel council members. At that session, information on the process for hiring new personnel, how the human resource department would work collaboratively with the SDWTs during the hiring process, and the federal regulations affecting hiring were discussed.

After this session, the team conducted all of the interviews for new hires and selected individuals by reaching consensus using a rating system developed by the human resource department. The unit manager participated in the interviews but refrained from participation in the selection of a new employee. The process worked well. Although candidates stated they felt intimidated by the group interview, they all acknowledged they clearly understood the requirements of the job and what would be expected of them as a result of the group questions.

On one occasion, the team made a choice that the unit manager felt was a poor one because she believed the candidate was the least qualified for the job. Out of curiosity, she questioned the selection. The team's response was not a good one, but because the team's selection followed federal guidelines, the decision held. Several weeks later, two members of the team came to the unit manager and announced that the new employee's performance was not acceptable. They wanted the manager to take care of the problem. The manager questioned the adequacy of the new employee's orientation. The team members realized they had not been fair to the new employee and decided to call a team meeting to discuss the situation. They returned later that day with a revised orientation schedule. They rearranged their schedules and redistributed responsibilities so the two could focus their efforts on the orientation of the new employee. Three weeks later, the new employee was functioning appropriately and contributing positively to the team. This scenario is proof positive of the importance of the team's accepting the responsibility for follow-up on their decisions and how the unit manager must support the decisions of the group and act as a coach in the resolution of problems. It also suggests that the team saw something in the new hire that the manager did not; because the new hire would be working closely with the team members, their vision probably was more valid.

One of the unique activities the Personnel Council developed was a peer review system. Because they understood the importance of the difference and uniqueness of team members and how these factors make a team effective, they also developed a system for publicly recognizing peers for exceptional performance. Like the other groups, the individuals in the personnel role met monthly as a council and had a representative on the leadership council.

Persons in the *quality/service* role were responsible for evaluation functions. These persons were responsible for the evaluation of customer satisfaction, the department's adherence to policies and procedures, quality assurance/improvement, and the teams' compliance with their own identified goals and objectives. They were also responsible for the evaluation of direct and indirect aspects of patient care provided by the team, as well as ensuring that the indicators for satisfaction were identified, data were collected and evaluated, interventions were identified, and a plan for correction was implemented. Some of the activities that were monitored included staff, patient, and physician satisfaction; falls; medication errors; nosocomial infections; and laboratory errors. All monitoring reports were presented and reviewed monthly at the leadership council meetings and then were shared with the hospital quality improvement committee. Each month, the quality/service persons from each SDWT met together as the quality/service council. One person from that group also served on the leadership council.

Managing Boundaries Early in the transition, we found that when too much room was given to the teams, they felt abandoned; and when not enough room was given, they felt stifled. We needed to monitor the teams' progress against the amount of autonomy they could assume. We learned that boundaries provide a reassuring link between what was happening and what we were trying to do. Orsburn et al. (1990) suggest that the purpose of boundaries is to ensure information flow and to manage accountability to encourage productivity and sustain high quality work. We found that boundaries provided a framework for our transition and thus were able to

1. Give each team a clear sense of its own identity
2. Harmonize team efforts with corporate objectives
3. Ensure the accountability of the teams
4. Ensure the teams conformed to fiscal, legal, and other critical guidelines

We learned SDWTs are not unmanaged teams; they are differently managed teams. Even high performing work teams operate within boundaries. We found that the teams could assume responsibility for managing the boundaries within the team while the managers monitored the boundaries between the teams and other departments and the organization.

Defining the Manager Role

All organizations face the challenge of changing leadership roles as they implement SDWTs. Manz and Sims (1989) suggest effective leaders teach team members how to (1) set goals for one's own work efforts, (2) practice work activities through mental or physical rehearsal before performing them, and (3) observe and gather data about one's own performance. They believe effective leaders encourage and coach others to internalize and self-manage much of the control previously imposed by managers.

After the definitions of the team members' roles were completed, the role of manager was defined. Clearly, the role of the manager is the same in an SDWT environment as it has always been with groups—to accomplish desired business results of the operating unit through others. To support employees' transitioning to a team-based model, our managers needed to learn new skills such as when to relinquish control, how to clarify responsibilities and roles, how to develop effective coaching approaches, how to approach discipline in a positive manner, and how to lead the change. Instead of chopping work into pieces, as in the functional model, managers had to learn how to reintegrate work processes.

We also knew that our managers needed to build the team members' skills and confidence. They also needed to gradually delegate new tasks, help employees set their own goals, evaluate performance, and take corrective action. Short-term goals needed to be reconciled with long-term organizational goals. Furthermore, the managers needed to learn how to seek out and distribute information needed by the teams, secure resources for the teams, and balance the interests of different individuals.

Orth et al. (1990) suggest coaching as a way of helping employees over time improve (change) their performance (behavior and results) to outstanding levels or at least to the highest level of which they are capable. The manager in the team environment must have the ability to get diverse groups of people to generate and implement their own best ideas. Switching from directing to influencing is a major change for a manager who has spent years telling people what to do. Transitioning from manager to coach was probably the most difficult of all individual changes that had to occur to bring SDWTs to their best performance.

Managers were active members of some teams and coaches and information sources for others, but they always needed to be closely aligned with what was happening within the teams that interacted within the department. Acting as a coach and fostering decision-making by the team was an important role for the manager, as was teaching teams to manage more of their own day-to-day work.

Giving people permission to do something differently is not helpful if they are not ready or able to do it. Ideally, managers and directors, like the team members, need to understand what they do and do not know and where they need additional training and education. This assistance was not available to us during this change, so the managers had to learn on their own.

When we began the PFC restructuring process, the manager acquired 100 direct reports. Because the organization expected a quarterly appraisal of all employees, it became very clear that we could not continue to operate as we had in the old model. Even though we were learning the CQI process and staff development was preparing a mentor system for managers, there was no other training available. We read a lot, learned by trial and error, and became part of a support network that had unique aspects. The physician champion for PFC, the evaluation consultant for the transition, and the chief executive officer were all available whenever the managers needed help, advice, or someone to listen. They all felt comfortable in offering advice, particularly if it looked like it had a positive outcome.

In the transition from a modified team approach to the SDWT approach, the role of the manager changed from that of organizer and manager of tasks to evaluator of clinical care and teacher and coach for team members. Staffing and assigning personnel are major responsibilities of most managers and were some of the first tasks targeted for transition to staff.

Some former head nurses and assistant head nurses whose positions had been eliminated were now members of the teams. They had already mastered the scheduling function and were asked to help their team members learn the task. They were happy to accept the responsibility; however, things did not go as smoothly as we had hoped. The former head nurses were accused of playing favorites and giving themselves the best schedule. They felt they had been placed in an uncomfortable position and wanted the manager to take back the task until all team members were trained. Instead, we gave anyone who voiced concerns about the schedule the job of preparing the next schedule. It took 3 months before the complaints stopped. Everyone who had prepared the schedule had a new respect for the process of creating an equitable one.

Just because we were in a self-directed environment did not mean employees stopped asking, "What shall I do?" Before SDWTs, we would probably have told them what to do, but in the new model, we had to stop, step back, and let them solve the problem themselves or help them through the process as best we could. We knew it would be quicker if we gave them the answer but that would not help them accept the responsibility they needed to assume. So unless a patient's life was in danger, we helped coach them through the experience of solving the problem or problems.

Coaching staff to confront one another was probably the most time-consuming task but one that had the most rewarding outcome. Several times a week, staff members would describe situations about another staff member or department that in their opinion required a manager's intervention. We would listen and suggest different ways they could approach the situation until we found one that they could accept. Then we would role play the situation until they were comfortable with the action. Usually the team member had no idea his or her behavior was a problem, and when confronted with this information, he or she was willing to work on a different way to behave or was able to defend the behavior. After several months, the staff realized their strength as a team was in the diversity of its members and that it was acceptable and often desirable to do things differently. We began to notice a significant difference in the way the team members cared for each other, which in turn strengthened the way in which they cared for the patients.

As the teams matured, the members could not believe how open they had become with each other and how less stressful work had become because an issue was addressed when it happened instead of letting it fester for weeks before someone went to the manager for help. However, not all conflicts were easily resolved, and not all individuals were willing to take that first step. As Wellins et al. (1991) point out, with any developmental process, one should be prepared to accommodate those who are ready for greater responsibility as well as those who are having difficulty keeping up with the team's progress. It is essential to match aggressive team members with external challenges and responsibilities and provide one-on-one coaching for those who lag behind. One highly specialized team had resisted the move to PFC and was resisting the implementation of SDWTs. An outside facilitator was hired to help them work through their problems, which made their transition period much longer.

The CQI process was widely used in the organization, so the steps we used for problem solving were similar to that process. We would identify the problem, the causes for the problem, the expected outcomes, and the options for solutions. Given those data, we were able to devise solutions and to develop an implementation plan and a process for evaluating the effectiveness of the plan.

There were several individuals who helped us personally during the changes. One of those persons was a faculty advisor from a local college that had a graduate program in nursing. She was working on a doctoral degree at the time, and her doctoral dissertation was about PFC using a grounded theory approach. Because of her frequent observations and discussions with the staff, she quickly developed a good relationship with them that continued through the process of SDWT implementation. It was healthy for the staff to be able to vent to an outsider, and it was beneficial to us to have an outsider's perspective. She noticed that we were spending a lot of time with a small group of the staff who were not getting on board with the new way. We wanted everyone to understand what we were attempting to do and to like it. She advised us to save our energy and to focus on the staff who were demonstrating the desired behaviors. She reminded us that we were giving 90% of our time to 20% of the staff and neglecting the other 80% who were doing a magnificent job. When we gave positive reinforcement to those who were making the effort to change, they moved even further. When the resisters saw what wonderful things the others were doing, resistance stopped and the entire group moved forward together.

The individual hired to evaluate the outcomes of the changes in the organization was a behavioral psychologist. She was also very helpful to the staff. While she received resistance from many staff and several physicians throughout the organization, our department was very interested in developing outcome measures, so we invited her to our leadership council meeting and asked for her help. She helped us see the power of information and of feedback to the employees. She also helped us develop reports for team use, and she advised us on behavioral issues. The managers and directors met formally and informally with her on a weekly basis. She also helped us personally by showing us ways to balance our lives as we progressed through the implementation process.

One physician, who was a champion for PFC, was very interested in the success of our department, so he gave us special attention. He always asked three questions: "How have you added value?" "Do you believe you are making a difference?" "Are you having fun?" We asked those questions of ourselves daily. He also played an important role as facilitator. He helped remove physician resistance by teaching them how to work with the SDWTs. Many physicians wanted to return to the old way and to communicate with the head nurse rather than a team. They also had trouble understanding the manager's new role. He helped them learn how to work with the team and to relate to the managers in their new roles. The transition was very difficult for the physicians because they were not an integral part of the education and training that was under way. Thus, this physician was extremely helpful, and we doubt whether we could have succeeded if he had not been there to work with the physicians.

The educational consultant for staff development had a special interest in SDWTs. She was a member of the design team and was involved in educating team members. Because the formal classes for management had not been developed at this time, she met with us weekly to determine where we were in the process and to identify the resources we would need.

Because we were a department with a pilot project and because PFC was not yet fully implemented within the organization, there were many barriers to our progress. Department members did not know how to work with teams and did not want to meet with teams to resolve the problems. They wanted to speak with the manager. The manager always agreed to meet with those department members but only if the team was also invited to attend. This helped to educate the other department members to the SDWT concept. When department members would not meet with the teams, the chief executive officer was notified, and he stepped in to help us improve communication.

Deeprose (1995) identifies the characteristics of good team goals as those that

- Contribute to organizational objectives
- Respond to customer needs
- Reflect the teams' key responsibilities
- Contain measurable standards
- Generate doable action plans

In our department, the managers helped the teams translate their common purposes into specific performance goals that were related directly to the organization's goals of increased satisfaction and improved cost of care. Decentralization and a flattened structure forced the managers to assume a new role. The challenge we faced was to maintain accountability for the department while empowering the teams to work within prescribed boundaries. The manager had to learn the right combination of withdrawal and involvement.

Relinquishing traditional management duties expanded the employees' knowledge and allowed the manager to concentrate on leadership responsibilities. According to Hammer, who is quoted in *Fortune* (1993),

> Coming up with the ideas is the easy part, but getting things done is the tough part. The place where reform dies is down in the trenches (p. 18).

Our managers were able to work with the employees so the changes were implemented in the trenches with the managers acting as coaches.

Education and Training

We learned during the implementation of PFC that the distress people experience during a transition to something new is directly related to the amount of education and training they receive and the timing of both. Education and training was a key concern for the design team. A subgroup of the design team developed the roles of the team members, while another subgroup developed education and training for team members, managers, and the shared leadership roles.

The first step was to identify the knowledge and skills the team members would need to be successful. Once identified, the curriculum was developed with the assistance of the staff development department of the hospital. All courses were designed in 2-hour blocks of time at the request of the staff. Staff members also agreed to cover for each other during class times so all education and training could be accomplished during the regular working hours. As the team members worked together, the curriculum was refined and new courses were added.

One of the areas in which the design team believed the team needed help was interpersonal relations. They identified the following eight skills that needed to be covered in the curriculum:

1. Effective listening
2. Giving and receiving feedback
3. Group decision making through consensus
4. Basic problem solving
5. Creativity
6. Constructive disagreement
7. Conducting effective meetings
8. Evaluating team effectiveness

We also learned early that trust and open communication were important aspects of successful teams. We knew that trust and openness occur in a team environment when members know they can speak freely and that their ideas and opinions will be valued and listened to. We knew that the team members needed to be able to accept and support each other and that the team must be a place where they could take risks and grow. To prepare the staff for functioning in an open and trusting team environment, the design team identified four areas that needed to be a part of the educational program for the staff:

- Team building
- Conflict resolution
- How to develop goals and objectives
- Scheduling

The purpose of the team-building class was to enable team members to function as motivated, skilled, and committed members of the team. The content for this session included the differences between teams and groups, the characteristics of successful teams, the difference between a ground rule and the norm, and the stages of team development.

The conflict resolution class was established to improve the team member's ability to resolve conflict within the team. The sessions included strategies for discussing conflict within teams, alternative ways for handling conflict, and the appropriate steps for conflict resolution.

The goals and objectives class was designed to assist the team members in the development of realistic goals for the work team. Content for this class included defining goals, objectives, and tactics and understanding how they are different; identifying the sources of information needed to establish goals and objectives; how to write measurable and realistic objectives; how to write tactics that are clear and concise; and how to develop follow-up measures for performance evaluation.

The purpose of the scheduling class was to help the SDWTs learn how to schedule the work hours of the team members. The class covered the appropriate sources for information about "personal leave," sick time, and employment status; the correct time for posting schedules; and the staffing requirements for the team. Scheduling games were developed so the participants could practice their ability to write work schedules that took into consideration the preferences and idiosyncrasies of the staff.

In addition to the core courses, modules were developed for ways to lead meetings and strategies for focusing on customers. Simultaneous with the development of the curriculum, design team members were learning how to teach the core courses, which were prepared in a syllabus format so the content would remain consistent and be useful to any instructor.

Factors That Enabled Successful Implementation of Self-Directed Work Teams

There were many factors that enabled us to succeed in the establishment of SDWTs in our hospital. The literature cites many success stories about SDWTs that flourished because of a "top-down" organizational approach. There also are stories about SDWT success from a "bottom-up" approach. Our experience was based primarily on a "bottom-up" strategy because we believed the establishment of SDWTs in our institution would work best if they "bubbled up" throughout our organization. We think we were right!

Regardless of whether the implementation of SDWTs is top-down or bottom-up, there are critical factors that are key to their success. A clearly defined organizational mission, vision, and value statement are essential because they serve as the foundation for all decisions that must be made. What the organization stands for, its purposes, and the behaviors that are expected from the employees must be clearly stated, easily understood, and communicated everywhere. Round-the-clock scheduled departmental meetings were held with the chief executive officer so we were sure we knew we were on the right track. Review and clarification of the organization's mission, vision, and values were extremely important steps because this sent a clear message throughout the institution of the chief executive officer's support for the SDWT approach. The unconditional support of the chief executive officer and the executive team was a key factor in our ability to move to a team culture.

An important factor that facilitated our success was the development of a system to measure our success. A baseline measure of our "old world model" was established, and a valid and reliable methodology was developed for measuring key outcomes of cost and quality of the new model. Outcome results were monitored frequently and shared openly with all team members. This sharing of data provided the perfect forum for identifying opportunities for improvement and celebrations of our success.

Another important factor that enabled us to be successful with this venture was feedback from our patients and their families. A large segment of our patient population was chronically ill and required frequent hospitalizations. We got to know these patients and their families and counted on them to share their comments and feelings with us. The feedback we received indicated there was a significant improvement in our ability to provide care after the implementation of SDWTs.

The teams themselves were the most important reason for our success. The significant investment in education and training sent the positive message to the staff that they were valuable to the success of the organization. Open communication with all team members facilitated the exchange of ideas and information and was an important reason we were successful. Team meetings, lunch sessions, monthly communication meetings, and the departmental newsletter not only kept everyone informed but also demonstrated how important these people were to the success of this major renovation of care delivery. We valued the teams' efforts, and they knew it. The more we praised them by our attention to what they did, the more they wanted to do for the institution.

In an empowered culture, there is a need to establish boundaries. Boundaries served as a checklist for team decisions and provided a control mechanism that supported their success. The boundaries for our unit were established in three areas: legal statutes, licensure regulations, and the budget. Team members knew they could not violate state or federal laws or function beyond the scope of their practice or exceed the budget. In summary, the following factors contributed to our success:

- Clearly defined mission, vision, and boundaries
- Chief executive officer support
- Criteria for measuring success
- Education and training
- Patient and family evaluation
- Open communication
- Continued focus on quality and improvement
- Boundaries established by statues, regulations, and the budget

Factors That Acted as Barriers or Obstacles to Our Success

Even in organizations in which there is support, there always are obstacles or barriers to success that must be dealt with. In our experience, the most significant obstacles were the difficulty in transitioning to a new role, the transfer of accountability from managers to the teams, personnel conflicts, and insufficient education. Another obstacle we had to mount was the readiness of the organization to accept and support our new departmental initiative. A lack of knowledge about SDWTs was prevalent throughout the rest of the institution. This lack of knowledge about SDWTs often created difficulty for the teams in carrying out their tasks that required interdepartmental interaction, such as ordering supplies. Looking back on the experience, we should have conducted an organizational readiness assessment before implementation of our SDWTs. We thus would have been able to discover what was lacking to bring the organization up to a level of readiness and spared ourselves this particular problem.

The literature indicates that other common barriers to the implementation of SDWTs include such things as lack of management support, first-line supervisory resistance, and misalignment of organizational systems. We had none of these problems; however, several months after SDWTs were established in our department, we reached a point where we seemed paralyzed. Staff members were walking around with the "deer in the headlight" stare, and the managers were tiptoeing around, trying to stay out of their way. Finally, a meeting was called by the manager to discuss the issues.

During the first 45 minutes of the meeting, nothing much was said. Finally, a licensed practical nurse spoke up, "In the old world, when we did not like something or when there were problems, we blamed you . . . not because it was your fault but because you were the manager and you were responsible. Now when we do not like something or things do not go well, we have to blame each other or ourselves because we are responsible, and this is very hard." We were all used to a functional team approach to care delivery and needed time to learn the new way.

The lesson we learned from that meeting was that we were transitioning skills to the team before they were adequately prepared to accept them. We were pushing change too fast, and we learned we needed to make responsible participation a cultural priority. If the team needed additional training, then we took back some of the tasks for a while and transitioned the responsibility when the team was ready. We also learned to work together better and to make the most of what everyone had to offer. We learned people need to be shown, convinced, and empowered to accept responsibility.

Many authors have described what is key for the successful implementation of SDWTs. Some have said it would have been nice to have a list of specific problems they would encounter (Berwick, 1989; Dumaine, 1993; Parker, 1994). It would have been nice to know what we might encounter, but charting a new course is always fraught with the unknown. It is this challenge that continues to inspire pioneers seeking to create a better work environment to achieve better results with less. Champy (1995) states, "We must dramatically improve business results now, and do it while earning the hearts and minds of our people. To make things still more difficult, 'now' has no tradition, no precedents, and no time-tested formulas. Now has never been seen before" (p. 9). In summary, the barriers we identified during our transition included

- Role transition difficulties
- Personnel conflicts
- Transfer of power from managers to the team
- Insufficient training and education
- Misalignment of organizational systems

Overall Results of the Establishment of Self-Directed Work Teams

PFC, SDWTs, and CQI were the embodiment of perpetual change in our department. They melded together, creating a culture in which staff members were continually striving to make things better. This model had an immediate and sustained impact on satisfaction and turnover of the staff. Realizing that it is impossible to hold an entire staff in a steady state to introduce a new model and measure its outcomes, it is difficult to achieve an accurate evaluation of the effect of change in its ideal sense. However, the vacancy rate before implementation of this model was more than 10%. One year after implementation, the vacancy rate was less than 4%.

Job satisfaction appears to be a key element for measuring staff morale, productivity, and retention. Using the Brayfield and Roth Nursing Job Satisfaction Inventory, staff members were surveyed every 6 months during the transition until the change was status quo. The inventory consisted of 28 items, and the subjects were asked to rate each question on a 1 through 5 Likert Scale. The staff on the unit consistently rated job satisfaction higher than did staff on other units not implementing the SDWT model.

Patient satisfaction was also considered an important variable for evaluation.

Patient satisfaction surveys were given to each patient dismissed from the unit. The scale used was selected for its published high reliability and validity scores (Atwood and Hinshaw, 1980; Risser, 1975). Each time it was administered, the scores were higher on our unit than those for other units in the hospital.

Some interesting outcomes of the implementation of SDWTs on our unit were the following:

- Caregivers doubled the time spent in caring directly for their patients.
- Additional professional skills that were acquired allowed the caregivers to take a leadership role in the care of patients.
- The time spent on medical documentation, scheduling, and coordination by caregivers was reduced considerably.
- The redesign of the physical plant reduced the workload and transport time for caregivers and patients.

To support the SDWT concept, the organizational culture needs to be one that prepares employees for additional responsibilities, understands how SDWTs function, promotes trust, broadens experience through the sharing of information, and provides necessary resources. An opportunity to test whether we had prepared our staff with these supports occurred. The manager saw a way to share some of our inpatient staff with our two outpatient units that would meet the needs of all three departments without hiring an additional staff member. She asked for a volunteer for the assignment; however, no one came forward. So she persuaded five individuals to try the assignment for 6 months. The results were very positive. Our inpatient staff had the opportunity to care for patients in the outpatient setting and found that following the patient throughout the continuum of care was a very rewarding experience. The knowledge and skills acquired from the outpatient unit were transferred to the inpatient unit, and care was improved. This example suggests that sometimes staff members need to be encouraged and pushed to assume additional responsibilities. Managers who know their employees well can promote the experience in a way that neither stifles nor scares the employees. Once there are positive results, everyone wants to participate.

Sometimes team members lack confidence to tackle something new. They may be privately afraid that they do not have the ability to deliver, and they do not want their failure to be made public. Rather than admit their insecurity, they simply refuse to participate. The lesson we learned is that if you desire high-performing work teams, you must commit to making each employee the most employable person she or he can be. Teaching team members management skills is one way of doing that; giving team members a broad base of work experience is another.

There were other activities we needed to address that we had not expected when we launched into SDWTs. DRGs and CQI activities had to be addressed and were tackled by the SDWTs in an aggressive fashion. With the onset of DRGs and other reimbursement and contract arrangements, we recognized the need for specific goals to sustain our high-quality clinical care standards while adapting to constant change. Care paths were developed for the top 20 DRGs for the hospital, which was organized around specialties. The department manager and medical director were accountable to the chief executive officer for length of stay and cost per case for the DRGs associated with their department. Monthly meetings with the pharmacist, social worker, utilization review personnel, and the SDWTs to review the length of stay and costs resulted in improvements in care that achieved the expected cost and quality outcomes.

CQI projects created improved processes that saved time and money while sustaining or improving quality. A CQI team evaluating beeper communications created a process that decreased the waiting time on hold from 3 minutes to 15 seconds.

A SDWT evaluating patient assignments developed a method to assign new admissions to staff based on acuity, actual census, and staff skill level, which resulted in more even workloads for staff and safer care for the patients. Another SDWT evaluated the steps involved in ordering medications and was able to reduce the number of steps in that process from 13 to 5 without increasing pharmacy support. Normally, three to five CQI teams were in process at any given time in our department.

Overall, the staff continually learned and applied new knowledge to improve performance. We knew we had created an organizational environment in which the operating principles could be implemented in a high-quality, continuously improving, teamwork-oriented, and performance-driven environment. We all believed we worked in the best place in the world!

SUMMARY

Gilmore (1990) says that improving performance while saving cost is "like trying to ride a bicycle and build it at the same time" (p. 37). He certainly is right, as we discovered when we implemented SDWTs as a new, improved, and cost-contained way to deliver nursing care. Staff members were entrenched in their jobs while trying to learn a new way of doing things. We were trying to change the culture while living in the old one.

Changing our culture required constant, deliberate attention to the behaviors of all those involved, and as Parker (1994) points out, there are considerable obstacles that have to be overcome when cultural change is attempted. Turf wars, weak leadership, and confusion about autonomy and authority acted as deterrents to the team members' efforts to work together and produce results. We also experienced resistance from every level during the process of transition, partially because of the time such an initiative takes. So how did we cope? Why were we successful?

Listed below are what we learned from this experience, which we offer to others who may want to embark on a journey similar to ours and which partially answer these questions.

- Persistence and patience are essential for the successful implementation of a change of this magnitude. We spent considerable time detecting the need for training and retraining and for anticipating and removing barriers so the teams could succeed. The transition from a functional team model to SDWTs did not occur overnight. It evolved. It was a long successful journey that required an unbelievable time commitment from everyone involved.

- When the task is something that is wanted, it is easier to accomplish than when it is mandated. The move to PFC was an organizational directive. The implementation of SDWTs was our choice, and one that from the beginning we believed would be successful.
- Lack of knowledge about an initiative is not necessarily a negative; it can be the unifying element of the change process. When we began the process, management knew nothing about SDWTs. The staff knew we were not going to tell them what SDWTs were or how we were going to implement them because we did not know. This lack of knowledge that everyone had was a unifying factor that created ownership of the process by everybody. We began the discovery phase together with no preconceived ideas.
- Empowerment of the staff can be the driving force for success. Despite an implementation period that included position eliminations, job restructuring, and leadership turnover, the staff in the pilot project remained positive and grew professionally because they felt empowered and accepted the accountability that went along with the added responsibility.
- Seeking advice and help is essential. Most of the stress we as managers experienced was due to the realization of how much we did not know. We were smart enough to seek out individuals with skills and knowledge to complement ours. We never considered that the project might fail.
- Understanding the history of the organization, knowing the staff, and accepting your own limitations are important elements when cultural change is attempted. We knew the staff and what they could do; we had been at the institution long enough to know what obstacles we would meet; and we knew our own strengths and limitations.
- Using patient-centered thinking, learning what each discipline can contribute, practicing safe delegation, and thinking collaboratively are also important considerations for the successful implementation of SDWTs.
- Being able to accept criticism is necessary even when it is hurtful. Not everyone was supportive of our endeavors, and it was demeaning to receive criticism from our peers who had not yet taken on change of this magnitude. We learned to accept their criticisms as a part of the change process. Although hurtful at times, those comments caused us to think through the process and helped us avoid pitfalls.

This chance to design and implement a new care delivery model was a professional challenge and a privilege. It was a rich opportunity that taught us that change can be thoughtfully and sensitively orchestrated. Although we did not know it at the time, this experience prepared us, as well as the staff, for the next phase of our careers.

One of the benefits of this experience was the opportunity to share what we learned with colleagues from other hospital systems. Frequently, we provided structured presentations and tours of our facility to hospital executives interested in implementing PFC and SDWTs. We soon discovered we enjoyed the experience of guiding others through the process; that prepared us for a career change.

Not long after the implementation of SDWTs was complete and in operation, we were offered the opportunity to develop a consulting practice for a large architectural firm that specializes in building and redesigning health care facilities. We now consult with people searching for a new way of delivering health care in institutions around the world.

Looking back, we now see that during the design and implementation period, no one ever told us what to do, yet we worked harder and learned more than in any other period in our careers. We are confident the implementation of SDWTs contributed to the creation of an enriched environment in which autonomy, a new identity, and a vision of the whole became the norm rather than the exception. It was an environment in which people knew they made a difference and in which we were able to provide the lead in a very different way. Leaders at all levels can benefit from what we learned.

REFERENCES

Alderson, W. T., & McDonnell, N. A. (1994). *Theory R management: How to utilize value of the person leadership principles of love, dignity, and respect.* Nashville: Nelson.

Antai-Otong, D. (1997). Teambuilding in a healthcare setting. *American Journal of Nursing, 97*(7), 48–51.

Atwood, J. R., & Hinshaw, A. S. (1980). Job Satisfaction instrument: A program of development and testing. In WCHE, Communicating Nursing Research: Papers Printed by WCHE. Boulder, Colo.

Barnum, B. S., & Mallard, C. O. (1989). *Essentials of nursing management.* Gaithersburg, Md.: Aspen.

Berwick, D. M. (1989). Continuous improvement as an ideal in health care. *New England Journal of Medicine, 320*(1), 53–56.

Booz, Allen, & Hamilton, Inc., (1989). Clarkson Futures Program, Bishop Clarkson Memorial Hospital, Omaha.

Champy, J. (1995). *Reengineering management: The mandate for new leadership.* New York: Harper Business.

Davidhizar, R. (1993). Leading with charisma. *Journal of Advanced Nursing, 18,* 675–679.

Deeprose, D. (1995). *The team coach.* New York: AMACOM.

Donovan, M. (1989). Employees who manage themselves. *Journal for Quality and Participation, 12*(1), 58–61.

Dumaine, B. (1993, February 22). The new non-manager managers. *Fortune,* 80–84.

Gilmore, T. N. (1990). Effective leadership during organizational transitions. *Nursing Economics, 8*(3), 135–141.

Hammer, M. (1993). Now hear this. *Fortune 128*(8), 18.

Hammer, M. (1996). *Beyond reengineering: How the process-centered organization is changing our work and our lives.* New York: HarperCollins.

Harper, A. & Harper, B. (1992). *Skill-building for self-directed team members.* New York: MW Corporation.

Howard, A. (1996). *Handbook of business strategy.* New York: Faulkner & Gray.

Izzo, J., & Klein, E. (1998, May/June). Changing values of workers: Organizations must respond with soul. *Healthcare Forum Journal 41*(3), 62–65.

Lambertsen, E. C. (1953). *Nursing team organization and functioning.* New York: Teachers College, Columbia University.

Liedtka, J. M., & Whitten, E. (1998). Enhancing care delivery through cross-disciplinary collaboration: A case study. *Journal of Healthcare Management 43*(2), 185–205.

Loveridge, C. E., & Cummings, S. H. (1996). *Nursing management in the new paradigm.* Gaithersburg, Md.: Aspen.

Manz, C. C., & Sims, H. P., (1989). *Superleadership: Leading others to lead themselves.* Englewood Cliffs, N.J.: Prentice-Hall.

Marram, G. D., Schlegel, M. W., & Bevis, E. O. (1974). *Primary nursing: A model for individualized care.* St. Louis: Mosby.

Moffitt, G. K., McCullough, C., & Sanders, D. (1993, Fall). High-performing self-directed work teams: What are they and how do they work? *Patient Focused Care Association Review,* 8–12.

Morris, T. (1997). *If Aristotle ran General Motors: The new soul of business.* New York: Holt.

Orsburn, J. D., Moran, L., Musselwhite, E., & Zenger, J. H. (1990). *Self-directed work teams, the new American challenge.* Homewood, Ill. Business One Irwin.

Orth, C. D., Wilkinson, H. E., & Benfari, R. C. (1990). The manager's role as coach and mentor. *Journal of Nursing Administration, 20*(9), 11–15.

Parker, G. M. (1994). *Cross-functional teams: Working with allies, enemies, and other strangers.* San Francisco: Jossey-Bass.

Peters, T., & Austin, N. (1985). *A passion for excellence: The leadership difference.* New York: Warner Books.

Risser, N. (1975). Development of an instrument to measure patient satisfaction with nurses and nursing care in the primary care setting. *Nursing Research, 24*, 45–52.

Swansburg, R. C. (1996). *Management leadership for nurse managers,* 2nd ed. Sudbury, Mass.: Jones & Bartlett.

Teschke, D. A. (1991, October). Nebraska hospital brings services closer to patients. *Healthcare Financial Management,* 118.

Wellins, R. S., Byham, W. C., & Wilson, J. M., (1991). *Empowered teams: Creating self-directed work groups that improve quality, productivity, and participation.* San Francisco: Jossey-Bass.

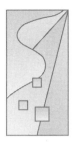

Chapter 6

Taking a Risk

Laura R. Mahlmeister

This chapter is about risk taking. It is about recognizing risks, the process of taking a risk, and the theoretical framework underlying risk taking. Most of all, it is about my experiences at taking risks and how those actions moved my career forward. I never thought of myself as a leader, but clearly the risks I have taken are like those of every leader, and so from that perspective I am a leader. No one providing leadership can avoid risk taking, so all nurses must at some time learn to take a risk.

The first thing I learned about taking a risk is that it is not jumping off the side of a mountain because it looks exciting and everybody says you can't do it. It is not thrill-seeking for its own sake, or looking for something new and different to do that has little chance of working out. It is not risking your reputation because someone challenges you to do what they are fearful of doing or deems won't work. Risk taking is a calculated conscious decision to do something that you are not totally sure will work. It is following your dreams with your eyes open. It is knowing the obstacles to the success of your risk taking and the potential outcomes, both positive and negative, of your actions.

Risk taking is anxiety-provoking and not for the timid. However, it is the most exciting thing I have ever done and has paid off for me in many ways. Fear and timidity have stopped many nurses from taking a risk when that is exactly what they should have done, so timidity should not stand in the way. There are ways that the anxiety of risk can be reduced, and there are ways for nurses to overcome their fears about taking a risk. My story is written to help those who are afraid to take a risk and for those who want to take a risk but do not know how to begin or proceed.

My life has been filled with risk taking. Sometimes the risks I took paid off and sometimes they did not. However, failure because of my choices has never stopped me from taking another risk, and that is another aspect of risk taking. Because one risky action does not work does not mean the end of risk taking; rather, it means the risk taker is more careful the next time and follows the process I describe in this chapter. I once heard it said that you are more likely to regret having said "no" to life's opportunities than saying "yes." Acquiring skill in risk taking will make it possible to say "yes" with greater confidence and with a greater likelihood of success.

In 1981, my husband and I pulled up roots and moved from Miami, Florida to San Francisco, California. We had both given up wonderful teaching positions in the community. We left our close friends behind so I could fulfill my goal of becoming a maternal-newborn clinical nurse specialist by attending a master's degree program in nursing. Some of my colleagues thought I was insane for leaving Florida. I had a secure teaching position in an associate degree nursing program. I was the senior faculty member in maternity nursing and made an excellent salary, and my lectures were all developed, requiring only minor yearly updating. My husband had a similar position. We had every summer free to pursue personal goals and traveled extensively. Life was very good.

I had not been accepted in the master's nursing program before we moved to California. We needed to establish residence in the state so I would be eligible for a significant reduction in tuition. Even working full-time, I would need the lower tuition fees to attend school and adjust to the much higher cost of living in the state. I did not have a job when we left Florida because of one of the periodic declines in employment for nurses. My plans were frequently questioned by well-intentioned acquaintances. "Why would you risk everything that you've achieved here?" "What if you don't get accepted in the master's program?" "Why not go to school here? "How will you survive if you don't find a job? "You've got so much to lose!"

I did realize how much I had accomplished, but something was missing. Although I loved teaching, I missed the daily contact with patients that I had enjoyed earlier in my career. I wanted the challenge of working with the highest risk maternity patients, providing direct care as well as teaching less skilled staff nurses. I needed the intellectual stimulation of working in situations where there were not always clear answers to the problems I faced. I yearned to create a leadership role in a clinically demanding environment.

Although I probably could not have articulated it at the time, the process of decision-making and the development of clinical judgment also fascinated me. I had already begun using case studies in my theory classes to delineate for students the process of problem identification, planning, and evaluation of nursing care. My course evaluations rose significantly, and students repeatedly noted the value of case studies in capturing the essence of the nursing process. I envisioned a long-term goal of continuing in staff development and nursing education. It was clear, however, that I needed additional graduate education to achieve my goal, and I wanted the best education possible. That meant moving to San Francisco.

Although the move was risky, my husband and I systematically listed our concerns and had planned carefully for this major life transition. We had started a savings account, which provided a financial buffer while I looked for work in California. My husband had secured a teaching position in San Francisco before we resigned from our jobs and left Miami. I had calculated that my chances were good for acceptance into one of the most prestigious schools of nursing in the world. In 1971, I had graduated with honors from an undergraduate program that was rated one of the top five schools of nursing in the United States. My education had prepared me well for higher education. I had practiced and taught nursing for 10 years and had excellent references. I continued to read the nursing literature, including the small but growing body of nursing research. I had prepared for and taken the Graduate Record Examination and had scored well.

A month after arriving in California, I was employed in a clinical and teaching position at San Francisco General Hospital in the maternal-newborn department. A year later, I had begun the master's program of my choice. My calculated risk had paid off. In the eyes of many of my Florida friends, I had been very lucky. In fact, it was more than "luck." I had planned carefully and accurately estimated my chances of success. My story does not end here. The decision to leave my well-ordered and pleasant life in Florida was just the beginning of a rocket ride to unknown areas and careers in nursing I could never have predicted. A chance encounter with one of my faculty members in the second year of graduate school changed the entire course of my professional and personal life. That meeting and my journey will be described later in the chapter.

My initial decision to leave behind a very secure and pleasant life in Florida exemplifies a risk-taking venture, the subject of this chapter. Risk taking is an act that implies choice. In choosing between or among alternatives, one is faced with the possibility of jeopardy, injury, or significant loss. Risking is often viewed as synonymous with "gambling," but it is not the same. Gambling is wagering something of value based on an estimated probability of loss or gain. In the gaming industry, the probability of winning or losing is preestablished and obviously skewed in favor of the house. Risk taking is a calculated process in which the anticipated losses can be controlled and the likelihood of gain can be significantly increased through careful planning.

A great deal has been written about risk taking in the management literature; successful risk taking is considered a hallmark of the effective leader. Nurses are exhorted to become skillful risk takers to achieve professional status and leadership positions in health care. Risk taking implies creativity, adaptability, informed decision-making, and courage—all essential traits of the accomplished leader. The assumption is that nurses have not traditionally taken risks, and this is not true. According to Dobos (1992, 1997) nurses have always been risk takers in their role as patient advocates. Since the inception of modern nursing, nurses have placed their personal and professional status in jeopardy to promote the health and well-being of patients.

Wolfe (1994) notes that nurses also take unacceptable risks, including exposure to a multitude of environmental hazards (chemical agents, toxins, biological hazards, physical threats) and psychological stressors (sexual and verbal harassment). Furthermore, the patterns of risk taking among nurses are more commonly based on assuming risks for others rather than for themselves. What nurses have failed to do is learn how to take *well-planned risks*, which increase the probability of success in their own professional development. It is only through professional advancement that nurses can become truly effective patient advocates without risking their personal safety, professional integrity, and careers.

A major inhibiting factor to effective risk taking is unreasonable or unwarranted fear. Fear is primarily stimulated by the potential for loss. Studies conducted in risk-taking behaviors indicate that the major driving force in not taking risks is loss aversion. Losses always loom larger in most people's minds than does potential gain (Bernstein, 1997). A key to successful risk taking is to control fear by minimizing real and potential losses—creating a "safety net." In planning for my move to California, I had to face my fears, which were primarily focused on loss. I would lose daily contact with close friends, interesting students, and cherished colleagues. I was giving up a secure job, a stable income, and a predictable lifestyle in a community I found exciting and stimulating.

Perhaps most important to me, I was surrendering the "expert" role I had achieved and would be exchanging it for that of student, a novice again.

The aim of this chapter is to explore the concept of risk-taking for nurses who aspire to lead. Essential characteristics of effective risking will be delineated and illustrated in the completion of my personal history. The issue of warranted versus unwarranted fear is examined, and a guide for confronting and managing fear is presented. A useful framework for viewing risk taking is the theory of transformational leadership. First articulated by Burns (1978) and expanded through the research of Bennis and Nanus (1985), transformational leadership recognizes the central role of risk taking for successful leadership. The transformational leader is willing to step into the unknown and to take risks through experimentation and introducing new ways of thinking and acting (Kouzes and Posner, 1988). I was first introduced to the theory of transformational leadership during my days in the master's program. The ideas, constructs, and relationships posited by proponents of transformational leadership have provided a sound foundation for the decisions I have made and the calculated risks I have chosen to take. This interesting and dynamic theory is shared with the reader.

WHAT IS RISK TAKING?

Risk taking on the part of professional nurses involves making a decision about a course of action that involves some degree of peril or threat to one's career and self-esteem. In the ever-shifting health care system, risk taking is a given and essential not only for survival but also for success. When nurses are asked to identify risk takers in the profession, they most often point to nurse leaders, managers, and entrepreneurs. They often fail to recognize their own risk-taking behaviors or to credit their skill in risk taking. In clinical practice, risk taking occurs when the nurse's advocacy role is activated by a problem that prevents the patient from achieving outcome goals, such as

- Physiological or psychological complications
- Provider orders that are unclear, inappropriate, or incomplete
- Inappropriate conduct of a health care provider
- Noncompliance with the informed consent process
- Violation of patient rights
- Environmental hazards

In these situations, the nurse must often make rapid, complex decisions that involve a significant degree of uncertainty regarding outcomes. Time and resources often are limited when a course of action must be chosen. The nurse may have to challenge authority and overcome other organizational barriers to assist the patient. Managers may not be available to guide the nurse, and specific patient care tasks may have to be delegated to other less skilled or unlicensed personnel to manage the problem. These situations are fraught with risk. Nurses often underrate their risk-taking abilities but in fact take legitimate risks every day spent in the clinical arena.

Midmanagers and nurse educators frequently fail to reinforce risk taking in nurses. I had the occasion to teach a leadership course for registered nurses seeking a baccalaureate degree. One class exercise required students to describe a work-related event that highlighted professional risk-taking behaviors. Many students described heroic efforts to save the lives of their patients. Others had placed their career in great jeopardy to maintain the patient's rights and dignity as a person. Sadly, only 4 of 46 nurses reported receiving any positive feedback from nurse managers or administrators for their efforts. Even when physicians came forward to state that the patient would surely have died had the nurse not intervened, nurses were not recognized by their nursing supervisors. In fact, five nurses were essentially told, "Don't do it again. You are setting a dangerous precedent. Nurses should not be challenging physicians or the system."

Nurse managers, leaders, and entrepreneurs are often engaged in high-stakes risk-taking behaviors. Health care systems are promoting nurses to the highest levels of the organization, often during periods of chaotic change. Risk taking is a given. The nurse manager's or leader's ability to anticipate, assess, and handle risk-taking situations will determine in great part how far he or she will rise and whether the organization will prosper or decline (Calvert, 1993). The areas for decision-making and risk taking are expanding exponentially for nurse leaders and entrepreneurs:

- Strategic planning
- Financial management
- Human resources
- Products and services
- Marketing
- Informatics
- Data management
- Risk control

Last, nurses at all levels of practice and leadership are challenged to take risks regarding professional development and advancement. The opportunities for nurses have expanded beyond our most imaginative dreams, but each step in the process of career transformation requires some degree of risk taking. Decisions regarding education and training, involvement in professional organizations, and political activism must be made, and for many nurses, decisions must be made quickly before the proverbial rug is pulled out from under their feet. Nurses must be willing to say, "This I can and will do to survive and thrive." Strategic planning can then be implemented to determine how the nurse will achieve the goal.

Too many nurses still hope to maintain the status quo and avoid taking risks. There is great resistance to attaining the BSN credential or graduate education to compete successfully in today's marketplace. "A nurse doesn't need to have a bachelor's degree to be a good nurse" is an archaic excuse for failing to act. In our information-based society, the message is clear. The minimum level of education required for successful career development in any business enterprise is a bachelor's degree. In health care, the handwriting is also on the wall. The master's degree will eventually be mandated for registered nurses who wish to assume leadership roles in collaborative, interdisciplinary health care systems and rise in an organization.

Nurses can begin by taking small steps in risk-taking behavior to advance their careers:

- Volunteering to participate in an organizational committee
- Joining a professional nursing organization and becoming an active member
- Attending programs about career opportunities and advancement
- Exploring all educational avenues available for nurses in the community and state
- Agreeing to present a paper or teach a class about an area of practice in which you are actively engaged
- Presenting your position as a nurse about a issue of public health before your town or city council
- Seeking out preceptors, coaches, and mentors to assist you in the process of career development
- Taking a course at a local community college or university that enhances your value and viability as an employee
- Finding out about preparation courses for the graduate record examination
- Enrolling in higher degree programs

WHAT ARE THE PHASES OR STEPS IN RISK TAKING?

Siegelman (1983) describes seven chronological stages in risking activities. The motivation to take a calculated risk begins with the *awareness of negative feelings* or a sense of dissatisfaction with one's work. Emotional awareness varies from a mild sense of discomfort about some aspect of work to anger or a sense of outrage, depending on the nature of the problem.

On reflection, the individual begins to *pinpoint a need for change* as essential to improving his or her emotional status and satisfaction with work. What this change requires and how it will be accomplished may be unfocused for quite some time. Each individual will move through this stage at a different rate of progress. Introspective people will tend to look for solutions within. They ask questions such as, "What will make me happy?" "Is it really the job, or am I dissatisfied because of other situations in my life?" "What do I envision myself doing to be fulfilled in my work?" Extroverts may look for answers from others they perceive as advisors or "experts." They may seek advice and consultation from family, friends, and respected colleagues. Extroverts may also attend career development workshops.

The third phase of risk taking is characterized by *feelings of uncertainty.* Once the need for change is articulated, a significant degree of ambivalence can be expected. The decision to risk, once real alternatives are identified, can provoke the greatest period of anxiety. This is a time when the focus is exclusively on the potential losses associated with change. The individual may be plagued by unwarranted fears and find it difficult to realistically assess the true risks and rewards. Those who do not find a systematic method for objectively evaluating potential gains and losses, and the chances for success, may never move beyond this stage in the process.

The time needed to resolve ambivalence varies greatly depending on the nature of the problem, its context, and the resources available to assist the risk taker in making a decision. The individual's formative stage of personal and career development will also influence how quickly movement through this stage occurs. Career decisions do not occur in a vacuum. Life events such as education, marriage, childbearing and rearing, and family crises will also alter the ability to resolve ambivalence and make decisions.

Once the decision is made to change, effective risk takers move through a fourth stage, during which *action is taken to control losses*. Attention is focused on preventing emotions, both positive and negative, from interfering with the work of risk reduction. Risk control may be directed at controlling social, emotional, personal, professional, and financial losses; however, the focus will depend on the nature of the project. The skilled risk taker will use all available resources to accurately appraise potential losses and limit them.

Seasoned risk takers often find that once a decision is made about a course of action, and risk has been limited, it is wise to step back and take a brief respite before beginning the project. This is the fifth stage of risk taking—*recharging one's batteries*. A person's energies are often depleted during the previous stages of searching for options and making decisions among alternative choices. Risking in itself requires full concentration and a great deal of stamina. It is unwise to begin a project in a state of low energy or exhaustion.

Taking the plunge is the sixth stage in risk taking. Novice risk takers and those less skilled in risking may wait too long to act, missing the important window of opportunity. Those individuals not fully committed to risk taking or overwhelmed by unwarranted fear may find themselves passively drifting along, hoping something will happen to make risking unnecessary.

The final stage in the risk-taking process is *evaluating the progress and outcomes* of the project. Periodically tracking the headway one is making is essential. At times, it may be wiser to stop midway through a project when it is evident that failure is likely and the costs of continuing are unacceptable. If success has been limited or there has been failure in the effort to effect change, a careful and objective assessment is necessary to learn from the experience. Even with the greatest success, it is advisable to carefully examine the conditions leading to the positive outcomes. As MacCrimmon and Wehrung (1986) point out, one of the greatest mistakes the risk taker can make is to develop a false sense of security about future endeavors based on a single success. The person who succeeds once must carefully consider whether the outcomes can be reproduced in subsequent projects.

WHAT ARE THE COMPONENTS OF RISK TAKING?

Calvert (1993) states that risk-taking activity includes four related factors:

1. Uncertainty
2. Loss
3. Gain
4. Significance

Because risk taking always involves some degree of speculation, it is fraught with *uncertainty*. Human beings are generally creatures of habit. We derive comfort from the regular rhythms of the seasons and the day-to-day sameness of our work activities. It is because of this predilection for certainty that many nurses find the present rapid changes in health care so disconcerting and painful. There are no longer any guarantees about nurses' future place in the health care system, where they will work, or what services they will render.

Global predictions have been made about the future of nursing practice and management, but they offer little solace for nurses who hoped to spend 25 or 30 years in one organization, working a 40-hour week and collecting a steadily increasing paycheck. Unfortunately, the expectation of predictable, well-compensated work has been reinforced in large part by technically oriented associate degree programs (ADNs). Students are often attracted to the 2-year ADN program because of the anticipated long-term payback (stable employment) for a short-term commitment. There has been little incentive for these nurses in the past to value or attempt risk taking. Now, during this period of extraordinary opportunity, they often find it difficult and uncomfortable to venture into new avenues and settings for nursing practice.

Risking by its nature also entails the potential for *serious losses*—personal, social, professional, and financial—and therefore is often viewed in a negative light. Health care managers interviewed by Parker (1998) perceived entrepreneurs who were risk takers as "pushy" and "irreverent toward cherished traditions." They also disclosed that bureaucratic organizations frequently apply pressure to suppress entrepreneurial (risk-taker) activities, even when the system would benefit from the changes that these individuals could implement. Nurses who experiment with appropriate risk taking may find themselves criticized, punished, or ostracized by their peer group.

Many nurses have fought vehemently against changing the status quo, fearing both the tangible and the intangible losses inherent in health care restructuring. Early reports of changes in health care published in the 1990s were often met with skepticism and disbelief: "I know it may happen in other places, but not here." As one hospital after another succumbed to redesign in the face of economic pressures, the majority of nurses continued to operate in a state of denial, fearing to take any action that would "rock the boat." Despite the rising tide of change, nurses refused to face reality. Hard and fast decisions needed to be made about career changes, the need for additional education and training, and planning for a financial future, but as many nurses said, "Taking risks is too risky!"

In reality, there is risk regardless of whether you act. And passively accepting and hoping to survive change may ultimately result in greater losses than taking calculated risks to improve your future career options. Aptly put by Calvert (1993):

> To risk, or not to risk, that is the question:
> Whether 'tis smarter in the end to suffer
> The slings and arrows of the status quo,
> Or to take arms against a sea of uncertainty,
> And by rising, achieve extraordinary goals (p. 10).

Although risk taking is always imbued with some degree of uncertainty and potential loss, the *gains* can outweigh these factors. When the positive outcomes are *significant*, the rewards can be substantial. Because research suggests that on average people will focus more attention on potential losses than gains (Bernstein, 1997), a concerted effort must be made to objectively evaluate both the potential losses and rewards and to place them in the proper perspective. Nurses can also learn to improve the reward/loss ratio. Kindler (1990) describes a variety of strategies to enhance the likelihood of positive outcomes in his textbook *Risk Taking: A Guide for Decision Makers.* Kindler maps out a technique very similar to the nursing process to limit loss and to improve the chances of success. A systematic process of diagnosis, planning, and implementing proactive strategies is recommended to improve the outcomes of risking.

WHY TAKE RISKS?

An underlying assumption of this chapter is that risk taking is a positive attribute of the nurse who wishes to take the lead. Taking risks has been identified for more than 20 years as essential for increasing both personal and professional power and for enhancing career development, work satisfaction, and patient advocacy in nursing practice (Crow, 1998; Stevens, 1983). In times of rapid change when major paradigm shifts occur, the opportunities for risk taking are increased dramatically, as are the potentials for gain and loss. The massive transformation of health care systems in North America, as well as in other countries, has initiated a need for nurses who have strong decision-making capabilities and are willing to assume the role of creative risk taker. New and almost limitless career opportunities exist for nurses across the spectrum of experience and education if they are willing to become intrepid risk takers (White and Begun, 1998).

Traditional career expectations for nurses are unraveling (Crow, 1998), and the predictable and stable world of long-term relationships between workers and employers is coming to an end (White and Begun, 1998). Futurists who have written about 21st century nursing practice describe the need for both nurse intrapreneurs (within the organization) and entrepreneurs. It is anticipated that an increasing number of nurses will render services as "free agents" in the new millennium. Even nurses affiliated with a particular health care organization may be viewed as independent contractors. The greatest commodity that nurses will possess and broker is information (Crow, 1998). An essential characteristic of intrapreneurial and entrepreneurial nursing practice is risk taking (Parker, 1998).

WHAT ASSUMPTIONS UNDERLIE THEORIES ABOUT RISK TAKING?

Calvert (1993) detailed critical assumptions that underlie effective risk taking; some of these assumptions are summarized in the following section. Every nurse should consider these propositions before initiating risk-taking behavior:

1. Risk by choice, not by necessity; chosen risk usually benefits you more than does forced risk taking.

2. Security is a myth; professional stimulation is worth the cost of risk taking.
3. A solution can be found for almost any risk-taking problem that allows you to survive even the worst-case scenario, should it occur.
4. Risk taking is typically fast moving, "make it up as you go."
5. No matter how many times your risking fails, there will always be another opportunity to risk and succeed; risk takers know that what counts most is the net value of wins compared with losses in an acceptable time period.
6. Luck always helps, but you create your own luck by taking risks and betting on yourself.
7. The bigger the risk, the bigger the reward, so go for the riskier choice if it offers a greater payoff; believe in your ability to produce results.
8. Failure and loss should be viewed as learning experiences and will pay off in the long term.
9. Achieving anything worthwhile requires venturing into unsafe territory; being satisfied with average achievements is a standard of mediocrity.
10. Being dissatisfied with anything less than outstanding is a standard of excellence and forces you to relinquish the safe, sure, and secure way.
11. Ambiguity and unpredictability always permeate and complicate risk taking; those able to cope with these constraints will do well at risk taking.
12. When you risk sensibly and boldly, you will sustain and expand your self-esteem even when you fail.

CAN ALL NURSES REALLY BECOME EFFECTIVE RISK TAKERS?

Studies indicate that the majority of workers in hierarchical, authoritarian organizations have been socialized to avoid risk taking, or at best to make low-risk choices with minimal payoffs (Singleton and Hovden, 1987), but times are changing. Calvert (1993) asserts that in today's economic climate, skilled risk-taking is inevitable, essential, and pervasive in all work settings. In restructured systems, nurses must make increasingly complex decisions with inherent risk, such as setting priorities, delegating critical tasks to subordinates, allocating resources and funds, and developing new or changing existing services. Today, the greatest rewards are accrued by high-stake risk takers who succeed.

Unfortunately, the majority of nurses in practice have been socialized to accept passive roles in authoritarian organizations. Appropriate risk taking was often met with punitive responses by physicians, managers, and administrators. Oppressed-group dynamics still operate within many health care systems, limiting the nurses' sense of autonomy and self-esteem (Roberts, 1997). These "institutionalized" nurses often resist change when new owners take over the organization and mandate sweeping transformations in its operations. Risk taking is an entirely alien concept for many seasoned veterans of nursing. As I began writing this chapter, an experienced, master's-prepared nurse manager who finds herself in a rapidly evolving health care system told me, "I hate the change. They won't give me any guidelines. All I'm given are options, and I'm told to make a decision about which option to choose when a problem arrives. If I make a mistake, I'll be held responsible for it!"

In light of these considerations, it may be unrealistic to expect that all nurses now in practice can become effective risk takers. In fact, some nurses have already left the profession, realizing they could not adapt to the growing demand for skilled decision-makers who welcome opportunities for risk taking. Education clearly is the key to preparing nurses for risk taking in 21st century practice and leadership. Preliminary findings suggest that both ADN and BSN students possess the same propensity for risk taking and that risk-taking capacity may be acquired during the educational process (Masters and Masters, 1989). These investigators discovered that the willingness to take risks was not influenced by nurses' experience; rather, personality traits and learning appear to play bigger roles.

Research in the realm of genetics supports a claim for a genetic tendency to risk-taking behavior. There also appear to be distinct gender-based differences (Pfaff, 1997). Mapping of the human genome has provided intriguing evidence that some individuals may inherit a predisposition to risk-taking or "thrill-seeking" behavior. These individuals are impulsive and easily bored with repetitive activities and continually seek new experiences. Risk-taking propensities in males result in exposure to hazardous situations that contribute to a higher rate of accidental injury and death in young men (Arch, 1993).

Arch notes that studies on risk taking also suggest that men and women respond differently to achievement situations that require intellectual risk taking, or risking in social situations. Females are more likely to engage in risk taking to support and foster egalitarian, cooperative group functions, whereas males take risks to assert the self, challenge others, and assert dominance in hierarchical organizations (Arch, 1993). Once free of the fetters of archaic hierarchical organizations, women are equally willing to venture risk-taking in the business world. In fact, empirical data suggest that women are taking risks in *greater proportion* to men in the start-up of new businesses and entrepreneurial enterprises (Gorgal-Eaton, 1994).

HOW CAN I TELL IF I CAN BE AN EFFECTIVE RISK TAKER?

Researchers studying risk have developed a variety of tools to assist human resource personnel and educators in assessing the risking attitudes and propensities of students and workers. Many of these instruments are simple and can be used by the individual nurse to rate his or her predisposition to take appropriate risks. The Risk Attitude Inventory (Calvert, 1993) is presented in Table 6–1.

The reader should be cautioned about placing too much emphasis on a core of personal risk-taking predilections. The decision to risk is a complex process, involving the individual's educational background, personality traits, genetic factors, organization structure, and available resources (Wolfe, 1994). Figure 6–1 illustrates the complex influences of these variables on the risk taker.

Even when an individual initially scores low on a risk-taking inventory, learning strategies are available to develop or enhance risk-taking behaviors. Kindler (1990) developed a Risk Taking Assessment Guide. This tool systematically moves the individual through a series of written exercises to aid in the identification of all components of a problem that requires effective decision-making with inherent risk.

Table 6–1. Risk Assessment Tool

Read each trait description. Assess yourself on the basis of the degree to which the trait description applies to you (most of the time) in your management work and circle the appropriate answer. Be aware that looking for hidden meanings will not improve the value of your self-rating. Your first reaction is probably your best. A guide for scoring your responses follows the exercise.

1. Taking management risks makes good sense only in the absence of acceptable alternatives. — Agree Disagree
2. I generally prefer stimulation over security. — Agree Disagree
3. I have confidence in my ability to recover from my mistakes, no matter how big. — Agree Disagree
4. I would promote someone with unlimited potential but limited experience to a key position over someone with limited potential but more experience. — Agree Disagree
5. Anything worth doing is worth doing less than perfectly. — Agree Disagree
6. I believe opportunity generally knocks only once. — Agree Disagree
7. It is better to ask for permission than to beg for forgiveness. — Agree Disagree
8. Success in management is as much a matter of luck as ability. — Agree Disagree
9. Given a choice, I would choose a three-thousand-dollar annual raise over a ten-thousand-dollar bonus, which I had about a one-in-three chance of winning. — Agree Disagree
10. I can handle big losses and disappointments with little difficulty. — Agree Disagree
11. If forced to choose between them, I would take safety over achievement. — Agree Disagree
12. Failure is the long way to management success. — Agree Disagree
13. I tolerate ambiguity and unpredictability well. — Agree Disagree
14. I would rather feel intense disappointment than intense regret. — Agree Disagree
15. When facing a decision with uncertain consequences, my potential losses are my greatest concern. — Agree Disagree

Give yourself one point for each of the following statements with which you agree: 2, 3, 4, 5, 10, 13, 14. Give yourself one point for each of the following statements with which you disagree: 1, 6, 7, 8, 9, 11, 12, 15. Calculate your total.

From Calvert, G. (1993). *Highwire management.* Copyright © 1993 by Jossey-Bass Publishers, San Francisco, CA.

WHAT ARE THE BARRIERS TO RISK TAKING?

The greatest single barrier to risk taking is *fear of loss.* Although a critical phase of risk taking must include an appraisal of the costs and potential losses, it must be a realistic and objective assessment. Seasoned riskers are able to step back and consider all aspects of the problem and to discern the differences between *warranted and unwarranted fears.* Irrational fears inhibit reasoned problem solving and planning. The ability to avoid distortion of the true estimate of loss is a function of three critical factors: the strength of the individual's self-esteem, the breadth and depth of resources available to assess the problem, and the person's ability to systematically evaluate risk. Common unwarranted fears are presented in Table 6–2.

ORGANIZATION STRUCTURAL/CULTURAL FACTORS

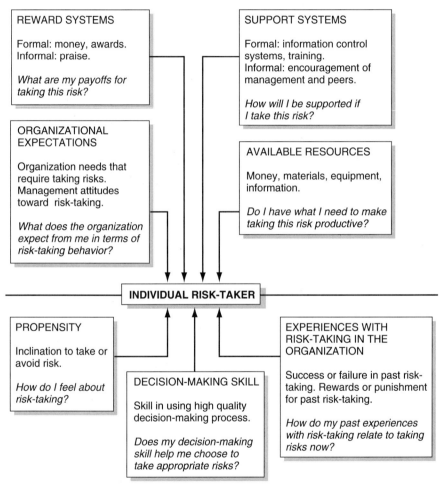

REWARD SYSTEMS

Formal: money, awards.
Informal: praise.

*What are my payoffs for
taking this risk?*

SUPPORT SYSTEMS

Formal: information control
systems, training.
Informal: encouragement of
management and peers.

*How will I be supported if
I take this risk?*

ORGANIZATIONAL
EXPECTATIONS

Organization needs that
require taking risks.
Management attitudes
toward risk-taking.

*What does the organization
expect from me in terms of
risk-taking behavior?*

AVAILABLE RESOURCES

Money, materials, equipment,
information.

*Do I have what I need to make
taking this risk productive?*

INDIVIDUAL RISK-TAKER

PROPENSITY

Inclination to take or
avoid risk.

*How do I feel about
risk-taking?*

DECISION-MAKING SKILL

Skill in using high quality
decision-making process.

*Does my decision-making
skill help me choose to
take appropriate risks?*

EXPERIENCES WITH
RISK-TAKING IN THE
ORGANIZATION

Success or failure in past risk-
taking. Rewards or punishment
for past risk-taking.

*How do my past experiences
with risk-taking relate to taking
risks now?*

INDIVIDUAL TENDENCY FACTORS

Figure 6–1. Organizational risk taking: contributing factors. (Reprinted with permission from Moore, M., and Gergen, P. [1985]. Risk and organizational changes. *Train Dev J 8,* 72–76.)

Table 6-2. Common Unwarranted Fears Experienced by Novice Risk Takers

When risk taking is well planned and executed, risk can be managed and losses controlled. The novice risk taker may envision catastrophic losses and unwarranted fears:

- Total loss of personal and/or professional reputation
- Loss of respect of peers and colleagues
- Loss of support system in work setting
- Ostracism
- Loss of position in organization; demotion
- Restrictions placed on future risk-taking activities
- Termination
- Total financial ruin
- Legal liability and lawsuits
- Personal losses: loss of respect of significant other or loss of significant other

HOW CAN ONE CONTROL AND ELIMINATE UNWARRANTED FEARS?

Self-confidence is an absolute given for risk-taking behavior. It engenders a firm belief that sound decisions can be made and that one can survive the inevitable challenges and losses that occur with risk taking. One of the greatest fears that arise when self-confidence is lacking is a fear of loss of "face," or reputation, if the project fails. At the core of this apprehension is a lack of self-esteem. The person anticipates intolerable personal and professional humiliation. This does not mean that self-confident people do not have some degree of anxiety as they consider the consequences of risking, but the fear that is experienced is a reasoned fear controlled by a strong sense of self-esteem. Individuals with a strong sense of personal competence do not unduly burden themselves with expectations of infallibility. When failure occurs, they transform it into a learning experience. They believe that if a project is well planned and executed, they will retain their self-respect even when outcomes fall short of goals.

Lachman (1998) provides useful recommendations for improving self-confidence and reducing acute anxiety in the leader-entrepreneur. The person who experiences inappropriate fear or anxiety can take positive steps to control this process. Perceptions can be modified by recognizing three types of distorted thinking that contribute to unwarranted fear: dichotomous and catastrophic thinking and stereotyping. The focus on loss should be carefully balanced with potential achievements and rewards. Self-help tapes are available to assist the motivated person enhance self-esteem. Daily exercises in positive thinking, spending time in the alpha (alert-relaxed) state, and seeking professional counseling are also methods Lachman suggests for improving self-confidence. Psychophysiology techniques such as biofeedback and yoga are often effective in reducing the physically debilitating effects of extreme anxiety. These activities heighten one's perceptions of well-being and personal capabilities.

Having *access to appropriate resources*—people and information—is the second factor essential to assessing one's ability to risk and control fears. The skilled risk taker consults close family and friends, colleagues, coaches, and mentors. Others can also help place fear in perspective and provide an invaluable source of support. Acquiring information is critical to appropriate planning. Information garnered through research, the use of experts, and other data sources helps place the problem in its proper perspective. Calvert (1993) recommends viewing problems that require risk taking with a microscope, telescope, or periscope; however, one danger for the novice risk taker is actually collecting too much data. Soliciting feedback from others should be limited to seeking out trusted individuals who have the ability to provide objective advice as well as encouragement. One must also set a limit on the amount of time spent and the information gathered. Living in the "information age" can actually be disadvantageous if one becomes swamped by the data.

Controlling unwarranted fears is also dependent on the person's ability to systematically appraise the potential risks and gains. Tools have been developed to assist individuals in this assessment process and can be particularly helpful to novice risk takers (MacCrimmon and Wehring, 1986). A focused assessment can eradicate negative circular thinking, a common component of unwarranted fear.

Calvert (1993) recommends the following five critical aspects of the potential risk taking be examined:

1. The scale of gains and loses
2. The time span over which gains and losses will occur
3. The permanence of gains and losses
4. The costs of gains and losses
5. The degree of control one has over gains and losses (p. 96)

The successful risk taker must learn to effectively control the unreasonable fears and anxiety that arise in situations that have an element of uncertainty. Improving self-esteem is the first step in this process. The nurse who is hampered by feelings of inadequacy must engage in self-help activities that boost self-confidence. Having a strong self-esteem makes it possible to discard unwarranted fears and to clearly evaluate the potential losses and gains of a project. Once the nurse feels confident about his or her ability to make rational choices, risk taking will become less threatening. Creative energy can then be focused on the project at hand; this also increases the likelihood of success.

TRANSFORMATIONAL LEADERSHIP: A FRAMEWORK FOR RISK TAKING

The nurse who wants to assume a leadership role must inevitably take risks. Transformational leadership is a relatively new theory that is a salient and useful framework that provides a rational basis for risk taking for nurses who want to take the lead. It is grounded in the central premise that meaningful change is more likely to occur in an organization or a situation when leaders and followers rise together to higher levels of motivation and morality (Burns, 1978). Typically, relations between leaders and followers are characterized by a mutual understanding that desired behaviors will be rewarded in tangible ways (e.g., salary, promotions, recognition). Transformational leadership principles move the leader and follower beyond this traditional relationship based on exchange theory.

Burns (1978) describes the transforming leader as one who is able to motivate followers to transcend their own self-interests for higher goals. The leader's commitment to a special vision is effectively communicated to and embraced by followers. The goal of transformational leadership is to achieve a collective purpose that benefits society. "Through articulation and role modeling, the transformational leader heightens the followers' awareness of what needs to be done to accomplish the shared goals" (Marriner-Tomey, 1993, p. 32). Under this premise, risk taking is often less "risky" for nurses. They are encouraged by colleagues and managers to be advocates for the patients, and they advance professionally in an environment supportive of risk-taking behavior. This is possible because of the mutually held higher vision.

The defining characteristics of the transforming leader have been elucidated by Bennis (1988); they include having self-knowledge, enthusiasm for learning and improving, curiosity and risk taking, and the ability to learn from adversity and failure. Other traits identified are being an effective decision-maker, intellectual stimulator, and mentor (Tacetta-Chapnick, 1996). Transformational leaders are both proactive and innovative. They can move beyond the confines and boundaries of traditional work settings. Because they do not fear risk, transforming leaders can design new roles for themselves and others to meet the needs of patients. They also create services to help health care organizations and related enterprises to meet their goals in new and efficient ways. They are true entrepreneurs. White and Begun (1998) define an entrepreneur as "a person who perceives an opportunity and assumes the risk of planning and creating the means to pursue it" (p. 44). Transformational leadership theory is particularly relevant as a foundation for risk-taking behaviors that are inherent in entrepreneurial nursing.

Crow (1998) asserts that the traditional career options for nurses are clearly unraveling. He says professional development and advancement will not occur in a predictable, stepwise fashion in the 21st century. The conventional social contract between workers and employers has been altered dramatically. Longevity and job security are no longer a given in any work setting. Retention will be based on client need and the value of services that the nurse provides. White and Begun (1998) add that success in the marketplace will be based on the ability of nurses to harness the power of knowledge, rather than on technical skills. Entrepreneurial enterprise will become the norm rather than the exception in nursing practice. These nurses must be prepared to taker greater risks developing innovative services if they are to compete effectively in the health care market.

MY STORY AND ITS THEORETICAL BASIS

Transformational leadership, entrepreneurial nursing, and risk taking were the three critical concepts that shaped the unfolding story of my personal and professional development. Siegelman's framework for risk taking is a useful perspective for relating the story of my progress toward entrepreneurship. The seven stages of risk taking are evident in my journey, and they offer others a yardstick for assessing their progress.

By 1982, I was able to achieve my short-term goals of moving to California, finding work, and beginning my progress toward the master's degree in nursing with a clinical nurse specialist (CNS) credential. My long-term goals were well outlined. I wanted to combine practicing on a part-time basis with clinical teaching in perinatal nursing. My focus would be the high-risk perinatal patient. I assumed that my role as a CNS would include staff development functions such as precepting new nurses and teaching selected classes for the nursing staff. I also hoped to maintain my connection with the academic world. I had taught nursing students for almost 5 years in Florida and particularly enjoyed the enthusiasm that they brought to the clinical setting.

Becoming Aware

It appeared that my future was nicely mapped out for me. It was predicated on the belief that the health care system I had been educated and worked in would remain virtually unchanged for the next 20 to 25 years. It was also a very traditional career trajectory, but I had not anticipated that my interactions with fellow students would upset my well-defined plans. The caliber of nurses attending the program meant that I had the opportunity to meet intelligent and highly motivated individuals from across North America and other parts of the world. Many were already employed in leadership positions and expanded practice roles. The greatest reward derived from attending the program was yet to come; within a matter of weeks, I discovered that some of my colleagues were already engaged in unique business enterprises. They were pioneering new roles in the profession that I had never envisioned or thought possible. I met childbirth educators in private practice and nurses providing home care nursing and support services for women with high-risk infants. I came to know other students who were combining the master's degree in nursing with previously acquired business credentials to start up companies that created products for pregnant women, new mothers, or infants.

Exposure to these entrepreneurial nurses astounded me. Although I read widely in the clinical journals about career options for the CNS and nurse midwife, I had not been exposed to the literature that described the nurse-in-business role. I do not believe that anyone was describing these activities as "entrepreneurial" endeavors. My colleagues in Michigan and Florida had been practicing nurses, certified nurse midwives, and educators. We had all been socialized in highly structured institutions and anticipated continuing our future careers within these establishments. In fact, my entire education and socialization had occurred in very rigid and structured settings. I had attended private parochial school for 12 years and then went directly into a nursing program. Although the university I attended in the 1960s had been one of the most forward-looking schools of nursing in the United States, it had not prepared me for the possibility of independent practice or a business career in health care.

Nurses who were carving out a unique niche in nursing fascinated me. What gave them the confidence to venture alone into the world of business? Could they really make a living? How did they deal with the issues of health and retirement benefits? What kind of obstacles did they face? Perhaps the question I asked myself most often was what would it feel like to be free of the constraints placed on me by my employer and the work setting? I began to ask myself if personality differences accounted for the unusual career development of these nurses, or could one learn how to become an independent businesswoman? My entire world view about possible career paths for nursing was suddenly challenged and changing, upsetting my general sense of certainty about where I was going and what I would do when I graduated from the program.

Sensing a Need for Change

Within 6 months of beginning the master's program, I found myself seriously questioning the established path I had set for myself. I was drawn increasingly to the possibility of creating a role that included at least some type of independent business practice. I searched the school of nursing catalog, hoping to find a class in developing business expertise. The school did offer a role development course for the clinical nurse specialist, and I quickly enrolled in one of the sections. I also audited nursing management classes, hoping that the faculty might address the topic of independent business ventures.

Unfortunately, the role development class focused mainly on preparing for the CNS or the evolving nurse practitioner role within the existing health care system. We did examine the process of establishing business partnerships, and this included a brief overview of financial considerations, but the discussion was primarily aimed at preparing advanced practice nurses for business ventures in physician offices. The nursing administration courses were squarely centered on nursing management within preexisting health care systems. I was, however. exposed for the first time to the theoretical concepts of risk taking, role development, and general leadership principles, and this was to form the basis for my independent research on the topic of small business start-ups.

By the beginning of my second year of graduate school, I had acquired no clearer sense of what I eventually hoped to accomplish. I did continue to have a strong sense of a need for change. The more information I obtained about potential business opportunities, the more confused I became. The nurses engaged in private business enterprises described long struggles to establish themselves. They often had difficulty in gaining acceptance and support from nursing peers, as well as from physician groups, in the community. All of the nurses were navigating in uncharted waters. Financial considerations weighed heavily on all of them. Third-party reimbursement was not possible at this time, and the nurses had to attract clients who could afford to pay out of pocket for their services. One of the nurses had a childbirth education company. She provided one-on-one classes for a variety of women who could not or chose not to attend traditional in-hospital programs. She had movie and television stars among her clients, as well as women with disabilities who were wheelchair bound, yet she needed to work a second job to realize the same income of the average staff nurse.

Experiencing a Growing Sense of Ambivalence

I was very concerned about changing proverbial horses in midstream. I continued to thoroughly enjoy the clinical focus of the program. My work in the maternal-newborn department of the city and county hospital was extremely fulfilling. I was continually expanding my level of clinical expertise. The incredible advances in perinatal and neonatal medicine occurring at that time fueled my speed of learning. The nursing care of high-risk women was changing dramatically with the development of technologies that increased the survival rates of very low birth weight infants. New drugs and therapies were introduced at a dizzying speed. I was challenged to master new skills while providing humane care. I was not ready to entirely give up my clinical practice.

In early 1983, a seminal event occurred that would eventually resolve the questions about my future and set me on the path of a business entrepreneur. A faculty member and I encountered each other on an elevator in the School of Nursing. She was aware that I worked in the maternal-newborn department at the county hospital and had more than 10 years of experience in perinatal nursing. "Say, I've got an interesting opportunity, and I think you might be the right person for the job. Why don't you drop by my office?" When I met with her later that day, she handed me a photocopy of a medical record. She told me that an attorney acquaintance had consulted with her about a medical malpractice case he was litigating. He was trying to find a practicing perinatal nurse who would review the medical record of a woman who had died of a postpartum hemorrhage. The goal of this review would be to determine if the nurses had met the standard of care and to articulate any identified breaches in the standard.

My immediate reaction was, "I've never done this before." How did one determine if the standard of care had been met? Would I be required to meet with the attorney or work through this faculty member? How much time would the review take? I was working and attending school full-time, and the prospect of taking on an additional project was not especially appealing at this time. At the back of my mind was another concern: Who am I to judge another nurse's actions? This question was one I would have to fully address in the future. At the time, I doubt if I really appreciated its importance in determining my subsequent course of action.

The faculty member was extremely helpful and encouraging. She had reviewed charts in the past when working as a manager and would be willing to mentor me in the process. Then she said the words that immediately allayed my initial reluctance and concerns, "The attorney is willing to pay $75.00 an hour for this work. He needs an expedited chart review and an opinion within the week." I would actually be compensated, and very well, for my services! I calculated that 1 hour of record review would be equivalent to 3 hours of pay for nursing services at the hospital. It was possible I could work fewer days at the hospital and devote more time to my studies. I was quite overcome for several moments while rapidly assessing the implications of this information. The value of the work had to be very great to merit such a generous payment. The quality of my work would have to be exceptional. Was I up to the challenge? I was willing to take the risk. I quickly accepted her offer of both the work and mentoring.

After leaving the faculty member's office with the medical record, I went directly to the library to do a rapid search of the literature on the topic of malpractice. There were several useful articles that I was able to locate in nursing journals that described the role of the expert witness. Expert witness—was that what I would be? Then I read that expert witnesses rendered opinions under oath in deposition and courtroom testimony. I was suddenly quite anxious. What had I gotten myself into? Reviewing the medical record did not appear to be too difficult a task, but formally rendering a coherent opinion about the standard of care under oath was an entirely different matter. I needed to speak to the attorney in this case before proceeding further.

Estimating My Risks

A part of me perceived this as a very risky venture. My professional reputation could be at stake. I believed that I was a skilled clinician, but I knew nothing about the law or the conduct expected of an expert witness. What if I couldn't determine whether the nurses had acted reasonably and met the standard of care? I would be paid $75.00 an hour to assist an attorney in developing his case. I was not so naive that I did not realize the outcome of this case would be measured in tens of thousands of dollars or more. Even in the early 1980s, there was considerable discussion in the literature about the cost of negligence for physicians, nurses, and hospitals. Would I be able to articulate the standard of care and breaches in that standard in a lucid manner and under some degree of hostile scrutiny?

Any seasoned risk taker will agree that success in risking is to some degree influenced by luck. Running into the faculty member on the elevator that morning was the first bit of luck. My collaboration with the lawyer litigating this case was the second fortuitous event. He was an experienced attorney, willing to work with a complete novice in this field, and incredibly supportive throughout the entire process. He guided me every step of the way, explaining all aspects of the malpractice case and my expected role. The nature of the case itself was the third advantageous component of this episode in my professional development. The facts of the case were quite easily delineated and clearly supported the contention that the hospital was, through its nurse, negligent in the immediate and ongoing management of a postpartum hemorrhage. Had my first case contained the complex elements of many subsequent cases I have reviewed, I may never have agreed to serve again as an expert witness.

Although luck is always part of the calculus in risk taking, the more important factors are competence and the resources available to analyze the problem and make rational decisions. Once I had completed my review of the literature and had spoken to the attorney, I began to reevaluate the risk I had actually assumed. I was a well-educated and experienced nurse and an active member of the professional association for maternal-newborn nurses (NAA-COG). I was familiar with the current literature and guidelines for practice and had used them in developing my teaching plans. I was a confident public speaker and had received excellent evaluations for my writing and expository skills. The natural confidence I had in my abilities began to reassert itself.

In addition to reviewing the literature about expert witness services, I sought advice and feedback from my spouse and close colleagues. They were also supportive, offering additional input about the project that helped me to place my fears in their proper perspective. As I began the process of reviewing the medical record, my reservations and fears were replaced by an intense sense of excitement and enthusiasm for the work. I had always loved reading mystery novels. The exercise of ferreting out clues, putting together the evidence, and developing a working hypothesis about the solution was a favorite pastime of mine. I found the examination of the medical record an almost identical process. I was building new skills on a solid foundation of past experience.

Balancing Gains and Losses

The difficulties I encountered in this first effort should not be minimized. I had questions about whether I was spending too much time reading the medical record and, later, the depositions of the health care providers involved in the case. I had logged in more than a dozen hours. How fast should I be working? How quickly would the average nurse complete the same amount of work? I had no frame of reference. The attorney also asked me to develop appropriate interrogatory questions in preparation for his depositions of the defendant nurses and physicians. This was an unfamiliar and painstakingly slow process for me.

I also was challenged by the sheer volume of data that accrued during the ongoing process of discovery. How could one keep track of all the information? There was nothing in the literature to guide me on this matter. On the suggestion of my faculty mentor, I devised a flowsheet format that I still use when reviewing medical records. Throughout the course of the case, I was confronted with new deadlines for completing additional work. I found that I had to be flexible to accommodate these short timelines. I was at the beck and call of my client—the attorney.

The defining moment came when I gave my deposition testimony in the case. I was well prepared by the lawyer, but I still approached it with a great deal of trepidation. I was forewarned that the defense attorney was an adversary who could be hostile, argumentative, and even rude. He was paid to discredit my opinion and would use whatever legal tactics he could to do this. Many nurses who pass through this test of fire resolve never to attempt it again. They find the experience anxiety provoking, distasteful, and generally too unpleasant to voluntarily undergo more than once. I loved every minute of it!

The defense attorney was extremely skillful. He put me through my paces. All of my opinions had to be carefully delineated and substantiated using national standards and guidelines for practice as well as the nursing literature. It was a long process meant to wear me down, but I found it invigorating. It was tremendously rewarding to explicate the essential aspects of nursing care and elaborate on the central role of nursing care in patient outcomes. I felt incredibly proud to be a nurse as I matched wits with the defense attorney. I was almost disappointed when it was over. The attorney who retained me provided very positive feedback. The case was quickly settled, and I found myself actually disappointed that it was over.

There were so many rewards accrued from this first experience, it is hard to enumerate them all. I found myself examining my own practice in great detail, asking questions about the process of nursing care and systems operations that I had never stopped to consider in the past. How did nurses identify problems and make judgments about their meaning and significance? What were the most common origins of error? How did nurses develop clinical judgment in the first place? There were so little data available in the nursing literature at this time to answer my questions. Luckily, Dr. Patricia Benner, a faculty member at the university, was just completing her seminal work on moving from novice to clinical expert (1984). I devoured everything I could find that she wrote on the subject. I was also incredibly lucky to be able to personally hear her speak on the topic.

During my work on the case, I was asked to review the hospital's nursing policies and procedures. This was an enlightening experience. I began to do additional reading about how effective policies and procedures were developed. I sat down and really began to look at the policies that guided my own practice. Eventually, this led to my volunteering to help in the revision of my unit's policies and procedures. Questions arose regarding the chain of command policy in the facility in this maternal death case and whether nursing staff had experienced previous problems with timely response by ancillary departments (laboratory and blood bank) during emergencies. This prompted me to read the literature regarding the use of incident reports and the role of risk management in controlling loss. I subsequently asked questions about the services at the hospital, more fully familiarizing myself with departments I had previously taken for granted. My own practice was transformed by my exposure to this first case.

Within 1 month of the first case's being settled, three additional attorneys contacted me. The lawyer I had worked with had given them my name and a strong recommendation regarding my abilities. Because there was no immediate deadline in any of these cases, I agreed to review all three. Each case involved questions regarding perinatal nursing care, but each one was different in terms of the problems and outcomes of care. By the time I graduated from the master's program, I had reviewed a total of 10 medical records. With each case, I found the work more interesting and rewarding. Several of the attorneys told me that with the completion of my master's program I would be an even more valuable witness, whether working for plaintiff or defense firms. This feedback reinforced the value of my graduate education. It appeared that I could combine the best of two worlds—clinical practice and independent consulting work that was extremely gratifying and paid well.

Unexpected Opportunities

As I look back at my career trajectory, I think of another assumption proposed by Calvert (1993): "Risk taking is typically fast-moving, make-it-up-as-you-go" (p. 43). Other events in the second year of the master's program were moving me in directions I could never have anticipated. The faculty praised my scholarly work; I was told my strong ability to write well contributed to my success in the rigorous course work. Two instructors were incredibly supportive, and each in her own way became a mentor. One was my faculty advisor. We spent many hours discussing my quandaries about career options. She began to strongly encourage me to consider doctoral education; in 1983, the university was developing a PhD doctoral program. The first class would be admitted in 1985. "You would be an excellent candidate. You love to teach, and you have the ability to reach the top in any academic setting should you choose that career path," she kept telling me.

My second mentor was one of the second generation of researchers beginning a career in nursing academia. She was engaged in qualitative research and was studying fathering behaviors. She helped me envision a career that could combine both clinical practice and scholarly work. "You're so tied to practice, you could be a clinical researcher, and a teacher, and even continue with your legal work." She pointed out that the most sought-after physician expert witnesses had a track record in academia, clinical practice, and publication. It would be logical that the same would hold true for nurses.

I had to make a very quick decision about applying for the doctoral program, and if accepted, I would begin just 1 year after finishing my master's degree. Both of my mentors thought it would actually benefit me to return to school in just 1 year. "You won't be rusty when you return to school. Give yourself a year to regenerate your batteries and then go for it!" they said. The big question was how pursuit of a doctorate would fit in with my hope to develop some type of business venture. There were so few role models—nurses with doctoral degrees engaged in independent consulting. In 1985, the majority of nurses with the credentials were employed in academia or nursing administration. I spoke with as many nurses with a doctorate as I could, trying to determine how the credential would benefit me.

I also spent some time discussing the pros and cons of the plan with my husband. He has always been my greatest coach. "Another 4 years of school? The time will fly! It's not a matter of if you can do it, but how much fun you will have achieving another goal. Go for it" he said. My immediate family was also supportive. Colleagues had different perspectives on the matter. My coworkers at the hospital couldn't fathom why anyone would want to spend another 4 years or more in nursing school to obtain a doctoral degree. Classmates in the master's program were often horrified. "Oh my God, the work! Your head will be ready to explode by the time you're through." Of more concern were the comments from individuals who believed I would not be able to maintain my close affiliation with the clinical arena.

Ultimately, I believed that I could only benefit from the rigorous training in scientific methods that the doctoral program would provide. I would have the opportunity to work with and learn from some of the finest nurse scholars in the world. The ability to critically review scientific literature and construct logical arguments would assist me in my legal work and make it easier to maintain a formal relationship with an academic setting. It would enhance my poise as a speaker. My greatest concern remained whether I would be able to continue practicing on a part-time basis, and I was determined to make that happen. I made the decision to apply.

It became evident that I was picking up the pace in risk-taking behavior and making crucial decisions about my life's work. It had taken me almost 5 years to make a final decision about pursuing a master's degree. I had resolved to apply for the doctoral program in a matter of months. I had come to believe that the greater the risks, the greater the potential rewards. If I could accomplish this goal, the sky was the limit.

Taking Stock of My Progress

I spent the year between the master's and doctoral programs assessing my progress toward independent consulting. I was happily juggling three work roles at this time. I continued to work with attorney firms. A steady stream of cases continued to come my way, and I was offered my first defense case. It was clear that I was well suited for legal consulting, and the rewards continued to accrue. I had also accepted a clinical instructor position at a college of nursing and was still employed part-time at the hospital. With my master's degree in hand, I began to expand my clinical role in the maternal-infant department, teaching classes and assisting with revision of unit standards and policies. Once school began, this mix would have to change. There was no doubt I wanted to continue my legal consulting, but how far was I willing to take this work?

Pushing the Envelope

The potential for work kept snowballing. During 1985, I had my first opportunity to testify in trial. It was a heady experience. Our team won the case—in this instance, a jury verdict for the hospital and its nurses. It was another defining moment for me. Testifying and being cross-examined in court were no more difficult than the process of deposition. I was also offered the chance to teach a class in the "Basics of Electronic Fetal Monitoring" for attorneys in a large law firm. I was told, "We speak legalese quite well, but we can't decipher this medical terminology. We need the help of a health care professional, but physicians are just too busy to help us out." The class was a great success, and other offers for teaching attorneys came my way.

As a consequence of my expert witness work, I found myself sharing the experiences and my observations about nursing accountability and legal liability with work colleagues. A nurse manager who had been a classmate in the master's program approached me. She asked if I would come to her hospital and speak to the staff nurses for about 1 hour about my legal work and the insights it gave me about nursing practice. "We can only offer you lunch as compensation, but I know we'd get a big group together." The presentation was well received. The following year I was invited back to conduct a half-day program for physicians and nursing staff, and I received an honorarium for the presentation.

One more opportunity came my way in 1985. One of my mentors was an editor of a new maternity nursing textbook. She invited me to write several chapters on the low-risk and the high-risk neonate. "It will be good practice for the doctoral program," she said. I had authored something for publication only once in the past, a short paper on the relationship between student and staff nurse in the clinical setting, so I accepted and moved quickly through the project; the chapters received excellent reviews. As a consequence of writing the chapters, I was increasingly asked to speak at programs, this time on the topics of neonatal physiology and nursing care of newborns. Whenever possible, I interjected comments on the legal aspects of nursing care.

Managing Unwarranted Fears

While I was making excellent progress in creating an independent practice, I was initially quite anxious about expanding my services into new areas. The same refrain replayed in my head: "You've never done this before. Will you be up to the challenge?" I discovered that the fears associated with the unknown were much greater than the anxiety I actually experienced when I finally made a foray into new territory. I began to accept that a small degree of anxiety is quite normal and may actually spur one on to do the best possible job. The unwarranted fears associated with the possibility of failure or loss of face actually interfered with my ability to think clearly. I resolved to put aside unwarranted anxiety.

I learned one of the most important lessons during this formative period in my career. I was not alone in being offered the chance to venture into uncharted waters. Many of my nurse colleagues spoke of interesting opportunities that were theirs for the taking, but the same concern was voiced over and over again: "I've never done that before." This was, of course, my response in 1982 when asked to review my first medical record. I had learned quickly that failing was not the worst fate: stagnation and mediocrity are far worse. Not achieving one's highest potential is the greater loss. I am reminded of Calvert's assumption, introduced early in this chapter, that security is a myth and professional stimulation is worth the cost of risk taking. I would encourage neophytes in risk taking to remember the adage "Nothing ventured, nothing gained."

Forging Ahead

In retrospect, it is hard to believe that I was able to juggle the responsibilities of a full-time doctoral student and my ever-expanding career as an independent consultant. Without the continuous support of my husband and close friends, it would have been an impossible task. Because the first 2 years of doctoral study (1985 through 1987) consisted of formal classroom work and research assistant responsibilities, I reduced the total time spent in reviewing medical records for attorneys. I focused on continuing my regular weekly practice at the hospital and accepted more opportunities to speak about legal issues in nursing practice and professional accountability. My knowledge of the laws and regulations governing nursing practice was also expanding. This added to my value as a speaker and consultant.

Concomitantly, I refined the use of case studies in teaching clinical topics and began a formal review of the nascent literature on critical thinking and professional judgment. I strongly believed that the way undergraduate theory courses in nursing were taught contributed to the nurses' lack of critical thinking skills and nursing practice errors. I entirely eliminated the lecture format from my teaching repertoire, developing interactive approaches to teaching the art and science of nursing. I emphasized group process to support adult learning and continued to develop an entire syllabus of clinical topics using case studies.

In 1988, I began my dissertation research, which focused on the outcomes of pregnancy for women engaged in strenuous work. I was particular interested in the rates of preterm labor and delivery among pregnant women who continued to perform heavy work. My sample was the group of women I encountered as a practicing nurse at the hospital. I was simultaneously engaged in cross-training the postpartum nursing staff at the hospital in the care of pregnant women admitted and treated for preterm labor. It was a fortuitous combination of events that made both projects easier and more fulfilling. My knowledge base about preterm labor added to my value as a consultant for preterm labor prevention projects and in medical malpractice cases involving premature labor and delivery.

In 1989, as graduation approached, I spent an increased amount of time consulting with attorneys, I continued to teach classes for law firms, and I spoke nationally on issues of professional accountability. I was continually presented with new opportunities because of my unique combination of talents: current practice skills, knowledge of the medical malpractice process, and teaching expertise. The doctorate credential added another dimension to the marketability of my services. For the first time, a hospital risk manager asked me to critique a maternity department's policies and procedures and unit-based standards. The department was converting to single-site maternity care, cross-training the entire nursing staff to provide labor/delivery/recovery/postpartum care. I was also asked to evaluate the process of cross-training and adequacy of competence testing for the new unit. This consulting contract expanded my expertise in assessing systems operations. I found myself reviewing the growing body of literature on risk management. This first consultation in a labor/delivery/recovery/postpartum care setting quickly led to additional work as word spread that I was available to provide this new service.

Holding Back and Recharging My Batteries

On graduation in June 1989, my husband and I sat down to explore my options. He strongly urged me to develop my own consulting company, a sole proprietorship. He believed I would be able to generate an income comparable to any salary I would earn as a full-time employee of a larger company marketing redesign consulting services or as a faculty member in a school of nursing. At this time, I was sure I could provide quality services to a wide range of clients, but I had been too busy during the doctoral program to fully explore the financial aspects of owning my own business. I had many questions about setting up my pension plan, dealing with tax laws, and securing sufficient liability insurance for a business. I resisted the urge to take the final plunge for one more year. I was determined to answer all the important questions before cutting loose.

During this 18 months of planning, I forged ahead. I had accepted a teaching position in a school of nursing at another university. Building on my prior successes with case study format at the hospital, I began teaching theory classes using the same techniques. I jettisoned the lecture format for maternity students; I was the first faculty member in the nursing program to do so. The acting dean was another mentor of mine during this time. She was extremely supportive of my efforts to foster critical thinking in the undergraduate students and encouraged me to continue my work as a consultant and speaker. She also promoted my active participation in the school's chapter of Sigma Theta Tau International (STTI). I was nominated for and elected chairperson of the research committee. Although the dean hoped I would find the lure of academia too strong to resist, she also realized my tenure at the university would most likely be very short.

We both left the university the following year—she to assume the position of dean at a university in Memphis, Tennessee, and I to launch my company. Our association would, however, continue through the coming years.

During 1989 and 1990, I spent every free minute acquiring the knowledge I needed to start my business. I systematically answered each question on the very long list I had generated about this enterprise. I prepared a home office and created a logo for marketing materials and stationery. I began to speak with valued colleagues about their interest in working with me on select projects. My husband was incredibly supportive and began talking about joining me in the enterprise at a later time. He was a respiratory care practitioner and director of clinical education in a respiratory care department. He was also approaching the point in his career when he would be eligible for early retirement. As an active participant in the redesign of his department, he believed the experience would prepare him to assist other facilities with this process. By combining forces, we could offer a wider range of services for redesign; in fact, many health care facilities were beginning to combine respiratory and nursing services at this time. A name was chosen for the enterprise—Mahlmeister and Associates.

I maintained a grueling pace during this last year before taking the plunge. I was teaching full-time at the university, continued to practice part time at the hospital, accepted speaking engagements, and reviewed medical records for attorneys. A new professional nursing organization was created to represent the interest of nurses who were engaged in a growing range of consulting services for attorneys; the American Association of Legal Nurse Consultants was launched in 1989. I became an active member and continue to serve as a director at large for the Bay Area Chapter.

I was ready to launch my business, and then the second shoe dropped! One of my mentors approached me with a proposition. I had written several chapters on the newborn for the first edition of her textbook. The first author of that book declined to participate on a second edition. My mentor asked me if I would become the second author of the textbook. I would be able to incorporate legal aspects of practice into the content and write as many chapters as I wanted. I would have editorial responsibility for the remaining chapters in the second half of this textbook. The publisher believed that a strong selling point for the book would be the combination of an academic credential and my current practice in maternity nursing. I jumped at the chance. I believed I could both begin my business enterprise and work on the textbook.

Taking the Final Plunge

In 1991, Mahlmeister and Associates was launched. I resigned my position at the university and opened my doors for business. It was a very uneventful transition. I was already engaged in several projects that I had accepted earlier in the year. My work was increasingly taking me beyond California. I had more offers than one person could handle, and the biggest decision I had to make was how large I wanted the company to grow. My husband unexpectedly required surgery in 1991, and that in part formed my decision not to expand my services by hiring additional full-time associates. I had tripled my income in the first year of operations and had no worry about finances. My biggest challenge remained choosing from among a growing number of exciting offers. I had frequent opportunities to interface with other practice disciplines as health care redesign swept the country. It was clear that there would be work for my husband when he was ready to join me, when he finally did in 1993. Mahlmeister and Associates became a partnership.

Evaluating the Outcomes

Mahlmeister and Associates continues to thrive as we approach the millennium. My husband and I choose to work only on the projects that appeal to us most and enhance our professional development. Our earnings have been healthy, and our income had grown steadily with the value of our services. We could continue to expand, but we find our current pace of work satisfying. I have stayed true to my resolve to maintain a clinical practice.

I am still employed at the hospital. I am approaching my 20th anniversary as a staff nurse in the maternal-newborn department. My primary practice is in our new birth center, caring for women during labor and delivery. I set aside time each week to provide direct nursing care and find this the most gratifying aspect of my professional work. My nurse colleagues call me "doctor-nurse" and provide a constant source of support for my career choices. Doing clinical nursing adds a dimension to my consulting services that cannot be matched by other nurses who have severed their ties with the clinical arena. My ability to continue practicing is also due in great part to the nurse leader of our department. She is a true transformational leader. She allows me great flexibility and latitude in my schedule, which is essential for my consulting work.

I continue to review medical records as my consulting work permits. My mentors were absolutely correct when they predicted that the combination of academic credentials, clinical practice, and publications would enhance the demand for my services as an expert witness. My work in the realm of medical record review has extended to insurance companies. I am now asked to review critical incidents and identify practitioner and systems issues that may have influenced the outcomes in particular cases. I have joined the American Society for Healthcare Risk Management and engage in collaborative projects with risk managers.

I write, speak, and conduct workshops on clinical issues and the topics of professional accountability and legal liability for nurses. By the mid-1990s, my coauthored book was in its third edition, and it has received wide recognition for its unique legal and risk control perspective in perinatal nursing practice. I have also maintained my connection with academia. In 1992, I was invited to fill a chair in nursing excellence at a university in Memphis, Tennessee, during the spring semester. My role included assisting faculty with the development of case studies and other interactive approaches to stimulate critical thinking in student nurses. This experience led to consulting work with faculty in schools of nursing across the United States in the development of case studies. Finally, I continue to intermittently precept student nurses from the universities in our birth center at the hospital, and I am invited to speak to student groups around the area every semester.

The past 2 years have brought new challenges, and my finely honed risk-taking abilities have helped me prevail. Both my husband and I have assumed leadership positions in professional organizations. I have just completed a term as president of the Beta Gamma Chapter of STTI. The former dean and past president of STTI was a mentor to me with my active participation with the organization. Her guidance and advice have been invaluable.

My husband is finishing his term as president of the California Society for Respiratory Care. We both serve on several editorial boards, and many days find us editing our own manuscripts on a range of clinical and professional topics. We have learned to work effectively together in our company ventures. It was a challenging adjustment to learn new roles in our long-term relationship.

I am currently collaborating with an extremely knowledgeable nurse attorney. We have published a definitive article on consent for perinatal nurses and are now working on a textbook for perinatal nurses. The focus will be legal issues and standards of practice for perinatal nurses. She is a former critical care nurse, and we complement each other quite well. She has added immeasurably to my knowledge of jurisprudence, and she now knows more about perinatal nursing than she ever hoped to!

Words of Wisdom

I am a voracious reader of the literature about nurse entrepreneurs and recently came upon an article that perfectly summarizes the critical aspects of starting a business for nurses. "Ten Common Mistakes to Avoid as an Consultant" was authored by Marilyn Hua (1997). She is an independent occupational health nurse consultant and owner of M. L. Hua and Associates. Every nurse who is considering this career path should read her observations. These guidelines have been described in the business journals for the past 40 years, but rarely have they been delineated so well in the nursing literature. Listed in the following section are Hua's recommendations and an additional commentary by this author:

1. **Chose a consulting venture that has a good probability of being profitable.**
Research should indicate that there is an adequate client base for the service and that they will be able to pay for it (insurance or individual payment). There should be evidence that the market in your community is not saturated with others providing the service.

2. **Adequately estimate the time needed for start up of the business.**
You will need to have additional resources to see you through the period when you are building your client base. Most ventures experience "dry spells." Also consider how much time you will need to spend with each client or each project. Honestly examine whether you are willing to put in some 80-hour weeks to meet critical deadlines.

3. **Develop a comprehensive business plan.**
Establish a mission statement, describe your product or services, and identify your target population. Hua states, "If you don't know where you're going, you won't know when you get there." Place this in the context of our constantly changing health care environment. Your goals may have to be revised as market-place forces alter the way health care systems operate. Planning for where you

will set up your office and capital acquisition is an easier task, but plan well in advance.

4. **Establish your fee for service or price for products**.

Hua observes that new consultants often undercharge for the time and quality of their work. Knowing what to charge will depend on knowing the average fees for services or products in your community, the state, or the country. I am often asked by fledging legal nurse consultants if it would pay off in the long run to undercut the competition in the community. This is an unwise practice. Significantly undervaluing yourself sends a message to the potential clients about the value of your work or product.

5. **Develop a sound marketing and promotion strategy**.

Desktop publishing programs and other computer software have made it possible for many business entrepreneurs to develop their own marketing materials.

It may be beneficial to consult a graphic designer to create a logo or letterhead for your business. Research the literature on marketing and promotion, and determine how you can best reach potential clients.

6. **Specify carefully the limitation of your services for clients**.

Hua states that overgeneralization can result in spreading the business too thin. This must be balanced against the rapidly changing health care system. The entrepreneur must be flexible and may consider an offer that takes the business off on a tangent if it appears the project reflects a new and important trend. Other services may have to be scaled down or eliminated.

7. **Consider all the legal ramifications of the business**.

Tax law, liability insurance, and contract language are all factors that must be considered to avoid legal disasters. Protecting one's intellectual property and products created by the company is also an important consideration. Seek the advice of attorneys who are specialists in business law, copyright and patent law, and contract language as needed.

8. **Determine the nature of the business for tax purposes**.

Hua discusses in detail the benefits and disadvantages of sole proprietorships, partnerships, and corporations. The input of a business attorney and or a tax accountant may be useful in making decisions about how one determines the structure of the business. Remember that 9 of 10 small businesses fail in the first year (Marder, 1991).

9. **Anticipate market changes**.

One of the greatest challenges is to keep ahead of the curve. The nurse entrepreneur must anticipate changes in technology, health care, the economy, nursing, and client needs. As noted, a sudden change in the clients' request for services may herald a real shift in the marketplace. Be sharply attuned to these often subtle changes.

CONCLUSION

The story of my journey from fledging consultant to president and co-owner of Mahlmeister and Associates is a tale in risk taking. Risking is inherent in establishing an independent consulting or business enterprise. The stakes are often high and the outcomes are always unpredictable in any commercial endeavor. The nurse who is determined to set out on a trajectory that diverges from the traditional career path must have a solid understanding of the theoretical underpinnings of risk taking. Nurses have the educational foundation necessary to refine risk-taking skills and to use them in the provision of new products and services. The role of patient advocate prepares nurses to be seasoned risk takers. It is hoped that this chapter will encourage nurses to capitalize on these underlying skills and take the first step toward new forms of leadership.

REFERENCES

Arch, E. (1993). Risk taking: A motivational basis for sex differences. *Psychological Reports, 73*, 3–11.

Benner, P. (1984). *From novice to expert.* Reading, Mass.: Addison-Wesley.

Bennis, W. (1988). Ten traits of dynamic leaders. *Executive Excellence, 5*(2), 8–9.

Bennis, W., & Nanus, B. (1985). *Leaders: The strategies for taking charge.* New York: Harper & Row.

Bernstein, P. (1997). How we take risks. *Across the Board, 34*(2), 23–26.

Burns, J. M. (1978). *Leadership.* New York: Harper & Row.

Calvert, G. (1993). *Highwire management.* San Francisco: Jossey-Bass.

Crow, G. (1998). The entrepreneurial personality: Building a sustainable future for self and the profession. *Nursing Administration Quarterly, 22*(2), 30–35.

Dobos, C. (1992). Defining risk from the perspective of nurses in clinical roles. *Journal of Advanced Nursing, 17*, 1303–1309.

Dobos, C. (1997). Understanding personal risk taking among staff nurses: Critical information for nurse executives, *Journal of Nursing Administration, 27*(1), 12–13.

Gorgal-Eaton, D. (1994). Perinatal home care: One entrepreneur's experience. *JOGNN, 23*(8), 726–Hua, M. L. (1997). Ten common mistakes to avoid as an independent consultant. *AAOHN Journal, 45*(1), 17–23.

Kindler, H. (1990). *Risk taking: A guide for decision makers.* Los Altos, Calif.: Crisp Publications.

Kouzes, J. M., & Posner, B. Z. (1988). *The leadership challenge.* San Francisco: Jossey-Bass.

Lachman, V. D. (1998). Care of the self for the nurse entrepreneur. *Nursing Administration Quarterly, 22*(2), 48–59.

MacCrimmon, K. R., & Wehrung, D. A. (1986). *Taking risks: The management of uncertainty.* New York: The Free Press.

Marriner-Tomey, A. (1993). *Transformational leadership in nursing.* St. Louis: Mosby.

Marder, J. S. (1991). Surviving the start-up years. White Hall, Vir.: Betterway Publications.

Master, M., & Master, R. (1989). Risk taking propensity of nurses: ADN and BSN. *Journal of Nursing Education, 28*, 391–396.

Parker, M. (1998). The new entrepreneurial foundation for the nurse executive. *Nursing Administration Quarterly, 22*(2), 13–22.

Pfaff, D. (1997). Hormones, genes, and behavior. *Proceedings of the National Academy of Sciences, 94*, 14213–14216.

Roberts, S. (1997). Nurse executives in the 1990s: Empowered or oppressed? *Nursing Administration Quarterly, 22*(1), 64–71.

Siegelman, E. (1983). *Personal risk: Mastering change in love and work.* New York: Harper Collins.

Singleton, W. T., & Hovden, J. (1987). *Risk and decisions.* New York: John Wiley.

Stevens, K. R. (1983). *Power and influence: A source book for nurses.* New York: John Wiley.

Tacetta-Chapnick, M. (1996). Transformational leadership. *Nursing Administration Quarterly, 21*(1), 60–66.

White, K. R., & Begun, J. W. (1998). Nursing entrepreneurship in an era of chaos and complexity. *Nursing Administration Quarterly, 22*(2), 40–47.

Wolfe, P. (1994). Risk taking: Nursing's comfort zone. *Holistic Nursing Practice, 8*(2), 43–52.

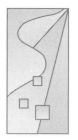

Chapter 7

Recognizing the Right Time for Action

Kathleen Rose-Grippa

> We are not born with maps; we have to make them, and the making requires effort. The more effort we make to appreciate and perceive reality, the larger and more accurate our maps will be. But many do not want to make the effort. Their maps are small and sketchy, their views of the world narrow and misleading (M. Scott Peck, 1978).

THE PRINCIPLES OF TIMING

Leaders require detailed knowledge of the systems in which they operate. The system may be that of a single individual, a group of people organized around a task, a health care agency facing reorganization, or a community coping with a flood. Knowledge of the system functions as a map. Embedded in this map's information is a sense of timing that guides the leader in determining which action is appropriate at what time.

Timing is a concept more frequently thought of in relation to a stand-up comedian than to a leader, but leaders are just as much in need of a highly developed sense of timing. A leader thinks, "I have used strategy A in comparable situations in the past. Do I stick with strategy A, or has the situation changed and strategy B is the better choice because it has a greater chance of success? When do I strengthen assets or minimize liabilities?" These are timing questions.

Stop and think for a moment about a comedian. Pick any one of your favorites (Jerry Seinfeld, Jim Carey, Woody Allen, Eddie Murphy). Think of a particularly funny routine. What do you remember most clearly? Perhaps it was the comedian's particular slant on life? Or the topic was so relevant that the entire audience laughed as one? Maybe the pace was memorable—as quickly as the laughter tapered off from one vignette, the next was being delivered? By the end of the act, you knew you had seen a superb routine. To use an old phrase, it had been "right on."

Now think a bit about the last time you or someone around you took the lead in a situation. It isn't necessary to think about a situation as complex as the reorganization of an agency; something as simple as starting a new Sunday school class in your church or organizing a fund-raising event for the high school band boosters will do. Remember the sequence of events? Something triggered a need for action: for example, new uniforms were needed because the band room had flooded. Initially, there was very little event-related activity. There was minimal eye contact. Some people looked at the floor. Others talked about tangential topics. Time seemed to be suspended. Then someone stepped forward, and activity began to happen. Someone took the initiative and used the necessary actions to get the group galvanized. Before long, there were new band uniforms. The timing was right, and action was taken.

Whether the focus is on enjoying a comedian or funding for new band uniforms, the situations share a reliance on timing. But what is timing? Is it as simple as fate combined with intuition? Does it just happen, so that being in the right place at the right time is the crucial variable? Or is there something that can be done to facilitate a sense of timing? Are there aspects of timing that can be learned?

The answers to these questions, and others about timing, are often found in the following three areas of inquiry:

- The origin of leadership characteristics
- Force field analysis
- Contingency theory

In the remainder of this chapter, each of these areas of inquiry is reviewed with some illustrative examples, followed by a discussion of the use of each in the development of timing.

Origin of Leadership Characteristics

Specific characteristics of leadership are easy to find. Many are listed in the table of contents of this book, such as self-knowledge, futuristic thinking, effective communication, risk taking, and mentoring. How do individuals come to possess these characteristics? Historically, two explanations have been offered as the source of leadership, and a single question highlights both perspectives. Are leaders born or made?

■ Leaders Are Born

The "leaders are born" perspective is the older perspective. In its pristine version, the leadership trait is passive and deterministic. Drucker (1968) stated, "Leadership is of utmost importance. Indeed there is no substitute for it. But leadership cannot be created or promoted. It cannot be taught or learned" (p. 158).

Leadership as an inherited trait is rooted in the thinking that "great men" shape history. Leadership is inherited; therefore, the qualities of leadership are part of an individual's personality. The key to becoming a leader is to choose one's family carefully. Examples of the "leaders are born" perspective would be the belief that

- The child of the person who designed the company would be the best leader for the company when the parent steps down.

- A prince, with his inalienable right, should rule as the monarch.
- The coach's daughter will be the logical winner in the tennis tournament.

Identifying the common characteristics of leaders is the first step in recognizing individuals who have inherited leadership traits. Such a strategy is exactly what the early investigators of leadership attempted to do. Hundreds, perhaps thousands, of studies have been designed to tease out the characteristic personality trait of leaders. The thought behind these studies was that if it were possible to specify the common characteristics of many individuals who were identified as leaders in a wide variety of situations, the personal characteristics that were common across all of these individuals would be those that were inherited. The only consistent trait identified through decades of research has been that of intelligence (Bass, 1981).

■ Leaders Are Made

The "leaders are made" perspective postulates that circumstances create leaders. According to this theory, the factors within a given situation become the dominant feature in determining leadership, and it is difficult to predict who will rise to leadership in any given situation. For example, the "leaders are made" viewpoint holds that events in 1776 were right for the American colonies to achieve independence; therefore, if George Washington had not become the general of the colonial army, someone else would have done so. The same thinking could be applied to the leadership of Ghandi in India, Martin Luther King, Jr., in the United States, and Nelson Mandela in South Africa. Leadership becomes a matter of the individuals' being in the right place at the right time. Within this perspective, leaders act no differently in one situation than in another. The environment changes in such a way that a given individual's everyday actions become those of leading.

Reality is neither black nor white; it is multicolored. Likewise, leadership is totally attributable to neither genetics nor the environment. It is multifaceted. There likely is some genetically inherited base that can be nurtured and strengthened during one's preadult years. Situations do provide the opportunity to behave as a leader; however, individuals must decide to cultivate any inherited talents and use them when the occasion arises. Thus, the cultivation of talents and taking action can be learned. Think about riding a bicycle; one cannot be forced to learn to ride a bike. A teacher of bike riding can point out the parts of the bicycle and advise the rider about things to attend to while attempting to ride a bicycle for the first time. However, this same teacher cannot force someone to sit on the seat correctly, to pedal, to run the risk of falling, to balance, and to brake unless that person is ready to learn those skills. The same is true for a sense of timing in leadership. *Timing,* or taking the right action at the right time, can be cultivated by assessing the interaction of self and the situation and acting on that information. Kurt Lewin's (1951) force field analysis and several social psychologists working with contingency theory can provide some guidance in learning the skills of timing.

Force Field Analysis

Force field analysis is the work of Lewin, a social psychologist whose influence began in the 1930s. Lewin's legacy is that a true understanding of behavior requires "not only a knowledge of the person (his past experiences, his present attitudes, and his capabilities) but also a knowledge of his immediate situation" (Deutsch, 1968, p. 418). In the post-Lewin period, it has become almost impossible to think of behavior without a reference to both the person and the environment.

Lewin was part of the Gestalt psychology tradition. Gestalt psychologists believe that understanding is based on a perception of the whole rather than an analysis of distinct parts. Lewin added to the Gestalt viewpoint an intense interest in the relationship between the abstract and the concrete and between theory and the application of theory in practice. Lewin believed theory is critical but that without the links between research and practice, theory is of little use (Lewin, 1947). Researchers should serve as this link and can do so "only if, as a result of constant intense tension, [they] can keep both theory and reality fully within the field of vision" (Bennis et al., 1969, p. 4). Thus, Lewin is credited with coining the term *action research*, which is research performed with an application to a known problem.

Lewin borrowed the concept of *field* from physics. Study in the area of electromagnetic forces late in the 19th century allowed scientists to realize that "it was not the charges nor the particles but the field in the space between the charges and particles which is essential for the description of physical phenomena" (Deutsch, 1968, p. 413). Lewin extended this concept of field to that of human behavior, so the characteristics of the individual and the factors of the situation are viewed as interactive.

Remember the trait-driven world where all characteristics are viewed as inherited? In that world, a statement such the following would not be uncommon. "John was able to dunk the basketball because of his height." "Margot's sensitivity caused her to cry." "She wore a brocade dress to her mother's funeral because she was stupid." "She rose to leadership because of her ability to get along with people." The behavior is tied directly to a specific trait within the individual.

How do we know that John's height is the only factor that allowed him to dunk a basketball? What about the other four team members who cleared John's way to the basket? What about the hours John practiced? We cannot fully understand John's ability to dunk basketballs without some information about the specific basketball-dunking situation. Likewise, judgment about the girl's inappropriate attire at a funeral cannot be made without other situational-specific information; perhaps the dress was the last one made by the mother before her death. Expanded explanations that include situational information are also needed to understand the other examples.

Lewin used the concept of field to develop his notion of the *life space*, the *psychological field*, or the *total situation*, "which consists of the person and the environment viewed as one constellation of interdependent factors" (Deutsch, 1968, p. 417). Human behavior is a function of the life space, which in turn is a product of the interaction between person and the environment.

Both *life space* and *psychological field* worked well when discussing individuals, but they were less suited for discussions of formally or informally structured groups of various sizes with differing goals. Eventually the term *field* came to be used as the more appropriate concept (Lewin, 1951).

There are several constructs within the concept of field, and a basic understanding of a few of these is useful in illustrating how field theory can be helpful when thinking about timing and leadership. A field contains *regions, cognitive structures,* and *driving and restraining forces* that create movement within the field. Additionally, field theory is bound to the present. It is not concerned with the past or the future.

■ The Present

Behavior can be considered only in the present. The past may influence the present but only through present perceptions of those past events. Past events do not directly influence present events. If the past influences the future, it can do so only through the interaction with events in the current situation. The statement "She abuses her children *because* she was abused as a child" has minimal validity. The past abuse of the mother may very well be an influential factor in the current mistreatment of her children, but other factors enter into her behavior. Change any one of the factors operating in her current life space (e.g., the presence of another adult in the room), and for today, child abuse does not happen.

Stop and think a minute about the following illustrative example. A student is studying in the library stacks. Hunger attacks, and the student remembers the Hershey bar left from lunch. The hungry student takes out the candy, eats it, and puts the empty wrapper in the backpack. Later that same day, the student is at home. The student opens the backpack and is hit with the odor of chocolate. Suddenly, the student is intensely hungry.

Did eating the Hershey bar earlier create the present hunger? Is that odor going to make the student eat another Hershey bar? No, but the odor triggered the memory of it and focused the student's attention on the present and the recognition of the present hunger. The hunger and what to do about it are in the present. The chocolate fragrance may provide a choice to add to the list of actions that will take care of the hunger, but it has not caused the hunger.

■ Regions

Fields also contain regions. A region is any distinct part of a field (i.e., regions are subsets of fields). There can be a multitude of regions within a given field. Contained within each region are the contemplated activities that may resolve the focus of a particular field. Let's return to the scenario of the hungry student.

We left our student ravenously hungry after inhaling the chocolate smell created by the wrapper left in the backpack. The field consists of "thinking about taking care of the hunger." The student considers the following possible alternatives, which are equivalent to regions:

"I could eat another Hershey bar."
"I could order a pizza."
"I could eat with my parents."
"I could cook something."
"I could go to sleep and forget about being hungry."

There may be other choices to consider, but let's pretend these are the only ones. To get from point A (student is hungry) to point B (hunger is addressed), the student must move into one of these regions. To get to one of the regions, the student must contemplate the requirements of each region, which in turn will be regions themselves. Thus, "going to parents" requires (1) using the telephone to see whether the parents are home, (2) checking to see whether the parents have eaten, (3) determining whether the planned meal is liked, (4) going to the parents' home, and (5) eating dinner with the parents. These five regions create a path within the hungry student's field. The student's observable behaviors (e.g., using the telephone, talking to parents, asking about the menu, traveling to the parent's house, and eating) parallel the movement from region to region along the path (Deutsch, 1968, p. 424). As the student grows in experience, knowledge, or sophistication, additional alternatives to dealing with hunger (and other situations) present themselves. New regions will become part of any given field; this process is labeled *differentiation*.

■ Cognitive Structure

Although the term *region* corresponds to one's being in a field, a *cognitive structure* is the individual's rational organization of that field. Cognitive structures are sets of ideas that can be brought into conscious awareness. One needs cognitive structures to know how to proceed in specific situations. If our hungry student had never before experienced hunger, eating the candy or ordering a pizza or going to parent's house for dinner would not have made sense and would not have been considered. There would have been no cognitive structure for how to deal with this internal sensation we label "hunger." The student would not have known how to proceed. New experiences lack cognitive structures, thus individuals tend to be more anxious, act cautiously, and feel conflicted. This is why timing decisions, which are usually unexpected during new events, are so hard to make. However, as one's life space or field becomes more differentiated, additional cognitive structures are built, so more choices exist within given situations.

■ Driving and Restraining Forces

Psychological fields are not static entities. They are dynamic. Think about a single human cell. There is movement in and out of cells. Material within the cells moves around. If a cell gets squeezed on one side, it can move contents to the other side so the cell is not destroyed. It can move electrolytes across the cell membrane to maintain the necessary chemical structure. The cell strives to maintain a dynamic equilibrium. In fact, Lewin's early sketches of the concept of a psychological field were not unlike artistic renditions of a single cell.

Lewin used the term *psychological forces* to discuss the energy that keeps a field in equilibrium. There are two basic types of psychological forces—driving forces and restraining forces. When the sum of the driving forces balances the sum of the restraining forces, the system is in equilibrium. Any time the equilibrium of a psychological field is disturbed, these forces are operating.

The *driving forces* are the forces moving the system toward a goal, and *restraining forces* are those that work to maintain the status quo. These two forces constitute the dynamic nature of any psychological field. They pull in opposite directions within the situation with the full intent of maintaining the stability of the system. The balance between these two forces defines any established level of behavior whether the subject is an individual, an organization, or a community. *Equilibrium* is the state that occurs when the countering forces in both directions are balanced (i.e., when a push in one area is balanced by a pull in another area).

Consider the following situation. A registered nurse completed her prelicensure nursing education 10 years ago. She is satisfied with her managerial position with a local home health agency. Her husband's teenage daughter from a previous marriage provides occasional after-school child care for the three younger children. Her husband is a troubleshooter for a computer company and often is out of town 2 or 3 days per week. Family routines are working. There is time for homework, time for work, and time for play. Life is good. The horizontal line in the figure below illustrates this stable current level of functioning.

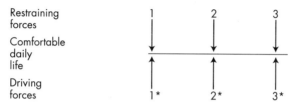

The vertical lines represent the driving and restraining forces; these are the forces at work to keep this family's life in this pleasant state. The forces that would push to create more "happiness" are balanced by those that work to keep life as it is.

The driving forces (1*, 2*, and 3*) are the vectors that could push for change in the current state of affairs. Driving forces could include such things as (1*) encouraging the husband to be home more to share in this happiness, (2*) the teenage daughter's making the high school volleyball team with after-school practices, and (3*) the television set's breaking.

The restraining forces (1, 2, and 3) are the forces that encourage the family to continue to function as they are doing. Restraining forces in this situation could include such things as (1) a daily schedule that goes smoothly, (2) a decrease in income if travel days are reduced, and (3) the cooperation of all family members.

When a system is percolating along in balance, it is described as being *frozen*. The system is not frozen in the sense that nothing is moving; it is still functioning. The system is just continuing to do things the way it always has done them. The registered nurse and her current state of affairs are frozen, but when some event occurs for which the system has had little experience (i.e., a change is required), the tried and true behaviors no longer achieve the desired equilibrium.

Let's rearrange the personal psychological field of the registered nurse described above. Assume the home health agency has had a change in ownership. Now add that the registered nurse is thinking of returning to school for another degree (whether the degree would be a BSN, an MSN, or a PhD is not relevant at this point). She has wanted this particular degree for as long as she can remember and is confident that further education will improve her professional practice. The horizontal line once again represents the current pattern of behavior (i.e., continuing to work in the home health agency with satisfaction,

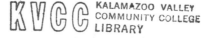

enjoying her blended family, sufficient income, and so on). However, additional driving and restraining forces (arrows) have been added.

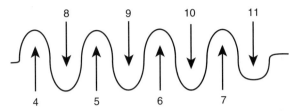

Driving forces that would support the decision to return to school could be personal fulfillment (4), delivery of better health care (5), career options if the operation of the agency deteriorates (6), and increased income (7). Restraining forces would include less time with family (8), the need for assistance with child care (9), added stress due to classwork (10), and doubts about whether she can succeed (11). If the driving forces are stronger in total than the restraining forces, she will return to school. If the restraining forces are more powerful, she will decide not to return to school.

These additional forces create an imbalance. The system's equilibrium is altered. The stability is disrupted. The pattern of behavior is unfrozen. The move from a stable (frozen) state to a fluid (unfrozen) state may be the result of a change in magnitude of any single force, a change in the direction of any force, or the addition of a new force. Tension is created. System members ask, If a change is needed, does that mean we have been doing things incorrectly? A threat exits. There is discomfort. If the restraining forces are more powerful for the registered nurse (she decides not to return to school), the family's stability will be restored but not necessarily at a level identical to the previous one.

The new driving force creates the "right time" for the family to think about the registered nurse's return to school. When the idea of returning to school was first considered, there was no cognitive structure for "mom/wife in school." Going back to school did not fit. No one knew how to incorporate this new region into the system's field. Ambiguity and uncertainty were the result. As the family system works with the possibility of adding the activity of school, different strategies for managing the needs of the family would be considered. New regions and new cognitive structures would be added to the family's field.

Facing something new is anxiety provoking because it is unknown. The system does not know how to proceed. The existence of this fluid state, of some level of tension, or of some level of discomfort is a necessary step in the process of change. Change includes those actions taken to reestablish equilibrium. The new level of behavior then refreezes until something occurs to create a new and different imbalance. This process repeats itself over and over.

Leaders recognize and capitalize on this process at two points with well-timed behavior. The most obvious time to act is when the system is fluid. The system (be it an individual, a group, or an organization) wants direction. Leaders will provide it. Timing in this case rests in being well prepared. The leader needs to know the desired direction and have strategies in place to move in that direction. A leader prepared to fill the void has time on his or her side.

The second strategic point for action occurs earlier in the process but is neither as obvious nor so easily implemented. This action point occurs when the system is comfortably stable. There is no discomfort. The most commonly heard expression during these times of stability is, "If it isn't broken, don't fix it." However, a system that is perpetually comfortable does not grow. So occasionally, it is the responsibility of a leader to create a little discomfort or a little tension, to shake things up a bit. Look around you. Is the system in which you work, study, or live making steady progress toward one of its stated goals (it doesn't have to be gargantuan steps—just slow, steady movement)? Is the system out of sync with what is going on around it? If one answers "no" to the first question or "yes" to the second one, it is time to throw some pebbles onto the smooth surface. Creating a different (new) situation by disrupting the existing one will force new patterns of response.

Lewin's force field theory provides a mechanism for determining when to act. The guidelines are simple:

- Stay in the present.
- Assess all of the operating factors.
- Determine the magnitude of the forces maintaining the status quo and the magnitude of the forces that are not satisfied with the status quo.
- Determine what regions and cognitive structures are available for use in the situation.

Lewin's force field principles provide a heuristic device for understanding how situations unfold and for recognizing their dynamic nature. The next step would be the provision of some specific guidelines for leaders who choose to operate within such a framework. Contingency theory can point to some factors to be considered.

Contingency Theory

"Contingency is the term that best describes social outcomes, and implies social forms are neither pure happenstance or pre-determined" (Itzkowski, 1997, Preface). As stated earlier in this chapter, there was a long period in history during which human behavior was believed to be predetermined; therefore, little credence was given to environmental influences. This was followed by a much shorter period during which environmental influences were considered to be the dominant component of any human condition, and by structuring the environment a specific way, it was possible to overcome inborn characteristics. Both lines of thinking have the same problem; they attribute human behavior (including leadership) to a single set of forces.

Contingency theories modify the single-attribute focus by postulating that the behavior of individuals, groups, or organizations can best be structured and guided through an understanding of the interaction among various factors operating in the situation. The birth of contingency theory, as described in the following few paragraphs, illustrates the interaction of theoretical principles and situation specifics.

Contingency theory was born through the merging of classic management theory and the human relations movement. Classic management theory postulated that the best structure for any organization was hierarchical and highly formalized, with organizational life governed by detailed plans and systems laid down centrally (Donaldson, 1995). Many believed that organizations so structured would be successful, but not all were.

The hypothesis of the human relations movement of the early 1960s was that the lack of success in hierarchical designed organizations was due to a lack of participation by the workforce. The human relations vision of the organizational world was much more decentralized and informal. Organizational effectiveness, it was believed, would improve through a focus on individuals and the use of communication as a mechanism of participation and influence within the organization (Likert, 1961). Some organizations that operated within this framework were effective, and others were not.

Each school could point to research that supported its particular perspective. Eventually, the two research streams were melded to form the contingency theory of organizational structure. Further analysis identified the specific contingencies of size, operational technology, and rate of environmental change as critical elements in the structure of an organization. Alterations in these contingencies led to different structures for different organizations (Donaldson, 1995).

Donaldson's description of how this process was supposed to work evokes echoes of Lewin's force field analysis:

> A change of the contingency variables moves the organization out of fit into misfit—and hence from equilibrium into disequilibrium .... The cycle is one of an organization that is initially fit, a change in a contingency produces misfit and reduces performance, and the organization's structure is changed which leads to a new fit which restores equilibrium and performance (p. 33).

Thus, a classicist or a traditionalist relies solely on documented principles (or theory) when acting in a situation, whereas a contingency-based actor modifies those principles based on the idiosyncrasies of the given situation. For example, assume that an individual is experiencing cardiac irregularities. The principle is to eliminate caffeine. On this individual's birthday, colleagues bring a surprise—pizza and Pepsi. Given the contingencies of this particular situation (e.g., the working relationships, the kindness of and appreciation for colleagues, and how little caffeine has been consumed lately), our individual decides to ignore the principle and to drink the Pepsi.

Now think about possible contingencies in the realm of leadership. Leadership began to be analyzed when Lewin and Lippitt (1938) distinguished the autocratic leader from the democratic leader. During the past 60 years, other writers have conceptualized leadership styles in a variety of ways. Common variables addressed in a majority of the discussions of leadership styles are the leaders' attention to tasks and to relationships and the resulting effectiveness.

One end of this continuum describes an autocratic leader who is much more concerned with getting the task accomplished than with the involvement of the individuals working on the task. This leader creates and initiates the structure of the task, controls the flow of information, and controls the giving and denying of rewards. Picture Ebenezer Scrooze in the *Christmas Carol* as the stereotypical autocratic, task-centered leader.

At the other end of this continuum is the person-centered leader. This individual seeks information from followers and their participation in decision-making. The resulting organization is decentralized. The term *participatory leadership* was coined from this perspective on the continuum.

Across these typologies, the focus is on the leader or the individual occupying the leadership position—a version of the "great man" theory. A sense of determination infused this thinking. After evaluation of one's style of leadership, there was not much else one could do. An individual led in his or her style and hoped it worked in most situations or moved from position to position until one's niche was found. For example, a task-centered leader would be very successful in producing a funding request for a project, whereas a person-centered leader would be more successful in revising the organization's mission statement and 5-year goals. A massive personality restructuring was viewed as the only way to alter one's style.

Because attempts to change leaders were less than successful, factors in the situation began to be analyzed. Maybe the situation held some clues to why leaders differed in their effectiveness. Eventually, the presence of interactions between the situation and the leadership began to emerge and gave rise to contingency models of leadership.

Fiedler (1967) is the earliest contingency theorist associated with the behavior of leaders. He developed the "least preferred coworker" (LPC) instrument, which asked individuals to identify the characteristics of the person with whom they would least like to work. Low scores indicate a person who is task oriented, and a high score indicates one who is relationship focused. The effectiveness of a leader could be determined once one knew the individual's LPC score and the value of three other variables (contingencies):

- The degree of leader/member liking
- The degree of task structure
- The position power of the leader

Individuals who are more concerned with good human relations than with the absolute accomplishment of the task are more effective in situations where the value of these three factors is somewhat ambiguous. A situation is favorable to the relationship-oriented leader if (1) the leader is esteemed by the group being led, (2) the task has minimal structure, and (3) the leader has position legitimacy and power.

As the value of the three contingencies shifts, the situation begins to favor the task-oriented leader. Focusing on the task becomes effective when one of three conditions is present:

1. The task is very clear or very unclear.
2. The members have either strong positive or strong negative feelings about the leader.
3. The power of the position is either very strong or very weak.

Simply put, task-oriented leaders are best suited for situations that are at the extremes, whereas person-centered leaders are more effective in situations between the extremes. With this information, Fiedler (1967) originally emphasized the need to place individuals in those situations for which they would be best suited. Thus, a task-oriented leader should work in situations that were very favorable or very unfavorable, and a relationship-oriented leader should need to work in situations that were not polarized.

Fiedler's later thinking about leadership focused on training leaders to modify their preferred style of leadership or to modify the situation to increase the likelihood of success. Leaders would identify whether they were task or relationship oriented. Next, they would learn how to analyze and classify leadership situations in terms of situational control. Finally, they would learn strategies that were most effective given the fit between the situation and the style. Leaders could choose to alter their leadership style or change the situation to achieve the best results.

Fiedler's model has the largest body of relevant research, which has led to both support and criticism of the underlying concepts. Other contingency models characterize leadership in different terms and identify different contingencies to be considered in each situation. Vroom and Yetton (1973) focused on decision-making within groups under an autocratic, a consultative, or a group style of leadership while addressing eight situational factors. House's (1971, 1974) path-goal model specified that once the goal is determined, the leader ties rewards to the successful completion of steps along the path to the goal. The relevant contingent factors are the "personal characteristics of the followers, and the environmental pressures and task demands subordinates face in accomplishing work goals" (Hollander, 1978, p. 37). Hersey and Blanchard (1988) considered the readiness of followers when determining the balance of task and relationship skills needed by a leader in a specific situation.

The literature addressing contingency models continues to grow. The important concept to carry from this body of literature is that there are several factors at work in any given situation (e.g., leader's characteristics, follower characteristics, organizational goals, task goals) and that these factors do not operate independently. One must take into consideration each of the factors and how that factor interacts with the other factors.

Summary

Contingency models of leadership and Lewin's force field theory are easily linked. Both bodies of knowledge rely on the interaction of forces within a given situation to achieve a goal. But how do we use such concepts as contingencies, cognitive structuring, and driving and retraining forces to develop a sense of timing to guide our actions? A few generalized suggestions in response to this question follow.

■ Get Involved, Observe, and Think

Remember that much of the tension and discomfort in situations come from the lack of *cognitive structures* to guide the handling of the immediate situation. A variety of experiences build a variety of cognitive structures. The regions within your field that parallel the cognitive structures provide paths of possible action. A well-differentiated field (i.e., the presence of many cognitive structures) is very useful when a situational analysis based on one of the contingency models indicates the need for the leader to provide structure for a task. It is much easier to rely on an existing structure than to be forced to create one on the spot.

- *Get involved*—volunteer to join committees. Every school of nursing or health care organization begs for committee members.
- While working on the committee, *observe* the leader or leaders.
- *Think* about the following:
  1. What is the committee trying to do?
  2. What specific behaviors did the leader exhibit?
  3. What was the result?

As you repeat this exercise over and over (volunteer, observe, think), you will develop the cognitive structures that parallel regions within the field. You will be prepared for that day when you choose to step forward and become the leader. You will have a set of internal structures that will guide you in developing the necessary regions that will move the group along the path to its goal. Remember, having relevant cognitive structure minimizes anxiety and discomfort, which allows you to think more clearly and act more easily.

■ Assess the Strength of Forces Operating in a Specific Situation

You can start practicing this assessment now. There is no reason to wait until you are identified as a leader. Pick one of those committee meetings for which you volunteered. Identify the goal of a specific situation, and map out all of the factors that are operating.

For example, assume that the periodic review of the nursing curriculum stimulates a discussion about whether nursing care plans should continue to be taught. One force (restraining) supports continuing with the teaching of nursing care plans. The reasons offered include the consistency across faculty and the ease of generalizing from problem solving and the nursing process to care plans. A driving force expresses the minimal use of nursing care plans in health care agencies and the growing use of clinical/care pathways as evidence for eliminating the teaching of nursing care plans.

Determine the magnitude of the forces maintaining the status quo (care plans) and the magnitude of the forces that are not satisfied with the status quo (no care plans). Sometimes these forces are more easily identified by their given names, e.g., Kristin or Bob, but if you look beyond the personalities you will find different versions of the same force. Sometimes the expressions are restraining, such as "X has a long tradition here," "Y will be difficult to implement; students, faulty members, or administrators won't like Y." Sometimes the driving forces are expressed, such as "B is really hot—we should implement it," "We need to be at the forefront of this movement."

Review the options you have accumulated through earlier observations. You have heard enough in the hallways and during lunch to realize that a big part of the discussion in support of traditional care plans is concern about available resources for teaching clinical/care pathways content.

You attend the next faculty meeting and listen intently. A comment is made about clinical/care pathways being implemented in Smith Hospital. You choose to act. You nudge the discussion toward the inclusion of clinical/care pathway instruction with comments like "Their [Smith Hospital] library has some excellent resources. They have offered to lend them to us. I'll be glad to arrange it if you like." The faculty's discussion moves to the use of these resources rather than additional debates regarding the inclusion or exclusion of care plans.

Your comments addressed one of the concerns (restraining forces) about a proposed change. The discussion shifted from the change itself to how to use resources. You chose the right action at the right time. The timing was "right on."

One cautionary note! Be wary of the twin traps: opposition (restraining force) equals wrong; change (driving force) equals right. Recognize both forces for what they are—forces that allow for continued functioning. Both are needed.

ONE LEADER'S EXPERIENCES IN ESTABLISHING THE BEST TIME FOR ACTION USING FORCE FIELD ANALYSIS AND CONTINGENCY THEORY

The first time within my nursing career that I considered the timing of an action to be relevant occurred during nursing school. It was toward the end of one clinical rotation, with the pediatric rotation being next. The pediatric instructors asked to meet me. I was no different from any other student. I immediately became anxious. What could they want? I hadn't even been on the unit yet. What had I done?

I met with the instructors. My fears were groundless. They had a proposal. Rather than being assigned to one pediatric unit for the entire time, they wanted to know if I would be willing to rotate through three units. I had to think about this request. One of the clinical expectations was the ability to manage care on the assigned unit. The hospital was a large teaching university and a regional medical center. The three units were large and usually had a full census. What was the risk? I stepped back to look.

The restraining forces were that (1) there was no really good reason to change the way things were going, (2) I would be risking my grade by exposing myself to the unknown pressures and stresses of learning the system on three units, and (3) the increased preparations necessary for a wide variety of clinical cases would result in a student's worse nightmare—more homework!

The driving forces were that (1) I wouldn't be as bored as I would be on one clinical unit, (2) I might impress the faculty, (3) the proposal was an opportunity to participate in some really interesting learning, and (4) the faculty must have had confidence that I could succeed or they would not have asked me to consider the possibility.

Strange as it may sound, I did think the situation through using a basic force field analysis. I considered all of the options and their relative weights (values). I was still vacillating. I talked it over with my roommate of 3 years; her comment clinched support for the driving forces. "Do it. You're dying to see if you can, anyway."

I agreed to participate. The other students agreed shortly after I did. I thoroughly enjoyed the challenge of the clinical experiences and learned much more about the problems confronting children and their families than if I had spent the entire rotation on a single unit. It was the right action at the right time.

The force field assessment led me to that decision by making it possible for me to list the driving forces (pushing me to take the challenge) and the restraining forces (wanting me to continue as I was doing). What I had not realized at the time was that my roommate's comment exemplified a principle of force field theory: It is more effective to strengthen a driving force than it is to minimize a restraining force. Her one comment reinforced one of the driving forces and had more value than multiple repetitions of "don't worry about your grade" and "you'll do fine," which would have had the intent of minimizing a restraining force.

A second experience that triggered questions of timing occurred during my second year as a registered nurse. I was working as an office nurse in a private practice of four physicians. The staff consisted of the four physicians, two registered nurses, an office manager, and an attorney/accountant who worked for several partnerships in the building complex.

I was the youngest and the least experienced of the group. The other registered nurse was in her early 40s. The office manager was in her mid-to-late 30s and had completed 2 years of a 3-year diploma program in nursing. The physicians were all in their mid 40s (two internists, one surgeon, and one obstetrician/gynecologist).

Two separate but connected incidents occurred that required action. I will share both simply because they occurred in the same professional situation and they provide a good contrast regarding timing.

The first incident involved the appearance of a radiologist at the office. He wore street clothes and began looking through some charts that were on the desk. I was seated at the desk working on other charts. I had never met this man and asked who he was. He told me he was Dr. So-and-so, the radiologist, and we each returned to work. Later I was called aside by the office manager and given two recommendations: (1) do not confront consultants, and (2) stand when physicians enter the room. Given the year this event occurred, this advice was not quite as ludicrous as it sounds now, but I still faced the same choices I would today. I could share my view of the advice ("This is preposterous!"), or I could shrug my shoulders and continue with the day. Some knowledge of contingency theory would have been helpful, but I had not heard of any such theory at the time this incident occurred. I had never before encountered such a situation and had no ready response. I remember thinking, "This is not the time to challenge this advice," so I muttered some inane comment and went about my business.

How would I frame the situation if I were operating from a field theory or contingency perspective? The field of this situation included the office manager, the employment environment, and myself. I had no previous experience with a comparable situation; therefore, I had no readily available cognitive structure. A preliminary assessment would have tallied the driving and restraining forces that would be operating (e.g., impose the logic of my reasoning about patient confidentiality [driving] or be out of a job [restraining]). A review of some operating contingencies would have fleshed out the above information. The following would have been included:

1. Although I had no intention of following the advice about challenging consultants given the same circumstances, the situation had a low probability of repeating itself. The radiologist in question was one of two who consulted with this practice. I had now met both of them and would have no need to ask either to identify themselves again.

2. The authority issue in this situation was not clear. The manager and I had had previous conversations about our respective backgrounds in nursing that were exacerbated by our current positions; the office manager had the authority that came with her position, whereas I was in a position of personal authority.
3. The goal (or task) of this encounter was clear. She needed to convey office expectations, and I had met my goal of protecting the patient.
4. The relationship between the two of us was one of toleration mandated by the work environment. There was a low probability that anything that I would have said would have been heard (i.e., the situation was in a frozen state).

I doubt that I would act much different today. My comments would be more easily heard because I am more skilled at being able to say "I hear you" without challenging the message. The timing was not right for a confrontation. The next situation (which occurred in the same office) highlights the right time for the confrontation.

Not too long after the advice-giving incident, a patient was seen by one of the internists. At the conclusion of the examination of the young man, the physician gave me instructions to prepare and administer a specified amount of intramuscular penicillin. I verified the dosage and mentioned that this dose would require two injections because our stock of penicillin would require 5 mL of suspension to reach the required dosage. The response was, "Yes, that is the correct dose. He has gonorrhea. But give it to him in one injection so he'll think twice about !x%!y#@!"

I thought fast. I was able to ignore the language. I had been a nurse in psychiatric settings for too long for the language to bother me. My goal? Medicate the patient in the most efficient and safe way, which would be one 2.5-mL injection in each hip based on the rationale that this would offer the best absorption given the amount of medication and the size of the muscle. His goal? Treat and punish. I could see no reason to risk the effectiveness of the medication or to provide an indirect punishment. The driving and restraining forces were

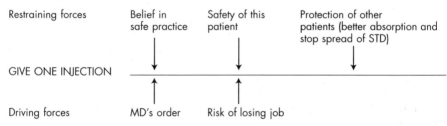

My response was to tell the physician I could not administer the medication in one injection. I would gladly administer the dosage in two injections, or I would bring him the supplies and he could administer the larger injection. He muttered, "Oh, all right" and stomped off. I prepared the two injections, administered them, and sent the patient on his way. I had acted in the best interest of the patient and thought the incident was finished.

The next day, the office manager requested that I stop in and see her. As soon as I was seated, she informed me that she was reprimanding me for my actions of the previous day. Further discussion revealed that the physician had shared with her the situation regarding the intramuscular penicillin. The office manager, not the physician, had decided that my behavior was insubordinate and warranted a reprimand. I explained the reasoning underlying my action and was told that my reasoning was not important; I was expected to follow orders. I signed the reprimand form after noting that I did not agree with its conclusions and that I would be seeking consultation in the matter.

I had to take into consideration the forces that were restraining me. What were those things that were telling me "don't rock the boat?" These were simple to list:

1. I had recently married, moved to California from the Midwest, and needed the job.
2. I was still a young, somewhat inexperienced registered nurse—maybe protocols had changed in the administration of penicillin.
3. Maybe the California nurse practice laws were different from the state where I had practiced previously.

On the other hand, the factors that were encouraging me to act were less easily articulated: (1) I made good decisions, (2) I was intelligent, (3) nurses are responsible for the actions they take, and (4) nurses are advocates for patients. The latter two tipped the balance for me. I was important in the health care delivery system and was not going to be censured until it was demonstrated to me that I was wrong.

I called the state nurses' association and eventually met with a recommended attorney. The opinion of the attorney was that my practice could not be reprimanded by a person who was not a licensed nurse or physician. This information was shared with the office manager, who refused to rescind the reprimand. I then initiated a meeting with the attorney/accountant who was the business manager and explained the situation to him. I explained that I was prepared to take whatever action was necessary to have the reprimand removed from my personal file.

Three weeks passed. Things were a bit cool in the office during the working hours. I had shared with the other registered nurse what was occurring, and we continued to work together well. Conversation between the physicians, the office manager, and myself were very brief and totally related to the care of the patients.

Finally, the business manager asked to see me. He had met with the partners, and the consensus was that the reprimand would be removed from my file. No mention of the existence of any such document would remain. I thanked him and returned to the office to complete the day's work. The next morning, I gave 2 weeks' notice of my resignation.

What was different about this second situation? Why was the time right for confrontation? The confrontation related to the patient was necessary because of my responsibility as a nurse. I had to control my practice within expected legal parameters. The timing of my resignation was right because the risk of being terminated had increased greatly. I had established my expectations of my practice, and they did not match the agency's expectations. There was no reason to believe that the environment in the agency was unfreezing (in Lewin's terms) as a first step toward change. For me to remain in control of my professional life, I needed to leave. So I did.

A third situation in which I actually used force field analysis and contingency theory occurred approximately 2.5 years after the incident in the physician's office. It is a bit more humorous than the last situation but still highlights the essence of timing. By this time, I had been employed in another agency in California, had completed a master's degree in community/mental health nursing, and had been hired as a faculty member in a school of nursing.

One other psychiatric nursing faculty member and I were hired for the same fall term. We were oriented, read course texts, prepared lectures, organized clinical experiences, and attended faculty meetings. Faculty meetings were all day on Fridays. No one taught on Fridays, so the only people in the area occupied by the nursing school were the faculty and the secretaries. Both of us, as new faculty, observed our environment, realized that we needed to learn the role of faculty member, and followed the lead of the senior faculty in our manner of dress on Fridays. We dressed as we would dress to teach or to participate in other faculty business (i.e., suits and dress shoes).

One morning in late fall, I was more tired than usual. The long days in trying to keep all of the bits of information together had taken their toll on me. I awakened late and knew that I had very little time to get to the faculty meeting. I did not want to be late. If I took the time to dress as I had been, I would be late. If I dressed more casually, I would be on time. I considered my options: Is this the time to take a risk? If I violate what I perceive to be an unwritten dress code, will I risk inclusion as a faculty member? Will I risk favorable evaluations on other activities? Will I risk a negative tenure decision in 5 years? If I am late and disrupt the meeting by walking in late, what will be the consequences of inclusion, evaluations, and the tenure decision? Weighing the contingencies (importance of total faculty involvement in team building during curriculum revision, no leadership status, a position with no power) led me to a decision. I pulled on my jeans, a sweater, and boots and went to the faculty meeting. I made it on time (barely); as I was looking around the room, I saw the other new faculty member also had on jeans and a sweater.

Later, as we discussed this coincidence, we found that we had worked through the decision-making process pretty much the same way and had reached the conclusion that it was the right time to act. We decided that we were far enough away from the tenure decision for the risk to be minimal. If the feedback was such that we knew we had overstepped the boundaries, we could mend our ways and dress in a less-casual fashion on future Fridays. We were both very task-oriented individuals with no positional power, which meant our choosing to dress differently was not going to create concern for any other faculty member. We realized that there was some disapproval, but to this day, we do not know if the disapproval was focused on the attire or on the thought that we had planned to dress comparably. Within 2 months, the majority of the faculty members were dressing more casually for faculty meetings. Leadership often comes in strange guises. We had not intended to initiate change, but our behavior that day created a new way of facing the work on Fridays.

The fourth experience with an element of timing that I would like to share occurred 10 years later. As a tenured associate professor, I had taken an active role in many aspects of the school of nursing. I also had participated in the university faculty senate and had just completed a second term of office when a vacancy occurred on the oversight committee for general education. I chose to be considered for the position.

The timing was right. The vacancy needed to be filled by a faculty member from the area of the university where nursing was administratively housed. The contingency factors were favorable for my being appointed. I was in a position of strong leadership within the college. My high profile through college-level committees and task forces had given me recognition power. The faculty in the college had strong positive feelings about me. The task was clearly within my domain. I had a strong interest in general education and had a strong preparation in literature and philosophy that would provide me with credibility on the committee. I was appointed to the committee.

With all of these factors screaming "act now," I still could have chosen not to act. I could have been silent and operated from the premise that was not uncommon. "Why would anyone want to serve on that committee? They had long committee meetings. Someone was always complaining about the decisions they made. There were enormous stacks of material to read." Again, I return to the analysis of the balance of the driving and restraining forces.

Here was an opportunity to create a small chink in the stereotypical perception of nurses as good-hearted individuals whose only interests are those of caring for the ill.

My experiences on the general education committee were successful and highlight a very clear example of timing. Take a personally held goal, mix it with a situational opportunity that has strong driving forces and a combination of contingency factors that best match one's leadership style, and act.

The fifth and final situation I want to share is of a slightly different nature. Not all actions taken by leaders are perceived by the individuals affected as being positive. Not all decisions to act occur in situations where all of the pieces come together to create an ideal time to act.

Nursing as a discipline has been found in institutions of higher education since the beginning of the century, but it has only been since the mid-to-late 1960s that nursing as a discipline has been located in colleges and universities in any number. As with all new endeavors, whether individually or discipline based, new behaviors need to be learned. Nursing faculties have had to learn how to balance a heavy teaching workload with the scholarly and service demands of being a university faculty. It was not, and is not, uncommon for the realities of these demands to clash with the university merit salary system. The designated leader can be caught in the middle of these two sets of expectations.

Imagine the following scenario. A small group of nursing faculty are teaching in a university with a historically strong undergraduate teaching focus. The institution is moving toward a more universal expectation that all faculty members will participate in all aspects of the academic role. For the faculty in nursing (and other applied disciplines), this means a shift in thinking and behavior. This shift is difficult to make and, given the other demands of the academic role, becomes low priority.

Annually, faculty members compile and summarize a dossier describing their activities of the preceding year. A personnel committee reviews the dossiers and gives the information to the school's administrator. Letters based on the data in these dossiers are sent to all faculty, summarizing the school's accomplishments of the past year and individual contributions to those accomplishments. These data are the basis for annual salary decisions with tenure and promotion decisions requiring a separate process.

Several annual letters had gone to the faculty encouraging them to increase both their professional service and scholarly activities. Minimal progress had been seen. Two years of allocating the university's standard salary increase for "satisfactory" performance had created no change in scholarly or service activity. A variety of other inducements had been offered, such as payment for travel to professional meetings, proposals of planned work that would lead to a term of lighter teaching load, restructuring the teaching load, collegial assistance, and so on. Activity still did not change. Obviously, what I perceived to be driving forces were not functioning in that manner.

Brainstorming, consulting with others, thinking, and more thinking produced no obvious change. In desperation, I decided that I would not use all of one year's available pool of funds in the school for salary raises. Some of the monies were returned to the college and allocated in other areas. The reasoning behind my action was to unfreeze the current situation. I believed that if the situation became more fluid, the probability for directed action would increase.

It worked. Individual faculty members actively pursued a variety of professional and scholarly tasks. The energy increased. However, the action and its consequences increased the demands on me. To carry out the action required a change in preferred leadership style. I had to be more directive than I prefer to behave with colleagues. I had to address some very specific concerns related to the relationship between workload and the merit salary system. The contingencies were still operating, but the polarization was the reverse of the earlier experiences I have shared. The task (workload) was not clear. The leader-member liking diminished. I, the leader, operated from a position of strength. One of the possible consequences of taking the right action at the right time is that the leader may increase his or her own level of stress.

CONCLUSION

Taking the right action at the right time is a complex task. Timing requires a leader to continually work on self-development. Gaining more experience creates cognitive structures that allow the leader to be more comfortable in a variety of situations. The increased comfort paves the way for a clearer and more accurate assessment of the various forces that are operating in a specific situation. Many of these driving and restraining forces are described in other chapters of this book (e.g., preferred level of risk taking or one's vision) and are to be included in the assessment of any situation. Additionally, a well-developed sense of self-knowledge allows the leader to recognize the match between leadership style and the contingencies of any given situation. This information will guide actions.

The key word in the preceding paragraph is "guide." There is no formula that will provide a leader with the perfect calculation of the right time to act. Thinking through the facets of timing that have been described in this chapter will increase one's chances of delivering the right action at the right time. Once this exercise in thinking has been completed, I add one more piece of advice: I consider the following from the *Talmud* to be important:

If not this, what?
If not now, when?
If not me, who?

REFERENCES

Bass, B. M. (1981). *Stodgill's handbook of leadership: A survey of theory and research*. New York: The Free Press.

Bennis, W. (1981*). Managing people is like herding cats*. Provo, Utah: Executive Excellence Publishing.

Bennis, W. G., Bennis, K. D., & Chin, R. (Eds.) (1969). *The planning if change*. (2nd ed.). New York: Holt, Rhinehart & Winston.

Deutsch, M. (1968). Field theory in social psychology. In Lindzey, G., & Aronson, E. (Eds.). *The handbook of social psychology*. Reading, Mass.: Addison-Wesley.

Donaldson, L. (1995). *American anti-management theories of organization: A critique of paradigm proliferation*. Cambridge, U.K.: Cambridge University Press.

Drucker, P. F. (1968). *The practice of management*. New York: Harper & Row.

Fiedler, F. E. (1967). *A theory of leadership effectiveness*. New York: McGraw-Hill.

Hersey, P., & Blanchard, K. (1988). *Management of organizational behavior: Utilizing human resources* (5th ed.). Englewood Cliffs, N.J.: Prentice-Hall.

Hollander, E. P. (1978). *Leadership dynamics: A practical guide to effective relationships*. New York: The Free Press.

House, R. J. (1971). A path-goal theory of leader effectiveness. *Administrative Science Quarterly, 16*, 321–338.

House, R. J., & Mitchell, T. R. (1974). Path-goal theory of leadership. *Journal of Contemporary Business, 3*, 81–97.

Itzkowitz, G. (1997*). Contingency theory: Rethinking the boundaries of social thought*. Lanham: University Press of America.

Lewin, K. (1951). *Field theory in social science*. New York: Harper.

Lewin, K. (1947). Group decision and social change. In Newscomb, T., & Hartley, E. (Eds.). *Readings in social psychology*. New York: Henry Holt.

Lewin, K., & Lippitt, R. (1938). An experimental approach to the study of autocracy and democracy: A preliminary note. *Sociometry, 1*, 292–300.

Likert, R. (1961). *New patterns of management*. New York: McGraw-Hill.

Peck, M. S. (1978). *The road less traveled*. New York: Simon and Schuster.

Vroom, V. H., & Yetton, P. W. (1973). *Leadership and decision-making*. Pittsburgh, Pa.: University of Pittsburgh Press.

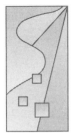

Chapter 8

Seeing Change as an Opportunity

Carol M. Rehtmeyer

Change! Who wants it, who needs it, and who asked for it? We usually are not prepared for it, cannot control it, and do not like it. Even though we know that change is inevitable and not based on our own personal needs, seldom are we prepared for many of the events that occur. What is happening to our health care system today is an excellent example of change that is hard to understand, hard to accept, and definitely not wanted. Nurses who want to take the lead must be able to see these changes as opportunities and not as threats and be willing to move even though there is risk. Understanding what is happening and knowing that some nurses have been able to see change as an opportunity help make the changes more tolerable.

Interest in and tolerance of change vary and depend on the approach's not being judged as good or bad; however, once change is viewed as an inevitable fact of life, then steps can be taken to learn how to view the change in a positive way. Changes in health care and the work environment, which must be dealt with and cannot be avoided, can be seen as opportunities that should be embraced, rather than as threats that must be avoided.

Because every change situation contains personal, professional, and organizational change dimensions, the nurse must be prepared to address these aspects of any change. To start, nurses must determine how much risk, change, and challenge they are willing to assume. For those who are motivated by change, there are plenty of opportunities in the health care environment that are both challenging and rewarding. For those who are less inclined to address change, there are skills that can be learned to help them. However, determining the degree of risk, the kind of risk (e.g., professional, financial, personal, and organizational), and how to effectively deal with the results of any change effort are paramount to the satisfactory outcome of any change venture, whether it is actively embraced or reluctantly pursued.

The stories told in this chapter focus on how a nurse made a change while having a growth-producing experience because she saw change as an opportunity. Even though some of the changes encountered and the risks taken were not expected or desired, the outcomes were positive. The nurse involved in the change and risk chose to use these situations as opportunities to learn and grow, to make long dreamt-about decisions to take entrepreneurial risks, and to change her working environment for the better.

BACKGROUND

Health care is one of the most volatile industries. Job satisfaction among health care workers is at its lowest level (Izzo and Klein, 1998). Some of the factors influencing job stress in health care workers include

- Increased economic pressure to maintain or reduce operating margins, which causes pressure to do "more with less"; this means fewer staff, fewer supplies, and less support but more demand for productivity.
- Tremendous pressure from purchasers of health care for lower prices for goods and services, better quality of service, more consumer-based information on available choices, and state-of-the-art technology
- Industry-wide anxiety as the health care environment struggles to become market oriented rather then politically driven by those in power (e.g., physicians, health care systems)

These changes have forced health care to operate more and more like a business, creating a climate that threatens the once unquestioned judgment of physicians. Health care has been placed into a cost/benefit framework in which the values for these parameters have not been identified, quantified, or agreed on. The work environment of nurses, physicians, and other professional health care workers has become that of a free market. For instance, because the cost of labor in health care (the largest single cost component) is subject to alterations in supply and demand, nurses receive bonuses for recruiting fellow nurses one month, then are asked to take off unpaid days to adjust for lowered patient census within the same calendar year.

My experience is a good example of how unexpected change can occur. One day, I was asked to resign from my position even though I had successfully accomplished all of the tasks and goals set for me. I had just been appointed chief operating officer of an independent physician group of nearly 180 physician members. Those who worked closely with me knew that my performance was exemplary. My boss, however, never gave me credit for what I did, and I learned later that he had even deceived me. On this day, he said, "It is either you or me and it is not going to be me." Although I took great satisfaction in telling him what I thought of him, I knew I did not have any interest in pursuing grievance actions. I told him I needed time to think about the situation and left after scheduling a meeting with him for the next day. The weeks that followed were spent negotiating a settlement.

This event changed my life in ways I never could have imagined. This personal and professional crisis provided me with opportunities and challenges that allowed me to (1) start my own business, (2) hire nursing professionals who are able to grow in areas they have only dreamed about, (3) provide services in the exciting new field of telehealth, and (4) receive one of the largest professional guaranteed small business loans ever awarded to a nurse. I know

now that unexpected change, although frightening, can be an opportunity in disguise.

But how do other nurses effectively cope with these unprecedented changes and remain dedicated professionals with the patient's welfare as their primary concern? And how can nurses take more control of their professional lives and provide the leadership for health so necessary in these times of dramatic change? The answers to these questions are what this chapter is all about; it is through a framework of personal, organizational, and professional empowerment that the responses evolve.

FRAMEWORK OF THE CHAPTER

The chapter is organized into three sections:

1. Personal steps to positive change: how to manage unexpected change based on the concepts of empowered risk taking
2. Organizational steps to positive change: the ingredients and actions essential for the creation of an empowered and proactive work culture based on the writings of Peter Senge, Margaret Wheatley, and Peter Block
3. Professional steps to positive change: one nurse's story about seizing opportunity using the concepts of individual empowered risk taking and the strategies necessary for the creation of an empowered work culture

Based on the concepts of personal empowerment and risk taking, the first section, Personal Steps to Positive Change, provides readers with a framework for placing their own times of turmoil and disappointment into a context of opportunity wherein growth and creativity can occur. For those who have not had a similar experience, this section is an opportunity for them to examine their lives in anticipation of the unexpected. Additionally, readers can complete an assessment of their current aptitude for the uncertainty inherent in new ventures, which would include looking at their strengths and areas for improvement.

The second section, Organizational Steps to Positive Change, describes the kind of organizational framework necessary for the creation of an empowered and proactive work group, an element considered to be essential in the development of a nurse business. The importance of a culture of stewardship, a strong vision and mission statement as the driving force, a customer service orientation, systems thinking, clear operational boundaries, respectful communication, a focus on group outcomes and processes, the reinforcement of personal accountability, and risk taking as a growth opportunity are discussed.

The third section of this chapter, Professional Steps to Positive Change, is my story about how I empowered myself to move forward in the development of an entrepreneurial endeavor. It includes how I used empowered risk taking (self-caring, reading the opportunity, taking the challenge, and recycling) and organizational empowerment (the ingredients and actions necessary for the creation of an empowered workplace) to establish WellComm, a telehealth business.

PERSONAL STEPS TO POSITIVE CHANGE: HOW TO MANAGE UNEXPECTED CHANGE BASED ON THE CONCEPTS OF EMPOWERED RISK TAKING

Having a personal feeling of empowerment and the ability to look favorably at situations regardless of the presence of risk are important skills for those facing change. *To empower* is to give power, strength, control, or authority (Oxford Dictionary and Thesarus, 1996). When people empower themselves, they fuel their own ability to direct their own lives. Being empowered enables the individual to take on challenging situations that might appear to others as risky. Accepting challenging experiences that require reaching beyond our previous experiences, to create something new or to try something where the successful outcome is not guaranteed, creates a feeling of empowerment.

Health care is challenging and full of situations in which the outcomes are not clear. Even when things lack clarity, the nurse can have control and feel empowered to take action. For instance, it is a personal decision nurses must make to determine how, when, where, and how much risk they wish to have in their lives. Furthermore, they have the right and responsibility to determine their "risk tolerance" and the best setting, job, culture, and level of responsibility they wish to pursue. Even when there are circumstances that limit choice, such as geography and family, the "risk tolerance" can be determined partially by these circumstances. Clearly, nurses have choices about where and how they can position themselves for success. They can decide to struggle with challenge with all of its unknowns, they can perceive themselves as powerless and let others make the decisions, or they can pursue the opportunity as a growth-producing experience. Empowered nurses choose the latter.

Should the nurse choose to be a leader, dealing with continual change is *not* optional. Whether the nurse feels empowered and takes on challenging situations or successfully pursues new and unknown activities that are risky and ends up feeling empowered, every nurse leader must view the pursuit of challenges as a critical skill for success, regardless of the outcome in these times of change.

Using the Four Elements of Empowered Risk Taking

Many well-known and highly qualified people have written about personal empowerment (Houston, 1998; Peck, 1985; Tracy, 1995). The number of books written about self-help and self-improvement testify to the tremendous interest in self-care. Self-care is a personal journey that allows people to acknowledge, honor, and support their own attributes. For example, some people have strong creative and leadership skills, whereas others are blessed with analytical skills. Experts in the area of empowerment suggest that this ability to care for self should be used to enhance the personal strengths of the individual so she or he can accept risk and actively face change. One way to do this is to pursue empowered risk taking by (1) caring for self, (2) reading the opportunities, (3) taking the challenge, and (4) continuing to cycle items 1 to 3.

Once the four processes of empowered risk taking are mastered, a plan for personal development must be undertaken. There is nothing more important for nurses in health care today than the need to take risks and to do so while promoting their own positive personal growth. Thus, the real issue is beyond learning about empowered risk taking; it is *doing* it.

■ Caring for Self

If one is lucky or undertakes a project that does not have an extended time frame between the establishment of the goal and its accomplishment, the need for self-care is not much of an issue; however, there are not many projects of this kind. Usually, if one accomplishes a major goal within a short period of time, another more challenging goal awaits attention. Lately, the challenge to do more with less and to devise ways to do new things without more resources has created stress for nurses. If the nurse has adequate self-esteem, managing these challenges is not a problem. However, many nurses do not have sufficient self-esteem to sustain them during these times of personal and professional stress. The ability to care for oneself (boosting one's self-esteem) during these periods of stress is paramount. Because we are all potential change agents, the most important skill in caring for self during continuous change is to "know self" (Quinn, 1996).

Self-esteem, which is the valuing of self, is an acknowledgment of our worth and a gift we give ourselves. According to Branden (1994), self-esteem is the practice of living consciously and purposefully, with self-acceptance, self-responsibility, self-assertiveness, and personal integrity. A healthy self-esteem provides one with the ability to be rational, intuitive, creative, independent, flexible, benevolent, cooperative, and humble and to be able to manage change. He also says:

> When self-esteem is low, we are often manipulated by fear: fear of reality, to which we feel inadequate; fear of facts about ourselves—or others—that we have denied. disowned, or repressed; fear of the collapse of our pretenses; fear of exposure; fear of humiliation of failure; and sometimes the responsibilities of success (p. 47).

Nurses and other caregivers are often not skilled at boosting their self-esteem. They receive rewards for their actions externally and know little about self-care. They obtain what self-esteem they have from patients who tell them how wonderful they are when they make them comfortable. Conversely, when nurses take risks, many of their colleagues or superiors are not comfortable with the actions and are not supportive, thus negatively affecting the nurses' self-esteem. Nurses embroiled in change who want to effectively manage the turmoil and take risks must be experts at boosting their own self-esteem. This kind of action can only come from self and often involves nurturing a healthy relationship with self. Branden (1994) supports this by saying,

> The alternative to excessive dependence on the feedback and validation of others is a well-developed system of internal support. The attainment of this state is essential to what I understand as proper human maturity. Innovators and creators are persons who can, to a higher degree than average, accept the condition of aloneness . . . they are more willing to follow their vision . . . unexplored spaces do not frighten them (pp. 54–55).

This chapter is not intended to be about self-help. It is about empowering self to move beyond circumstances that are limiting. If nurses look to others for empowerment, they will not have personal resources to call on but rather will have to depend on others. Just as it is not helpful to look to others for self-esteem, it is not helpful to look to others for empowerment. The Serenity Prayer of St. Francis of Assisi nicely underscores this need for self-initiation:

God grant me the serenity
To accept things I cannot change,
Courage to change the things I can, and
Wisdom to know the difference.

The term *codependence* has been used and overused, but essentially codependence speaks to the problem of needing others to feel good about self. Mellody (1989), one of the world's renowned experts in codependence (and a nurse), calls self-care "self-love"; she says:

When you don't love yourself, when you don't have good boundaries, when you don't know how to be political or interdependent, you'll experience a lot of stress . . . . Self-love is the single most powerful lesson . . . . self-esteem affects everything about your whole life. . . . How you feel about yourself determines what kind of people you associate with, what you choose to do, how well you take care of yourself and others. . . . Love starts with the thought: I'm enough, I matter in spite of the fact I'm imperfect (p. 242).

To be a risk taker in nursing, one must have a wonderful relationship with self. To have the courage to change or to face changes over which you may have little control requires a strong self-image that is supported by self-care.

■ Reading the Opportunity

Reading the opportunity often conjures up the image of a Native American scout or Daniel Boone reading the subtle clues in the environment that other less-experienced travelers miss. Such experts have developed skill over time through careful observation, listening to older and wiser people, and pulling themselves out of nasty scrapes. The same can be true for nurses who want to be empowered risk takers. The experience of those who have been in the forefront of health care change can serve as excellent role models of how to survive and thrive in somewhat treacherous territory. Nurses can learn a lot from people who have learned that change is opportunity and are doing new and innovative things.

Keeping informed is another way to read opportunity. Being isolated, out of touch, and closed to events puts the nurse at a disadvantage when change occurs. Although change can be frightening, closing oneself off, as a protection, only keeps opportunity from the nurse. Like the scout, the nurse must be alert to what is happening, informed about the possibilities (not closed because of fear), and willing to leap when opportunity calls.

Watching and sharing what is going on are excellent ways to read opportunity. Even though nurses are where change is occurring, they often are so busy they miss opportunity. The stresses of the job, a culture of competition rather than cooperation, and a lack of sharing accomplishments often block nurses' views of opportunities. In addition, nurses are so pressured to maintain productivity standards, to justify costs of care, to demonstrate outcomes to payers and providers, and to work in settings with limited resources that they are turned off to what is going on and do not see opportunity in the midst of these demands.

Reading opportunity does not mean waiting for opportunity; the nurse must also be prepared by knowing about how she or he would handle success or failure if opportunity arose. Knowing that every choice has a tradeoff or consequence can help the nurse determine how she or he might respond if the choice were offered. Being prepared can turn what otherwise might be disastrous into a challenging and enjoyable situation. The following story illustrates this point: My brother and his family live on Lake Michigan in Chicago and have a boat that they sail on the lake. The lake is notorious for its unpredictable storms and choppy water, which can make boating very dangerous. When I asked my brother if these conditions made him less likely to take out the boat, he replied, "As long as I am prepared for the bad weather, I have no worries. In fact, preparation makes the excursions even more enjoyable if there is bad weather."

Readiness for reading opportunity is paramount to being able to pursue something new and different during change. One method for defining personal risk and evaluating how to act if opportunity arrives is to have thought about the answers to the following questions:

- What is my personal goal as a nurse clinician/nurse leader/nurse educator/ nurse businessperson?
- What is the personal and professional risk or opportunity in which I am interested, whether it is in the form of an offer or is still an idea?
- What are the best and worse possible outcomes of this opportunity?
- What is the probability of each outcome?
- What resources do I need or desire to successfully address this opportunity?

According to Wheatley (1992), this time of questioning and reflecting often is very painful because a good solution or approach may not be apparent. She goes on to say,

> You have to get into the messiness of the data before you see what it means. . . .
> I have been in enough experiences with groups of people where we have
> generated so much information that it's led us to despair and . . . deep
> confusion. I know now that's the place to be if you want to be really open to
> new thoughts . . . you can't get there without going through this period of
> letting go and confusion, For somebody who's been taught to be a good
> analytical thinker, this is always a very painful moment. . . . It's not healthy if
> you stay in it your whole life, but it can be healthy if it's part of your process
> of moving on, of letting things reconfigure (p. 250).

To feel confused, overwhelmed, and not certain about what you want or can do if opportunity knocks is part of the process and must be endured and pursued. It is also important to take time to feel the confusion or encounter the panic that is natural and then to accept and reflect on it and to let it go when facing alternatives that seem risky. Giving the most comfortable course of action time to gel in your mind is difficult but necessary. Keeping a journal and testing your options against your values and goals are two simple but important ways to focus on whether there is a readiness for taking on the challenge.

■ Taking the Challenge

The nurse who wants to accept the challenge, according to Campbell (1976) and his followers, must envision the action as a part of a larger quest called the hero's or heroine's journey. In this quest, the hero leaves the secure environment of the "known"; travels to the unknown, where he confronts challenges that forever change him; and returns home, bringing his new persona. Bateson (1990) takes a more feminist perspective and suggests the driving forces for women are more qualitative or community oriented. However, both Campbell and Bateson stress that each of us is motivated to take risks and wants to venture beyond the known and that fulfilling this desire is the key to personal happiness.

Taking the challenge often rests on how closely the opportunity fits with our personal professional self. Sinetar (1987) emphasizes the importance of personal vision as a driving force for career decisions in her book *Do What you Love and the Money Will Follow.* Sometimes it seems impossible to maintain personal core values in the health care environment, but if the challenge or opportunity enhances or does not violate our values, then it is worthy of consideration. Taking challenges using empowered risk is much more likely when the challenge is in harmony with one's personal vision.

After the test of consistency between the challenge and one's personal vision is met, the next step is to set timelines for pursuing the opportunity. Timelines must be process oriented, so the necessary steps toward the goal are included. Many people use GAANT or PERT charts as a way to plot ways the challenge or opportunity can be pursued. However, Wheatley (1992) points out that a fixation on goals can sometimes be limiting or even inappropriate. She says the focus should, instead, be on what is changing in the organization. Using this focus in conjunction with one's personal vision can help the nurse appropriately take the challenge. An analogous situation might be the pilot or sailor who must fix his gaze on the horizon while also checking the navigational instruments and adjusting the course as needed so the ship arrives at its destination.

Because taking the challenge is a highly personal activity, it is often a frightening experience. This is not a reason to avoid the venture; it is the beauty of it, because the venture can be crafted to meet the nurse's needs and liking. The nurse will have to be able to realistically identify the risks, make a commitment, garner support, adjust priorities, and deal with disappointment and turmoil, all while maintaining a positive attitude

Taking the challenge should not rest with the risk taker alone. The nurse traveling a new pathway needs personal resources; one needs energy, optimism, stamina, patience, friends, and courage (Peck, 1985; Tracy, 1995). New ventures do not happen over night, nor are they immediately successful. This is where friends come into the equation. Having friends to talk with, check out assumptions with, and console you is very, very important. They also give honest, even blunt, feedback.

There are some limitations when others are used as resources. The first is

Table 8-1. Model for Acquaintance, Colleague, and Friend Support

Type of Relationship	Suggested Activities for Support
Acquaintance	Attend meetings together.
	Discuss areas of shared professional interest.
Colleague	Collaborate on projects.
	Lobby for support.
	Develop strategic partnerships.
	Include in business or professional ventures.
Friend	Discuss personal vision and risks.
	Examine core values.
	Discuss organizational climate, which includes political and personal agendas.
	Risk financial, personal, and professional security together through business or professional ventures.

that it takes time to develop a network of trusted colleagues. Second, not all colleagues can be used in the same manner; some we confide in, others are good for reflection, and others are good for advice. Third, it is not usually possible to find someone who can provide all of these kinds of help. It is better to examine relationships along a continuum and to relate to each colleague based on what she or he brings to the relationship. Table 8–1 illustrates how each colleague may be expected to provide assistance when the challenge or opportunity is considered.

Last, the challenge or opportunity must be judged in terms of the organization and the culture in which it rests and whether they are congruent with one's own values and personal vision. The degree to which taking the opportunity will work often rests with whether the organizational culture allows or blocks personal growth. Empowered risk taking allows the nurse to evaluate the culture to determine whether it is open to change and personal advancement or, if the culture is closed, whether the risk is worth the energy it would take to modify the culture.

Regardless of how the quest is approached, the nurse can keep a positive perspective toward the desired goal when it is understood that progress is a spiral rather than a linear process (Sheehy, 1976, 1981). Success with risk taking occurs by understanding the difficult task of beginning, keeping an eye on the goal, and not losing faith. Often, when time seems to be passing without progress, a sudden surge of activity occurs, such as a response from a long-awaited prospect, an offer of backing, or both.

Another element to consider when confronted with challenge or opportunity is to realize that "no one is coming." Empowered people do not wait for others to do things for them or for conditions to be just right because they know that neither will occur. Branden (1994) says it well:

> If I don't do something nothing is going to get better. The dream of a rescuer who will deliver us may offer a kind of comfort, but it leaves us passive and powerless. We may feel if only I suffer long enough . . . yearn desperately

enough . . . a miracle will happen, but this kind of self deception one pays for with one's life as it drains away (p. 115).

Likewise, to pursue goals that are unrealistic even though the challenge or opportunity looks promising is foolhardy and demoralizing. The payoff for learning this lesson is that one's self-concept is left intact and the sense of empowerment is preserved. The Don Quixote experience of fighting unseen enemies and defending unwanted goals leads nowhere; instead, it is wiser to deal with the disappointment early and move on to other opportunities that have a higher probability of success. Also, it could be that the goals are worthwhile and appropriate but the timing is not right (Brandon, 1994).

Last, when taking the challenge, one must have courage. "Courage is the resistance to fear—mastery of fear—not absence of fear" (Mark Twain, *The Tragedy of Pudd'nhead Wilson,* Hartford, Connecticut: American Publishing Co., 1894).

Because most challenges and opportunities offer a journey into the unknown, there is a certain amount of self-doubt in the person considering the options. What if the venture fails? What if I find I am leaving one poor circumstance only to find I have entered a worse one? What if I do not have the skills it will take to be successful? What if I fail in the job? This is when courage is needed the most. For some, faith and spiritual practices help; but for most, it is the ability to care for self, to accurately read the opportunity, and to accept the challenge using empowered risk-taking decision-making.

What is guaranteed of any change or risk is not success but a broadening of one's perspective and a growth-producing experience that propels us beyond what we know and can do. Given this perspective, there is no way one can really fail. Campbell (1976) describes taking the challenge by citing what a Native American elder speaking to a youngster said at the time of his initiation:

As you go the way of life,
You will see a great chasm.
Jump.
It is not as wide as you think (p. 275).

■ Recycling

Recycling means to keep in touch with what is happening, what needs attention, what must be changed or modified, and what needs to be discarded in the plan to take a risk or met a challenge. The process is cyclical and must be accomplished with the same diligence used in caring for self, reading the opportunity, and taking the challenge. This phase of empowered risk taking is about keeping going when making the dream a reality or dealing with the new challenge even when there may be snags or barriers to accomplishments. It is also a time for evaluating the resources to determine whether they are adequate or appropriate for the tasks to be done. Several questions can be asked at this time to acquire the needed data:

1. *Self-care.* Am I conserving or replenishing my personal energy and making good use of my resources and support systems? Am I using empowered risk taking to boost my own self-image?
2. *Reading Opportunity.* Using a scale of 1 to 10, how likely am I to be successful at this venture? Do I need to revise or rethink my goals or strategies? Is my assessment of risks and rewards accurate? Is what I hear about what I want to do? Do I have or could I get the skills necessary for this opportunity?
3. *Taking the Challenge.* Am I doing the tasks I need to do to accomplish my goals? Is there anything that is keeping me from taking action? Could I be procrastinating, letting negative self-talk increase my reluctance to act?
4. *Recycling.* Am I looking at the ways I am providing self-care? Are the issues necessary for reading the challenge being evaluated? Are the resources needed for taking the challenge being assessed? Have I gotten a realistic appraisal of my challenge from those who might share my vision and have more experience or expertise than I have? Have I looked at whether the challenge or opportunity is consistent with my personal vision and values?

The term *recycling* is a good one for this phase of empowered risk taking because it requires some personal, interpersonal, and environmental evaluation. As Sinetar (1987) puts it, "This period is when we must become good readers of our own situation" (p. 127). It is also absolutely essential if the task at hand is to be successful and the dream realized.

ORGANIZATIONAL STEPS TO POSITIVE CHANGE: THE INGREDIENTS AND ACTIONS ESSENTIAL FOR THE CREATION OF AN EMPOWERED AND PROACTIVE WORK CULTURE

Understanding the Nature and Benefits of Empowerment in the Workplace

Empowering employees is not a new idea. Some of the top firms in the world have moved to shared governance. The health care environment, however, has been slow to adopt the concept, partly because it requires a tremendous cost, a massive cultural reorientation, and nearly a generation to implement—while service must continue to be available. It is therefore more easily implemented in new, smaller, and more entrepreneurial ventures or in organizations (such as the automobile industry) where radical change was necessary to compete in the global market. However, it has been successfully introduced into health care organizations and thus becomes an excellent opportunity for nurses who are ready for change. What is the nature of empowerment in the workplace, and what are the benefits? As Jaffe and Scott (1993) state,

> Enhancing the capacity of employees and whole organizations to produce higher quality customer focused results is the goal of an empowered workplace. In this workplace people at all levels feel directly responsible for results, are continually learning and developing their skills, feel the trust to share their best ideas, and work together in teams that contain not one, but many leaders.

"Empowerment" has become a buzzword that represents a range of initiatives—training programs, motivational speeches, and structural shifts—that help organizations develop this new style of operation (pp. 139–146).

Essentially, an empowered workplace requires a deep transformation of management style. Managers must shift their attention from others to themselves. Workers are accountable for their actions and the productivity of their unit. Decisions are made by teams, and everyone—worker and supervisor—is responsible for customer service. Chapter 5 presents the experiences of two nurses in a unit in a large hospital who developed an empowered workplace.

Empowerment does not mean throwing away everything that currently exists. As Schneider and Bowen (1995) suggest,

Empowerment isn't just the act of "setting the front line free" or "throwing away the policy manual." It requires systematically redistributing four key ingredients throughout the organization, from top downward: (1) power, (2) information, (3) rewards, and (4) knowledge (p. 250).

Power must be distributed, information must be shared quickly and widely, meaningful rewards must be provided for proper behavior and in a timely fashion, and knowledge of empowerment must be provided to everyone from the top down.

Recognizing When Empowerment Is Possible

Some environments are perfect places for innovation. Others are not. However, during this time of rapid change in health care, most health care facilities are ripe for change. Until recently, most health care systems operated with a traditional 5-year plan, but with increased competition and the initiation of managed care, these same organizations are now hotbeds of opportunity with change occurring at a very rapid pace.

How would the nurse know when there is a good opportunity? To recognize opportunity, the nurse must not be afraid of intense turmoil, and change must not be avoided but rather seen as an excellent chance to take the lead. Because nurses are very skilled at dealing with clinical crises, they are well prepared for other kinds of crises. Nanus (1991) puts this into context when he says, "In this day and age, if you're not confused, you're not thinking clearly" (p. 84).

This context of rapid change with all of its turmoil is happening to everyone, not just health care workers. In fact, many experts on leadership and change (Senge, 1995; Wheatley, 1992) believe that this confusion serves a very important role in providing us with a process for sorting out information to arrive at innovative solutions and that this is why group process and work team approaches in hospitals have been so successful. Nurses need to seize the opportunity to use the confusion in the health care arena as a source for trying or taking new directions.

Assessing the Culture of the Workplace

Empowered risk taking is an individual activity, but it does not occur in a vacuum. People can learn to use empowered risk taking, but the environment or culture in which they work is also important if they are to use empowerment. Finding a work environment in which the nurse's aptitude, risk tolerance, vision, and goals will fit is essential, particularly if the goal is to use the skills of empowerment. However, nurses can create an empowered and proactive work culture if they have the motivation, support, leadership skills, and time to devote to the endeavor, even in places where empowerment has never been tried.

Organizations have unique characteristics. Most are traditional with top-down decision-making: managers govern, and workers perform the tasks. Although this model has been changing, with more decision power shared with the workers, many health care facilities are still organized in this hierarchical way, which is not conducive to worker empowerment. However, within smaller work groups in these traditional organizations, it is possible to develop and maintain a culture of empowerment; therefore, nurses must evaluate the work setting to determine whether empowerment is present or whether empowerment of themselves and others in the environment is possible.

Assessing the Focus of the Operation

An important aspect of an empowered workplace is the focus of the operation. Once the vision, values, and culture are established, the organization must translate its product or service into terms of value to the customer. Treacy and Wiersema (1995) present a model for addressing this issue using a systems approach. They suggest the product or service must be presented in terms of value to the customer on one of the following dimensions:

- Operational excellence
- Product leadership
- Customer intimacy

If one selects the operational excellence dimension, the organization puts its energies and resources into centralizing systems where standard operating procedures are refined, and decisions are made to improve the results. If product leadership is selected, the institution is fluid, and decisions are made by ad hoc structures. If customer intimacy is adopted, decisions are moved as close to the customer as possible, and individualized solutions are encouraged. Peters and Waterman (1988) describe this customer-driven and customer-focused model in their landmark book *The Search for Excellence*. They believe the important thing is to satisfy the customer, not to maintain the structure.

This focus on operation is important because it must be clear to the entire workforce where their energies are to go and it must be consistent with what the customer expects. For instance, the organization may be preparing products for customer intimacy (i.e., written postoperative instruction with follow-up telephone calls) when the customer in more interested in operational efficiency (i.e., clinic appointments on time and correct billing). Knowing what the customer wants is paramount to any business venture but essential when the organization shares its decision power with the entire workforce.

Customer service as a focus has long been missing in health care. It is not that health care workers did not care about patients; it is just that they never viewed the patients as customers, nor were the services provided with the customers in mind. For instance, what patient would select to have breakfast at 6:00 a.m. or surgery at 4:30 p.m.? These times were selected because they met the needs of the kitchen staff or the surgery schedule of the physicians. However, things have changed, and hospitals and other health care facilities are trying to focus on customer service.

Selecting the Leadership Style for the Development of an Empowered Workplace

The literature is full of discussion about the kind of leadership style that promotes an empowered workplace. These discussions agree that leadership, regardless of style, must provide the organizational vision and core values while fostering a culture of shared governance. Some propose that leadership be provided by a strong visionary or a group that sets the tone. Others, like Senge (1990), have proposed a "servant-leadership" model. Block (1996) suggests leadership occur through stewardship. Peters (1984) believes a worker should be treated with dignity and be valued by the organization.

According to Senge (1990), effective organizations continually learn or improve through the conscious use of systems thinking, personal mastery, shared vision, and team learning. These processes begin with the organizations' leaders but spread to each member of the organization. The function of leadership is to help workers understand the complex world by answering the following questions:

- How do we establish a direction?
- How do we build the capacity of a group of people to move toward a shared vision?
- How do we improve the quality of thinking—especially people's ability to understand increasingly complex and interrelated realities?

The overall goal of the leader, says Senge, is to be a servant-leader—to cultivate an environment in which there is participation in the leadership role. The leader offers the way of doing business based on the constants of change, good questioning, and the inner and outer powers of consciousness. People practicing business in this way operate from inner wisdom and make decision by consensus, instead of submitting to some arbitrary outside control.

Ray and Rinzler (1993) suggest that the leader in an empowered environment is able to create vision, culture, and core values, which are definable and observable, in concert with those people in the organization. In organizations in which empowerment is successful, the following criteria are met:

- Employees are included in the defining of the organization's vision, goals, and processes.

- Employees are empowered to solve their own problems.
- Employees are self-directed.
- Training is done by team process, consensus, and conflict resolution.
- Cooperation, feedback, and teamwork are encouraged.

Peters (1994) identified three distinctive "areas of competence" in successful companies—(1) superior customer service, (2) internal entrepreneurship, and (3) a belief in the dignity, worth, and value of every person in the organization. Cloke and Goldsmith (1997) believe a critical test of leadership, in an empowered culture, is how well the customer is valued, listened to, and made a part of the service-improvement efforts.

Nurses who are in leadership roles or who aspire to such positions and want to create an empowered workforce must assess their own style of leadership and the climate for change. They must determine whether the opportunity exists for change *and* whether they have the type of leadership behavior that will foster an environment of risk taking and positive change.

Being able to answer "yes" to the following questions by Weiss (1995) will indicate how ready the organization and the leader are for the development of an empowered environment:

- Do employees see themselves as members of a team?
- Do employees judge their successes in terms of team versus individual performance?
- Are ideas eagerly welcomed and entertained?
- Does management provide processes and guidance but not answers?
- Is implementation undertaken only after commitment is gained?
- Are individual goals aligned with organizational goals?
- Do leaders gain leverage by working across boundaries and turf lines?
- Do the leader and employees focus on the customer first, employees second, and shareholders third?
- Does the leader ensure jobs are rewarding by getting and giving feedback?
- Is the focus of work on outcomes and goals, not on input and tasks?
- Are all in the organization allowed to fail?
- Do people admit their mistakes and learn from them?
- Do the leaders continually develop themselves and others? (p. 95)

If more than five of these questions receive a "no" answer, the leadership provided is not empowering. Accordingly, Kay (1998) describes the key elements a leader should keep in mind as empowerment is introduced:

- Provide new values along with high-stretch financial goals.
- Create teams that are accountable for analyzing and reconfiguring operations to yield dramatic transformations and economics.
- Propagate the new values relentlessly, and incorporate them into the accountability structure (p. 155).

PROFESSIONAL STEPS TO POSITIVE CHANGE: ONE NURSE'S STORY

In this chapter, a framework for seeing change as an opportunity has been presented. Empowered risk taking and creating an empowered workplace have been explained. However, to best understand the framework, it must be supported by real events accomplished by real people; thus, the remainder of this chapter is about one nurse's experiences using empowered risk taking and how she created an empowered workplace.

My journeys into seeing change as an opportunity were exciting, frightening, and ultimately the most rewarding ventures I have ever pursued. Although the last one began with a shock, once I accepted the challenge and used self-caring and the principles presented in this chapter, I was on my way. I never had envisioned I would own my own business or realized how much I had to offer until I began to develop WellComm, a telehealth operation. The following scenarios are just a few of the experiences I had using the concepts presented in this chapter.

Caring for Self

Shortly after I began my venture of establishing my own business, I realized I needed something or someone to support me. I was scared. I lacked self-confidence, and I felt like I was a fish out of water. One of the things I did to reduce my anxiety and to determine whether I had what it takes to start my own business was to take a self-test I found in a book by D. E. Rye (1994) entitled *Winning the Entrepreneur Game*. It was a test to determine suitability for an entrepreneurial venture. The test contains 14 questions and is easily scored, with each correct answer worth 5 points. If you score above 60 points, you have the right entrepreneurial instincts to run your own business. If you score between 40 and 55 points, you have the potential to do your own thing. If you score below 40 points, you should not attempt to establish your own business (Table 8–2).

I scored high on the test, which indicated I was challenged by entrepreneurial situations. This test helped me find out if I was ready for the opportunity and whether I had the attitudes, beliefs, and understanding of what I was interested in doing. I discovered I liked a flexible work atmosphere, that I frequently juggle three or more tasks, that I know the key factors to starting my own business, and that I know what to do if I am successful or unsuccessful. I had no idea how good I would feel about myself after taking that test, but it clearly helped me to care for myself as I had removed one of the obstacles to my movement forward: self-doubt.

The second important thing I did to care for myself was to avoid situations and people who created anxiety and fear in me about my future. I learned early in my career that there are times when you avoid others because they create a negative environment. For instance, when I was working on my master's degree, I was anxious and afraid that I would not be able to succeed—thinking my whole career would be ruined if I did not get the degree. I used to study in the student lounge where other students gathered and often complained bitterly about the program and all of the work. One day, I decided not to spend any more time there because it made me crazy. It was difficult to do this, but it worked. By avoiding the complaining students, I took care of myself. I did the same thing after I lost my job and was trying to decide what to do next. Instead of being with people who were afraid and unsure, I chose to be with people

Table 8–2. The Entrepreneurial Test

Each correct answer is worth 5 points. Any score above 60 points implies that you have the right entrepreneurial instincts to run your own business. If you score between 40 and 55 points, you have the potential to do your own thing. If you're below 40 points, you may want to stay where you are. The answers most commonly given by entrepreneurs are summarized at the end of the questionnaire, along with a brief explanation of each answer.

1. You want to open a business because
   A. You want to be a millionaire.
   B. You hate your present job.
   C. You're obsessed with trying out a business idea.

2. The best work atmosphere for you is
   A. A flexible structure.
   B. A hierarchical organization.
   C. One in which you mostly operate solo.
   D. Strictly team oriented.

3. Which example best describes your work style?
   A. You delegate most tasks to subordinates.
   B. You tackle problems sequentially.
   C. You juggle three or more tasks at once.

4. Your colleagues at your current job
   A. View you as a team player.
   B. Think you are outspoken and share your ideas.
   C. See you as a 'yes' person.

5. If you lost your job tomorrow, you'd find the experience
   A. Depressing.
   B. Liberating.
   C. Mildly embarrassing.
   D. Instructive.

6. If you're caught in a traffic jam, you're likely to
   A. Search for radio traffic reports.
   B. Pull off the road and wait it out.
   C. Take papers out of your briefcase and work.
   D. Try alternative routes.

7. When should you launch a business?
   A. Only when the economy is growing.
   B. In a slow economy, when labor and office space are cheap.
   C. Toward the end of a recession.
   D. Any time in the business cycle.

8. You're planning to start a business. You should first
   A. Mail your business plan to venture capitalists.
   B. Hold a press conference to generate publicity.
   C. Consult experts in the market you want to crack.
   D. Keep quiet so that nobody steals your idea.

9. You should be willing to wait as long as it takes for your business to make a profit.
   A. True.
   B. False.

10. The economy has strained your company's resources. Several key employees are complaining about low wages. You should
    A. Tell them you can't afford raises now, but will make it up to them later.
    B. Look for employees who will work for less.
    C. Create an incentive plan that offers them a share of profits if productivity or sales rise.

Table continued on following page

Table 8–2. The Entrepreneurial Test *Continued*

11. A client who accounts for 35% of your sales cancels his order. You should
    A. Find out why you lost the account, and solicit new customers.
    B. Cut prices to get him back.
    C. Raise prices to make up for the loss.
    D. Cut expenses.

12. Your company has just survived its first year and you need a vacation. You should
    A. Keep working.
    B. Take a trip to recharge your batteries.
    C. Go to an industry conference.
    D. Do either A or C.

13. After just 3 years, your company suddenly becomes very profitable. You should
    A. Treat yourself to a new car.
    B. Invest in a friend's new business.
    C. Reinvest the profits in your business.
    D. Open a retirement account.

14. After 10 grueling years, your business is consistently beating the competition. Now is the
    time to
    A. Sell stock to raise capital.
    B. Introduce a new line of products or service.
    C. Franchise the business.
    D. Do any of the above.

Answers:

1. C. Most entrepreneurs are obsessed initially with trying out their new idea. They believe the
   rewards will follow if they succeed.
2. A. Entrepreneurs avoid rigid work styles.
3. C. Entrepreneurs know that they have to be capable of handling a number of tasks
   simultaneously.
4. B. Most entrepreneurs want to share their ideas so that they can seek creative solutions.
5. D. Entrepreneurs look for lessons learned from every setback they encounter.
6. C. Entrepreneurs hate to waste time and therefore always have something they can work on,
   regardless of the situation.
7. D. If the idea is good, it can be successfully launched in any economic environment.
8. C. Entrepreneurs know that impartial advice from experts can help them avoid costly
   mistakes.
9. B. Entrepreneurs set a deadline for financial success. If they don't make it, they are not afraid
   to close their business and start something new.
10. C. Key employees are your greatest resource. Give them an incentive to help you solve the
    problems.
11. A. Relying on a single customer can cause the demise of your business. Call your lost
    customer to find out why you lost the business.
12. D. The first years of a new business are too critical to take a vacation.
13. C. Don't get complacent. Plow the profits back into the company.
14. D. Look for innovative ways to expand your business, and make it even stronger.

who encouraged me and were positive about my future. Avoidance in this case
was the best option for caring for myself.

One other time I had to leave a position because I found that I had all of my
self-worth and persona tied to my professional role. I had a terrible time

accepting the fact that I was not indispensable. I really did not know who I was without my professional role. As a single parent with a wonderful son and a commitment to joint custody, I was not free to relocate to another city, so I chose to leave my position and try something entirely different. It took me 5 years to fully integrate myself, but it taught me how important self-care can be and that one can survive by leaving behind something that is comfortable but stifling for one's self-worth.

Another strategy I used was to surround myself with people who knew me and my talents and who encouraged me to accept opportunities. I learned this from a boss who was the president of the college where I taught. He asked me to be the vice president of academic affairs for the college, saying "You've got to take the brass ring because you don't know if it's going to come around again." He was supportive of me and wanted the best for me. Unfortunately, he didn't remain in his position very long, so I did not stay in that position long either. What I gained because of his support and trust in me has helped me through the years when I feel worried about the future and my ability to "make it" in something new and different. He had faith in me; that is very reassuring and helps me when I have self-doubt.

A pragmatic strategy I use now to provide self-care for myself since I started my own business is to reflect periodically on my dream and vision. Keeping in mind what I want to do and where I am going is very self-assuring. It gets difficult when I spend 18 hours on the job and worry about money. How do I do it? I keep focused on the dream and remember all of the things that others have done for me in the past. I remember the college president and what he said; I remember how I scored on the entrepreneurial test; and I remember what my network of friends have done for me when I have had a tough day. Most of all, I remember that I must take care of myself because many others who work for me need me to do the same for them.

Reading the Opportunity

I have been blessed in my professional life with plenty of opportunity, but before the past decade of my life, opportunity was fairly confined and socially defined. Those who loved and respected me told me my career should be secondary to a family and that a job was something to fall back on once the children were grown. Women were supposed to be teachers or nurses, and work was a way to supplement a husband's salary and to prevent the empty nest syndrome. Even though this perspective never felt right for me, I followed the rules.

My first job after college was in a prestigious general hospital where I was hired to work in neurology and then to progress to intensive care. I was excited about these areas and vividly remember on my first day being told by the supervisor who hired me that I would be working on a renal and urology unit. I was shocked, mad, and terribly disappointed. I distinctly remember the thought that went through my head—I can make a big deal out of this because the job market is very good, or I can wait and see if it has anything to offer. I decided to stay and started on the 3-to-11 shift, where I discovered a great opportunity in disguise. Sometimes the most unexpected events turn out to be the best opportunities.

While on the renal unit, I learned to care for transplant patients. One of my patients was a nun who was dying, and it was my task to keep her comfortable. Each day, another nun visited, and she would sit quietly and watch me. She always carried a black patent leather purse and wore black patent leather shoes and looked very regal. After about 2 weeks of observation she asked to talk with me in the hall. As I stood listening she said, "Have you ever thought of teaching? You're a good nurse, and I need a teacher for next semester. Come see me, and we will talk." I did go see her and she hired me.

For the next 13 years, I taught a variety of courses, became the head of the fundamentals of nursing course, was in charge of the first year of medical surgical nursing, developed two new programs, led the faculty senate, and was granted the teacher of the year award. I also completed my master's degree, receiving the highest award for my research. Looking back, I can see now that when I accepted the job, I was really blind to the demands of the position and to where it might take me. Because the nun had seen potential in me and because I had trusted her insight, I accepted the opportunity offered. The first lesson I learned was to trust those who make the offer because they may see something in you that you cannot see.

At another time in my life, I incorrectly read an opportunity. I had just received my doctoral degree and had been working in sales for 2 years. Even though I was good in sales, I missed the ongoing relationships I had developed with my students and the other faculty members of my previous position. As a favor to a friend who thought I was qualified because my doctoral degree was in statistics, I interviewed for a job in market research. I spent the next year or so in what was to be the most boring and frustrating job of my career. I was appointed director of market research for a midsized insurance company that sold its product via direct mail inserts in credit card statements.

What was wrong with the job? Several things were not right for me. First, change was not welcomed. I was given a lot of responsibility and was supported by one of the senior executives, but I was never really challenged because I knew my views about marketing were not supported by the managers, who had never worked outside of the company. Second, I missed people interaction. Third, I could see no future for me in the operation. It was an opportunity, however, where I learned a lot about insurance and marketing (something I needed to know for my own company later on). The most important thing I learned is that no matter how attractive the job looks to others, if you are not challenged or fulfilled, it is not the right job. Sometimes, however, you have to take the opportunity before determining whether it is right one.

By now, I realized that I was not following the usual and accepted role for women. I knew I was going to be working all of my adult life and that ultimately I would be a top executive. I also found my path was similar to the one described by Katherine Graham, the publisher of *The Washington Post*, in her memoirs (1998), in which she describes three things I had also encountered:

- She was enculturated into gender-specific roles: "Men do this, and women do that."
- Her father told her that women do not run companies even though she was smart and had demonstrated leadership talents.

- Earlier in her professional life, she accepted her roles without much consideration.

Until I left nursing, I was doing women's work; once I entered the business world, I knew I would never return to nursing but would probably stay in health care in some form. Once my father had said to me, "If you were a man, I'd ask you to run my company—you'd do a very good job." He did not live long enough to see me do so, but much of what I do I learned from him. He was an excellent mentor and role model. And over time, I have gotten better at reading the opportunities and take more time considering the options.

My last experience with reading opportunity occurred when I was reading the newspaper. After being terminated as the vice president of the physician group, I remember the excitement I felt when I read an article in the *Wall Street Journal* about the new and rapidly growing field of *telehealth*. I thought to myself what a perfect thing for nurses to do—provide information and support to patients. I tested this idea with my colleagues in business, health, and managed care. After a little more research, I was convinced the market (which two large, ineffective service providers dominated) was ready for a small, independent telehealth provider. The opportunity was there, and I read about it in the newspaper.

Accepting the Challenge

Accepting the challenge has never been hard for me. As you have read, I have accepted challenges all of my professional life. When I was reassigned on the clinical unit in my first job, I accepted the assignment even though I thought about not doing so. When I accepted the position in a school of nursing without any preparation for the job, I did so because the director of the program believed I could do the job, and I succeeded and then some. When I was offered the position as director of marketing research at the insurance company, I accepted the job and hated it. The difference in this instance was that I did not thoroughly assess the kind of company I entered and did not know what I could *not* do. I learned something from each of these jobs that has helped me establish my own business.

There was one incident when I was asked to take a job by a recruiter. After leaving the insurance company, I was approached by an executive recruiter I had known for many years. He asked me to interview for a job as general manager of a home care company that sold home oxygen and durable medical equipment and was trying to get into the home intravenous therapy business. I interviewed for the job and was told by the man who became my boss for the next 6 years that if I hadn't taken the job, the company would have probably closed the location. This opportunity was too good to pass up, and again, I learned a lot that has helped with my own operations.

The office of this company was not clean or orderly. Employees smoked at their desks. The general attitude was "We cannot afford it, so we do not do it." Fortunately, my boss and I were able to strike a deal. I told him what I needed in order to be successful, and he told me the time and resources he could devote to my plan. Fortunately, the employees knew things had to change and thus took my direction without too much difficulty even though I presented a very different perspective. Seven years later, my area of responsibility had grown from the original branch to three locations and from 10 employees to over 40. My territory was losing nearly $200,000 per year when I accepted the position and was generating $7 million when I left. We were awarded top honors in the company for revenue, profitability, employee retention, and clinical performance. Accepting this challenge paid off for the company and me.

I am glad that I took on this challenge because it taught me there is a valuable service to be provided to the public and a lot of money to be made in health care if one knows where the opportunities lie. When I decided to leave the company, it was for another exciting opportunity in health care that had the potential to be on the cutting edge of change; however, this opportunity did not proceed as I had envisioned, nor did I know that it would be my last venture before I founded my own company.

Looking back, I made several errors when I accepted the challenge of being a top administrative executive for the largest independent physician group in the area. First, I overestimated physicians' ability to work together. I also overestimated the purpose of the organization and believed what I was told. I did not have a sufficient understanding of the politics of the area to know that this venture was doomed from the start. Although physician groups had formed in California and the Pacific Northwest and had been very successful in their negotiations with hospitals and insurance companies where I lived, it was too early for such an arrangement; physicians were not ready for change and resistant to losing their stature. I also trusted my boss, and I should have paid more attention to what he was doing. Another factor that overshadowed my clear thinking about this challenge was the dissolution of a 13-year personal relationship that took a lot of my attention and energy. Accepting a challenge demands a lot of your time and all of your attention. If other things get in the way, the challenge can become a nightmare. However, if I had succeeded in this challenge, I would not be where I am today or telling this story about my success as an entrepreneur. Life does not stop when jobs fall apart. New opportunities are always just around the corner, if you look.

Recycling

Each time I have changed a job, I have repeated the cycle of examining my ability to care for myself and have assessed the opportunity before I accepted the challenge. Sometimes I was disappointed at the results of the decision, and sometimes I felt betrayed, but I always learned something even if it was a negative lesson. Did I stop trusting people because a few had let me down? No, because I realized that I had gained some excellent mentors and had expanded my network of colleagues who are always there when I need them. It would be magical thinking to believe that all ventures have happy endings. By recycling this process of self-care, assessment of the opportunity, and acceptance of the challenge, I have learned more about myself, improved my ability to see things clearly with all of their dimensions, and prepared myself for my latest career challenge—being an entrepreneur.

Empowerment in the Workplace

I learned from my father how to empower a workplace. When my father was in his late 40s, with children in private high schools and colleges, he and my mother sold everything they had and moved to another city, where my father had purchased a business. My father devoted most of his energies and time to making a failing business profitable. I worked for my father during the summers and over the holidays from the time I was 13 years old until I graduated from college. By that time, the business was extremely successful, and he sold it.

What I remember best is how he was involved in his business on a day-to-day basis, yet gave those who worked for him total responsibility and account-ability for their areas. He did whatever it took to solve the customer's problems, a value and behavior quickly modeled by the employees. I also saw him compete fiercely for business and deal with suppliers aggressively when orders for materials were not correct or were late.

On busy days, he would help pack items for shipping. No job was beyond his reach and too insignificant for his attention. When he died, the best testament to his leadership and success as a businessman was that people from all over the country came to town for his funeral. Customers, suppliers, and colleagues were there. To this day, his secretary says he was "the best boss I ever had." Giving the employees respect and being willing to help while still providing the employees with responsibility and accountability empowered his workforce.

I followed his lead when I was general manager of the home care company. I worked hard to empower the employees. Drivers who delivered the oxygen to the patients were given uniforms and told to do whatever it took to make the patients comfortable; thus, they felt professional and needed. The respiratory therapists and a nurse were asked to develop clinical standards, and the customer service and billing employees were sent to communication seminars. I also demanded that there be no smoking in the offices and that everything be cleaned up. They did what I asked and told me they felt much more like professionals and were proud of what they contributed to the operation. Clearly, these changes helped them feel good about themselves and willing to commit to the company's goals.

This experience helped me learn more about empowerment. I felt strongly that employees, no matter whether they were truck drivers or master's prepared nurses, could excel at their jobs if given the opportunity. I gave them the opportunity and held them accountable for the results, and they fulfilled my expectations and were proud of their accomplishments. Employees who lack empowerment are usually not ready if given the opportunity or are afraid to take a risk. I gave my employees opportunity and they took the risk.

These experiences with my dad and his company and my first attempts at the home care company helped me understand that the boss (chief executive officer) can make an operational, financial, and cultural difference in a business. I have tried in my own business to continue to follow his lead. I have empowered my employees to take risks for the customers as long as it is safe and legal and does not jeopardize the company financially. I treat my employees with respect and reward them with praise when they meet a goal. I also am in the trenches, doing whatever is needed yet keeping it clear that I am the helper. We are a team working together to make the business a success. Every employee feels a part of this endeavor and looks to me for the vision and direction. I was lucky to have a role model like my dad.

Wellcomm is a technically and clinically focused business. Every time we discuss client needs and how technology can help us provide better service, we must consider the following:

- Ways to respond to calls in a timely way
- Ways to route calls to available nurses
- Ways to alert the nurse to her or his next call
- How to time the calls
- How to monitor calls for quality assurance
- How to determine the correct problem and solution for the caller
- How to determine the severity of the caller's problems
- The kinds of home care treatments to suggest

The staff are involved in these discussions and thus are a major part of the company's operations. Without their expertise, the service could not be provided. They feel empowered because they essentially are the business.

SUMMARY

I have learned a lot about myself, the world of business, and how to succeed as an entrepreneur from the events I described. I saw change as an opportunity and used empowered risk taking to start my own business. Much of what I have learned during my professional life that helped me establish my own business can be summed up with the following principles:

- Women and men can do more than history suggests. There really are no gender-specific jobs anymore.
- Having a network of supportive people is essential if you are thinking about taking a risk.
- Opportunities are plentiful if you keep your eyes open and are willing to take a risk.
- Not all opportunities work out. Some opportunities are duds, but if you do not accept the challenge you will never know which ones will blossom into something great.
- Role models are important, both for you and for those you want to help.
- Everything takes longer than you expect, so do not get anxious if things do not work out right away. After 2 years, my business is finally making a profit.
- Keep focused on your vision and dream, especially when you are tired and things do not seem to be going like they should.
- Take care of yourself. Surround yourself with positive people, get plenty of rest, remember what others have taught you, and draw from your successes of the past.
- Keep informed about what is happening in your field.

- Enjoy each day and plan for the next one.
- Remember, change really is an opportunity!

REFERENCES

Bateson, M. C. (1990). *Composing a life*. New York: Dutton/Plume.
Block, P. (1996). *Stewardship: Choosing service over self interest*. San Francisco, Calif.: Berrett-Koehler.
Branden, N. (1994). *The six pillars of self-esteem*. New York: Bantam Books.
Campbell, J. (1976). *The hero with a thousand faces*. Princeton, N.J.: Princeton University Press.
Cloke, K., & Goldsmith, J. (1997). *Thank God It's Monday!* Chicago, Ill.: Irwin Professional Publishing Group.
Graham, K. (1998). *Personal history*. New York: Vintage Books.
Houston, J. (1998). *A passion for the possible*. San Francisco, Calif.: Harper.
Izzo, J., & Klein, E. (1998, May/June). Changing values of workers: Organizations must respond with soul. *Heathcare Forum Journal, 41*(3), 62–65.
Jaffe, D., & Scott, C. D. (1993). Building a committed workplace: An empowered organization as a competitive advantage. In Ray, M., & Rinzler, A. (Eds.). *The new paradigm in business*. New York: Putnam Publishing Group.
Kay, M. Z. (1998). Memo to turnaround boss. In Dauphinais, G. W., & Price, C. (Eds.). *Straight from the CEO*. New York: Simon and Schuster.
Mellody, P. (1989). *Facing codependence*. San Francisco, Calif.: Harper.
Nanus, B. (1991). *The leader's edge: The seven keys to leadership in a turbulent world*. San Francisco, Calif.: Jossey-Bass.
Oxford University Press. (1996). *The Oxford dictionary and thesaurus*. New York: Oxford University Press.
Peck, M. S. (1985). *The road less traveled*. New York: Simon and Schuster.
Peters, T. (1994). *Liberation management: Necessary disorganization for the nanosecond nineties*. New York: Fawcett Books.
Peters, T., & Waterman, R. H. (1988). *In search of excellence: Lessons from America's best-run companies*. New York: Warner Books.
Quinn, R. E., (1996). *Deep change: Discovering the leader within*. San Francisco, Calif.: Jossey-Bass.
Ray, M., & Rinzler, A. (Eds.). (1993). *The new paradigm in business*. New York: Putnam Publishing Group.
Rye, D. E. (1994). *Winning the entrepreneur's game*. Holbrook, Mass.: Bob Adams.
Schneider, B., & Bowen, D. E. (1995). *Winning the service game*. Boston, Mass.: Harvard Business School Press.
Senge, P. M. (1990). *The fifth discipline*. New York: Currency/Doubleday.
Senge, P. M. (1995) Robert Greenleaf's legacy: A new foundation for twenty-first century institutions. In L. Spears (Ed.). *Reflections on leadership*. New York: John Wiley.
Sheehy, G. (1976). *Passages: Predictable crises of adult life*. New York: Dutton.
Sheehy, G. (1981). *Pathfinders: Overcoming the crises of adult life & finding your own path*. New York: William.
Sinetar, M. (1987). *Do what you love and money will follow*. New York: Dell Press.
Tracy, D. (1995). *Take this job and love it: A personal guide to career empowerment*. New York: McGraw-Hill.
Treacy, M., & Wiersema, F. (1995). *The discipline of market leaders*. Boston, Mass.: Addison-Wesley.
Weiss, A. (1995). *Our emperors have no clothes*. Franklin Lakes, N.J.: Career Press.
Wheatley, M. (1992). *Leadership and the new science: Learning about organizations from an orderly universe*. San Francisco, Calif.: Berrett-Koehler.

READINGS

Byham, W. C., & Cox, J. (1998). *Zap! The lightning of empowerment: How to improve quality, productivity and employee satisfaction*. New York: Fawcett Books.

Covey, S. R. (1989). *The 7 habits of highly effective people.* New York: Fireside.

Dauphinais, G. W., & Price, C. (Eds.). (1998). *Straight from the CEO.* New York: Simon & Schuster.

Debashis C., & Senge, P. (1998). *Leading consciously: A pilgrimage toward self-mastery.* London: Butterworth-Heinemann.

Hall, D., & Wecker, D. (1997). *The maverick mindset.* New York: Simon & Schuster.

London, S. (1992). An interview with Margaret Wheatley. *Insight & Outlook.* San Luis Obispo, Calif.: Public Radio for Peace International.

Senge, P. M., Roberts, C., Ross, R. B., & Smigh, B. (1994). *The fifth discipline fieldbook: Strategies and tools for building a learning organization.* New York: Currency/Doubleday.

Spears, L. (Ed.). (1995). *Reflections on leadership.* New York: John Wiley.

Wilson, L., & Wilson, H. (1987). *Changing the game: The new way to sell.* New York: Simon & Schuster.

Wholey, D. (1997). *The miracle of change.* New York: Pocket Books.

Chapter 9

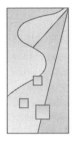

Being Proactive, Not Reactive

Robinetta Wheeler

A proactive response to questions and proposals and during planning is often contingent on how decisions are made. Each day, nurse managers, faculty, researchers, staff nurses, nurse entrepreneurs, and student nurses, to name a few, make many decisions. Decision-making is part of most nursing curricula, discussed in workshops, written about by many disciplines, and a topic of many speakers, yet we all continue to seek better ways to make decisions. The ability to make a wise proactive decision is a great asset for any leader in nursing at any level. Before discussing the topic of proactive decisions, a look at several decision-making perspectives may be helpful.

MODELS FOR DECISION-MAKING

A review of the literature indicates there are many models for decision-making. According to Keiser and Sproull (1982), early models of decision-making portrayed the process as rational—one that allowed decision-makers to make decisions that fit perfectly with the environment in which they operated. The newer models, says Jones (1993), recognize that although decision-making is an inherently uncertain process, decision-makers grope for solutions that they hope will lead to favorable outcomes. Decisions often have to be made at the spur of the moment, when least expected, and often when the stakes are high; the ability to initiate action using a decision model that reflects the world around us is an important skill.

It is important to distinguish problem solving from decision-making. According to Higgins (1991), in problem solving, the issue is to determine whether the decision made was a good one based on whether it solved a problem. In decision-making, there is a choice to be made after the generation of alternatives has been considered. It is a process of making choices from a variety of options; thus, decision-making does not necessarily include a problem and may or may not create a favorable outcome.

Jones (1993) describes five kinds of decision models that help us understand the evolution of decision theory:

- Rational model
- Carnegie model
- Incremental model
- Unstructured model
- Garbage can model

Rational Model

According to Simon (1960), the rational decision model is a straightforward three-stage process of (1) identifying and defining the situation, (2) generating alternatives or choices, and (3) selecting an action and implementing it. As Jones (1993) describes it, when using the rational model, decision-makers seek to identify problems that may interfere with the relationship between the organization and the surrounding environment. Recognizing potential opportunities or threats, decision-makers explore ways to maximize the organization's ability to take advantage of the opportunities or diffuse the threats. The possible consequences of these alternatives are then examined, and a set of activities that appear to predict the best outcome are selected for implementation.

The problem, says Jones, with the rational decision model is that it ignores ambiguity, uncertainty, and chaos, which typically plague decision-making. Other researchers have claimed that the model is unrealistic or simplistic because it assumes that all decision-makers (1) are smart, (2) have all of the information they need, and (3) agree about what needs to be done. In reality, says Jones (1996), most people have a limited ability to process information or the time to act that the rational model demands. And because the environment is inherently uncertain, not every alternative course of action and its consequences can be known. Furthermore, the rational decision model assumes that different people have the same preferences and values and that the same rules will be used during decision-making. According to Robbins and Coulter (1996), these assumptions are unrealistic.

Carnegie Model

In an attempt to create a decision model that better reflects the realities of decision-making, the Carnegie model (Larkey and Sproull, 1984) was introduced with attention placed on three factors: satisfying, bounded rationality, and organizational coalitions.

Satisfying refers to an agreement made by decision-makers to develop a certain set of criteria that will be used to evaluate possible actions. Instead of searching for all possible alternatives, they resort to the few that meet the criteria; thus, the generation of information for making the decision or decisions is much less costly and time-consuming.

Bounded rationality assumes that the decision-makers have limited capacity to process information and can process what they know about and value. This does not mean they will select the first acceptable alternative generated. They can sharpen their analytical skills and use technology to augment their decision-making skills. Bounded rationality acknowledges that decision-making is subjective and relies on the decision-makers' experiences, beliefs, and intuition.

Organizational coalitions exist, according to the Carnegie model, because the preferences and values of the decision-makers differ; hence, conflict among them is inevitable. Decision-making takes place through a process of compromise, bargaining, and negotiation by a *coalition* of decision-makers. The alternative selected must be approved by the dominant coalition, the collection of people who have the power to select an action and to commit resources to implement it (Cyvert and March, 1963).

Incremental Model

Because of the limitations of the Carnegie model, the incremental decision model was developed. "In the Carnegie model, satisfying and bounded rationality drastically reduce the number and complexity of alternatives that need to be analyzed" (Jones, 1993, p. 480). In the incremental model of decision-making, alternative possible actions that are only slightly or incrementally different from those used in the past are acceptable. This approach decreases the chance of error. Often called the science of "muddling through," the incremental decision model allows the decision-maker to make a succession of incremental decisions that eventually lead to a new course of action. Limited by reduced information and foresight, the decision-maker moves cautiously, one step at a time, to limit the chance of doing the wrong thing. A prime advantage with this model is that it can be used by the novice, and because the steps are small, any errors can be easily identified and corrected.

Unstructured Model

Because the incremental model works best in a stable environment, Mintzberg and his colleagues (1976) developed the unstructured model, which works best when uncertainty is high. Like the incremental model, the unstructured model recognizes the incremental nature of decision-making. The model contains three stages: identification, development, and selection. In the unstructured model, whenever there are roadblocks, the decision-makers reconsider the alternatives and resume solution generation. The process is not a linear and sequential but rather a process that "may evolve unpredictably in an unstructured way. For example, decision-making may be constantly interrupted because uncertainty in the environment alters managers' interpretations of a problem and thus casts doubts on the alternatives they have generated or the solutions they have chosen" (Jones, 1993, p. 480).

Mintzberg's model emphasizes the unstructured nature of incremental decision-making. Generally, people make decisions in a haphazard and intuitive way as they adjust to the uncertainties of an ever-changing environment. Uncertainty forces them to act in an unstructured way. The "unstructured model tries to explain non-programmed decisions while the incremental model tries to explain how organizations improve their programmed decisions" (Jones, 1993, p. 481).

Garbage Can Model

Decision-making as an unstructured process taken to its extreme is known as the garbage can decision model. This model starts the decision process from the desired outcome. In other words, decision-makers propose actions for hypothetical situations, for example, how to decrease the patient length of stay or how to empower the workforce. The organization then seeks ways to use existing solutions, such as an in-house home care team, the telephone triage program, or the organization's training department, to reach the desired outcomes. After plausible situations are presented, everyone one seeks ways to use the existing resources to implement them (Cohen et al., 1972).

Although the organization is faced with new hypothetical situations, it is also trying to deal with those generated by the environment. Consequently, people are competing for a priority position in decision-making and the allocation of resources. Decision-making becomes a "garbage can" with invented and real situations, proposed actions, and preferences all mixed together. Chance, luck, and timing are important aspects of what the organization decides to do because the situation with the most uncertainty for the organization will get first priority. As Jones (1993) states when using this model, "outcomes for the organization become more uncertain than usual, and decision-making becomes fluid, unpredictable, and even contradictory" (p. 481).

Conflict Model of Decision-Making

Another model of decision-making has been proposed by Janis and Mann (1977), and it is known as the conflict decision model. This model assumes that decision-making is stressful for most decision-makers. It is built on Lewin's psychological conflict theory that focused our attention on the influences of social pressures and other sources of erroneous judgments on decision-making and the tendency of people to withdraw from stressful conflict situations. Janis and Mann (1977) describe their work as "being concerned with . . . decisions . . . that affect the welfare of one or another member of the family, of the family as a whole, of the community, or of an organization with which the decision maker is affiliated—and not with the mere opinions of people" (p. 4).

A unique aspect of the conflict decision model is that it distinguishes decisions that have consequences from those that have inconsequential outcomes. Janis and Mann (1977) believe the psychological laws of opinion and attitude differ for decisions that require significant action. Their research has focused on how people make "important life decisions" such as career, marriage, health, and political affiliations. Because the stakes are high, decisions about these issues become "socially committing because they require efforts at implementation if the decision-maker is to fulfill his role in the community and maintain his public reputation as well as his self-image as a reasonably reliable person" (p. 4).

Decisions that affect one's fate and the fates of other people are often so stressful that they are postponed or avoided in an effort to prevent mistakes. Although the person is rewarded for making successful decisions, "gaining utilitarian and social rewards is not enough; the person has to be able to live with himself" (p. 9). Decision-makers in such situations use efforts to avert feelings of guilt or to enhance a sense of moral worth and self-esteem. This explains why some decision-makers make what appears to be an irrational choice.

As the result of research, Janis and Mann (1977) devised a seven-step process called *vigilant information processing* that leads to satisfactory decisions. Failure to engage one of these steps is a defect in the decision-making process; hence, as the number of defects increases, so does the likelihood of failure. The seven steps are listed:

1. Thoroughly canvass a wide range of alternative courses of action.
2. Survey the full range of objectives to be fulfilled and the values implicated by the choice.
3. Carefully weigh whatever is known about the costs and risks of negative consequences, as well as the positive consequences that could flow from each alternative.
4. Intensively search for new information relevant to further evaluation of the alternatives.
5. Correctly assimilate and take account of any new information or expert judgment, even when the information or judgment does not support the course of action initially preferred.
6. Reexamine the positive and negative consequences for all known alternatives, including those originally regarded as unacceptable, before making a final choice.
7. Make detailed provisions for implementing or executing the chosen course of action, with special attention to contingency plans that might be required if various known risks were to materialize (p. 11).

Janis and Mann (1977) believe that this version of conflict theory provides the detail necessary for knowing when decisional conflict is best handled by withdrawal. They also suggest that it is best used in situations where conflict is likely to occur and where typical responses can be expected. For instance, their research found that there are five coping patterns that affect the quality of decision-making. One pattern is to seek more thorough information; the other four are useful because they reduce time and emotional turmoil.

There are limitations for the use of this model. It is impractical for individual use because it requires details about an individual's stress level so that comparisons can be made when the individual is making decisions. It is, however, useful as a heuristic model for training decision-makers about broad categories of pitfalls and ultimate strategies for decision-making. Knowing that conflict is a major factor (i.e., stress) in decision-making is useful; if decision-makers can identify when they are in conflict, they may be able to sort through the conflict to make better choices.

Summary

The early models of decision-making were linear and suggested certainty as a conclusion. Later models described decision-making as an uncertain process that may or may not lead to satisfactory outcomes. The early models implied that decision-makers had adequate time to obtain information to make decisions. It is now known that decisions often must be made on short notice and with incomplete information. In addition, we know decision-making is influenced by the interaction between psychological and social factors. What is common about these models is their attempts to adjust for variances resulting from human limitations. The seven steps of Janis and Mann for the resolution of conflict during decision-making provided us with ways to monitor and improve our decision-making.

FOCUSING ON CHOICES: A WAY OF BEING PROACTIVE

Regardless of whether one decision model is better than another or better used in one situation than in another, each model demands that the decision-maker make choices. It is this process of making choices and how the decision-maker arrives at a choice that are the keys to effective decision-making for any model.

Making Choices

Making a decision means one has choices. *Choice* refers to the selection of one item from at least two; therefore, when there are two options (e.g., doing something or not doing something), there is a choice. All decision-making models include a step that requires making a choice, but one must have the perception there are choices. The following example illustrates this point. A new nurse is placed on unit A, a medical unit. Shortly thereafter, the nurse manager leaves, several other nurses change shifts, and the new nurse is left as the only full-time person on the day shift. The hospital staffing office decides to meet the staffing needs of the unit with part-time nurses who are also new to the organization. The nurse manager from an adjacent unit is asked to provide management coverage for unit A. Then, the new nurse is assigned as the assistant nurse manager. Later, when congratulated on the appointment, she says, "I had no choice." The nurse did have a choice, but she did not perceive that a choice was available.

People often believe they have no decision because they have not been presented with multiple choices. The fact is that when no decision is made, a choice has been exercised. "Riding it out," "letting the chips fall where they may," or "letting nature take its course" gives choice to others. Such statements indicate the choice was to "not act." Not deciding allows other people or events to determine the outcomes. It is important to remember that choice occurs even when all of the options are disliked and no action is taken.

Sometimes, the perceived lack of choice is due to the most desired choice's not being available. In other words, if I want to do X and that is a choice, then I believe I have a choice. However, if I do not want to do X and it is a choice, then it seems that I do not have a choice. Hence, an understanding of what choice means to the individual makes a difference in the way that person will act given choices.

Acting as though there are no choices fosters a habitual disinterested response that ultimately ends in a resentment of the activity, resulting in an increased unhappiness or dissatisfaction with the situation. For example, there are nurses working in environments they do not like who feel resentful because they believe they have "no choices." Actually they do have choices. They can leave the organization (resign), obtain the necessary education or experience to transfer to a different specialty, or leave the profession entirely. Although none of these choices may be appealing, they are choices.

Nurses are constantly making decisions while performing their duties. These decisions usually involve making clinical choices within their areas of clinical expertise. Many of the decisions are automatic; that is, they are determined by professional or organizational policies or procedures (i.e., nurse practice acts or hospital policies). Others are determined by the desires of the patient. Often, decisions are the result of group or team decision-making.

Choice becomes a conscious activity during decision-making when there is a deficit between the desired action and the means to implement that action. Ordinarily, individuals do not engage in discussions of choice except when there are overriding determinants that preclude alternatives, such as "Will the patient's insurance pay for the service?" If the answer is "yes," and it is medically indicated, then the choice is made. If the answer is "no," then decisions have to be made given a set of other choices. For example, what about the elderly patient who would benefit from 1 week of custodial nursing care but does not have additional insurance beyond Medicare? One option would be to teach the patient how to care for himself. Another would be to identify a family member, friend, or neighbor who could help. Probably, both options would be suggested, and a third one sought. In the current cost-conscious climate, increasingly patients are being discharged with a need for continued care. Health professionals sigh, lament the changes, and hope that the patient will fare well as they decide how to manage their care.

Nurses most often encounter choice when there is an ethical decision to be made. In ethical decision-making, the individual is faced with deciding what is morally right. Frequently, decisions must be made from a selection of equally undesirable choices. These are called moral dilemmas because "no matter which action is taken something of value will be compromised" (Purtrilo, p. 46).

A few years ago, ethical decision-making centered primarily with life-and-death decisions. Now, situations like the one described earlier are becoming the norm for ethical decision-making. The right or wrong of sending a patient into an environment believed to be detrimental to his health because of financial reasons has become the focus of ethical decision-making.

Proactive Decision-Making

A proactive decision model is a useful way for nurses to make a choice, but what does it mean to be proactive? According to the *Oxford Dictionary and Thesaurus* (1996), *proactive* means "creating or controlling a situation by taking an initiative" (p. 1188). Furthermore, the dictionary defines *pro* in three ways: as a noun ("a short form of the word professional"), as an adjective ("a favorable response"), and as a prefix ("in front of"). It is this third form that is used when proactive behavior is discussed. When an action is taken before an event or an anticipated event, it is considered a proactive act.

Proactive decisions are made in view of a vision or goal; therefore, proactive decision-makers must anticipate the future and they must embrace change. They must be able to look at developments in society and project into the future and envision what might occur to begin preparation. For example, I have had the vision of the baccalaureate degree as the criterion for eligibility for the nurse license since my education at New York University. Holding that vision prompted me to make choices that would support attainment of that goal. When I had the opportunity to teach educational courses that helped diploma and associate degree nurses obtain the baccalaureate degree, I eagerly accepted the position.

Being proactive is also akin to being a gardener. Often, one has to "sow a seed," await its germination, promote its growth, and nurture it to maturity. An example of this was when I wanted my staff nurses to conduct research. My vision of the staff nurses engaged in ongoing research was not too far-fetched because the unit on which they worked was devoted to medical research. However, the nurses had to see themselves as researchers. Thus, my proactive decisions included identifying their strengths and promoting them among the nurses. It involved providing opportunities for them to attend nursing research symposia, meet nurse researchers, and enroll in continuing education courses about conducting research and numerous other activities that culminated in their participation in a marketing research study. These activities occurred during a 5-year period of time.

Another example of proactive decision-making is when nurses, years ago, began looking at the impact of computers on nursing. They helped to develop the field called *informatics.* Other examples of nurses who acted from a vision or to support an idea before it was generally accepted were those who encouraged advanced practice areas (e.g., nurse practitioners, clinical nurse specialists) or expanded roles in nursing such as holistic nursing, spiritual nursing, and nurse entrepreneurs. By their preparation, these nurses were ready to administer to patients whenever opportunities presented themselves. They had to wait for changes in the political, governmental, and social conditions that would permit them to use their knowledge and skills. This was the case for nurses prepared as nurse practitioners who were employed as staff nurses. These nurses were prepared to enter nurse practitioner positions when they became available and thus were proactive in their professional choices.

Being proactive involves keeping abreast of new techniques and theories for improving the workplace. For example, Drucker (1986) writes about the three American teachers (Deming, Juran, and himself) who are credited with the economic turnaround of Japan after World War II. One of Drucker's contributions was teaching the Japanese to value their employees as a resource, which then required managers to help them evolve "to be responsible for their own and the group's objectives and productivity" (p. 220).

In the staffing example described above, the administrators knew about the planned reassignment of the nurse manager because they had approved the transfer. Although the nurse manager knew about her departure 2 weeks before the date of her departure, the staff learned about the changes only days before her announcement and were surprised about all of the changes. There were no formal announcements about the new assistant manager position, so the "rumor mill" bulged with predictions about who would or should be selected for the position. Several of the experienced nurses denied being asked to assume the assistant nurse role. The assistant manager was selected a few weeks later. These management decisions did not allow the staff to be responsible for continued implementation of the unit's "objectives and productivity"; consequently, both suffered during the weeks after the manager's departure.

Using a proactive approach, the former nurse manager and administration could have identified a potential nurse or nurses to act as an interim nurse manager months before her scheduled departure. Staff could have been informed and participated in the process of deciding the form and selection of the unit's interim manager. Instead, many staff members were angry because they had not been asked to serve as the acting nurse manager; others felt betrayed or believed the manager left because in some way they had not supported her. All of these feelings could have been avoided if a proactive implementation process had been used.

The remainder of this chapter is about being prepared to make proactive decisions. Proactivity requires keeping abreast of changes so that one is acting from an informed perspective. It is about how leaders make decisions in the present while considering the effects of the decision in the future. It is about creating a decision-making process that places the leader in a proactive rather than a reactive position when important decisions must be made.

THEORETICAL MODEL FOR PROACTIVE DECISION-MAKING: CONSIDERING THE CONTEXT OF THE DECISION

Being proactive in decision-making involves the ability to anticipate the "event" so as to act *before*. To do this, one must consider not only the decision to be made but also the context of that decision. There really are two aspects to be considered whenever the decision-maker makes a choice regardless of the decision model that is used. There is the consideration of the choice to be selected and the consideration about how the *context* of the decision affects the outcome of the choice. The model presented here for proactive decision-making includes this second aspect of decision-making: the context of the decision.

There are five primary areas (contexts) of consideration when determining choice and when making decisions. These contexts are called *arenas* and are conceptualized as concentric circles (Fig. 9–1) because there are relationships between the arenas. The first level, or personal arena, is where decisions pertaining to the individual occur. Decisions made at this level will not affect others. The second arena includes the family and significant others. These are the people and the intimate relationships most likely affected by the decision. The third level is the social arena. Business associates (e.g., coworkers and professionals) and close friends (e.g., social club members) are those affected in this arena. Their opinions and reactions to the decisions are important and of concern to the decision-maker. The next arena is the community. This arena contains the ethnic, religious, national, and cultural groups who will be affected by the decision-maker's choices. This group also includes formal relationships, such as elected officials. The last arena is the global or international arena. This arena is more often addressed at the philosophical, political, or financial level. For example, one might envision the earth as one large society and work with

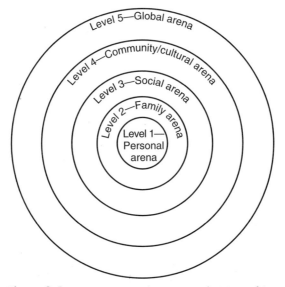

Figure 9–1. Arenas: contexts for proactive decision making.

international organizations to increase the number of world "citizens"; to strive to increase concern about the plight of children in third world countries; or to donate money to aid the sick or invest in developing countries.

Decisions become more difficult as more arenas become involved. For example, most single people can engage in career decisions that involve travel without feeling conflict unless a second or third arena is affected. Hence, a single person living alone would most likely experience less conflict when deciding to accept a job requiring considerable travel than would a single parent, a married person, or a person living with aging parents.

The first step in making a decision is to determine what you want to do. Next you need to identify which arenas are involved; this is not usually a conscious action. Rather, it becomes apparent when the person says, "I can/can't do that because . . . ." The responses that follow will give clues to which arenas are being considered.

■ I CANNOT DO THAT BECAUSE	■ ARENA	■ I CAN DO THAT BECAUSE
It is expensive.	Level 1	I can afford it.
I have children/family plans.	Level 2	There are no standing commitments.
My work schedule is full.	Level 3	I am off that day.
My religion banned the movie.	Level 4	I choose what I will see.

This example illustrates the importance of considering the consequences in relation to the concerned arena. Options and possible consequences are listed and decisions are made that create the least conflict between the levels. Potential consequences for an action may entail what needs to be done to manage the decision within the context of a given arena. For instance, once a nurse decides to act in a way that is expected to elicit an unfavorable response from other nurses, administration, and the family, the consequences of that decision can be weighed so the nurse is prepared for what will happen before the decision is implemented.

Determining which arenas are involved when a decision is made can help with the identification of the issue. For example, sometimes it is believed that the decision is about "whether to take the job," when the real issue is "how to manage the family." The person wants to take the job but does not know how to handle the resistance from the social and community arenas. The issue then is how to manage the resistance to the decision rather than whether to take the new job.

The following scenario illustrates this point. A patient had a 13-year-old nephew who was scheduled to visit her during the Thanksgiving holiday. Although she and her sister discussed the visit and made the decision during the summer, they were reluctant to inform her sister's in-laws. They did not know how to tell the grandparents that their grandson would not be there with them for Thanksgiving because they expected the grandparents to object. When the sister finally informed the grandparents of the changed plans, they thought the visit with his aunt would be good for him. The patient bemoaned the time she and her sister had spent on unnecessary worry. Clearly, they worried needlessly because they misjudged the grandparents' response. How many times do we focus on the insignificant aspect of decision-making or stall in our attempts to make decisions because we misjudge how others will respond? Remembering to consider which contexts the decision will affect helps the decision-maker avoid stalls and often focuses the decision-maker on the real issues.

How does this model help the nurse behave proactively? The model helps the nurse consider the total impact of decisions. After identifying the choices, the arenas affected by the choices are determined. The better the nurse can distinguish the arenas impacted by the potential decisions, the easier it will be to remain proactive. Use of this model requires the nurse to be aware of changes or shifts in attitudes or values within the arenas. For example, keeping abreast of changes within the organization where one works and of those made by the professional groups that influence the work setting improves one's knowledge of options if a job change is considered. Before making that job change, a proactive examination of the latest roles would help the nurse determine whether the job was desirable and whether the time was right for a change.

An example in a different arena might be helpful to highlight this point. Imagine that you live in a suburb and recognize that your teenager will not have the right to drive a car at age 16 because of new state laws. This knowledge allows you to be proactive about how you will manage the numerous activities associated with that period. You decide it is a good time to begin your child's use of public transportation, so you take trips together on public carriers. Your fears are allayed, your comfort level increases, and you note that your child's expectations change. These changes suggest that it might be a good time to start preparing for a job change. Will you need more or less flexibility in job duties?

What's predicted for your industry or specialty within the next 5 years? You decide it might be a good time to consider a job that keeps you "in the field," such as home health nursing. The flexibility of home health care would be compatible with the needs of your teenager, or perhaps it is a good time to plan for a job with travel because your child can manage a daily routine. What are your family members' thoughts about time together, support, and competition? Remember, it is important to be alert for shifting attitudes, values, and expectations within the arenas.

Summary

The previous discussion outlined a decision model that focuses on the context of the decision rather than on the process for making the decision. The advantage of this approach is that decision-makers can use their preferred decision-making model as long as the context of the decision is included in the consideration. It is also helpful in focusing the decision-maker on the *real* decision. Knowing what arenas are involved in the decision allows the decision-maker to be proactive because every aspect of the decision has been considered.

The following section contains scenarios of one nurse's experiences with proactive decision-making. They include both personal and professional examples to illustrate what a leader in nursing needs to know to make proactive decisions and to help others do the same.

ONE NURSE'S EXPERIENCES IN DECISION-MAKING USING THE PROACTIVE CONTEXTUAL DECISION-MAKING MODEL

Level 1— Personal Arena Decisions

My decision to run in a marathon (26.2 miles) in 1996 was a personal decision; however, after seeing the training schedule, it became apparent that the decision would also affect arenas 2 and 3. I needed to consider not only my work schedule and what my training would do to staffing but also how it would affect my time with my children. I worked the night shift (11:00 p.m. to 7:30 a.m.) and thus had to decide whether I would take the night off before the days I would train or work each night and run the next day. I also had to decide what I would do with the children while I was so preoccupied with running.

To address the level 2 arena (my children), I explained my reasons for participating in the training and run. I told them that I needed to get into better physical condition and that my running would contribute to the larger community (a level 4 arena) because the run benefited the Leukemia Society of America. I also took them to many training events so they could see others working as hard for similar reasons. I thought it would be good for them to understand how important involvement in worthy causes can be. I also enrolled them in runs that were available for children. They found these events enjoyable and were proud of their ribbons and tee-shirts. From a proactive perspective, it was better to explain my goals in the beginning and gain their understanding and cooperation than to spend precious time trying to convince them of the value of my running when I was running and not available.

Anticipating that my personal decision to run in the marathon might affect staffing where I worked, I decided to train after work. This meant that I would train after working all night; that was no particular problem because I usually stayed up for several hours after returning home before going to bed. I just continued doing the same thing but substituted running for other activities I would have done. What I did not anticipate was how I would feel after running. I learned after the first day of running that I felt a lot better and that when I did go to sleep, I slept better. By the time I was running more than 15 miles a day, I had adjusted my work schedule and had nights off before the longer runs. This worked better because the runs were usually not local and started early in the day. As before, I shared my goals and experiences with the staff before I began to train so I could gain their support for days off when I requested them. This was a proactive action that paid off.

My activity as a marathon runner had an unanticipated impact on the staff. After I had completed the marathon, several of the staff decided to run races and a few trained for triathlons; you never know when a decision you make may influence someone else's decisions and thus provide leadership.

Another personal decision that has affected other arenas, particularly arena 2, is my diet. Although I will eat dairy products (cheese, milk, yogurt, and so on), fish, and chicken, my diet consists primarily of vegetables. I eat animal protein at no more than one meal a day, and I will let 2 or 3 days pass without consuming any animal protein. Although this diet works for me, when the staff had potluck meals, it became a small problem because I did not eat much. In the culture of my work setting, food and the potluck meals symbolized an important social event. People considered it an honor to prepare special meals for their peers and even more for a supervisor. Almost every day someone brought in a special dish to share. Over the years, my peers have teased me about my weight and diet. At one work setting, the staff consciously tried to "fatten me up." Anticipating a possible response and not wanting them to feel insulted, I tasted all of the wonderful dishes. I just did not eat much. I had to be proactive and creative with my daily eating schedule, so I planned lighter meals during those periods.

I have found that when my peers get serious about changing their behaviors, they often come to me for advice. Perhaps my personal behavior has been a model for them, so many things that they previously thought were impossible are now considered possible. Eating sensibly and running marathons are ways that I have improved myself. Clearly, these personal decisions have affected arena 3 participants as I created proactive personal choices.

Another area of personal decision-making that has affected others is my interest in other cultures and other languages. Compared with many new immigrants and persons from other countries, we Americans are often ignorant about other cultures and languages. I have much respect and admiration for those who speak more than one language. I keep improving my Spanish language skills and recently refreshed my French language skills because one of my personal goals is to fluently speak another language. This I believe is a proactive approach because of the population changes within the United States;

the demographics suggest an increasing need for health professionals with bilingual skills.

Traveling has helped me discover that people are more alike than they are different. Everywhere, people are concerned about similar issues in their lives: raising their children, performing well on the job, having friends, and caring for each other. They are concerned about their future and their country. Some knowledge about culture and language is helpful when I have a patient who speaks another language, even ones I know nothing about. When given a choice, I volunteer to be assigned to the non–English-speaking patient. I am always glad at these times that I had the foresight to travel and learn. Again, my personal decision affected another arena, in this case arena 4. Other nurses have done similar things (e.g., volunteered to travel in other countries with health teams to provide free treatment) to improve their ability to relate to patients while providing the needed care.

As you can see, decisions that you think are only personal ones often affect other arenas; that is why it is important to consider what arenas might be affected before making a decision. It can be costly to change some decisions once they are made. From my examples, you can see that my decisions were proactive because keeping healthy and physically fit increased my effectiveness in work and provided better experiences for my patients, family, and friends, all arenas affected by my personal decisions.

Level 2 — Family Arena Decisions

I began proactive decision-making (although I didn't call it that) as a young woman, as the following examples demonstrate. Most people experience considerable pressure from arena 2 until they are at least 18 years old or move out of their family's home. Making decisions when I was a teenager was fairly easy because I was clear about my family's expectations. Raised Catholic, I was also clear about and had accepted the church's position on many moral decisions teenagers have to make; however, I must admit that my decision regarding sexual abstinence had more to do with a consideration of my own values than those of my family or the church.

I clearly remember the discussion I had with my mother about the consequences of pregnancy. She didn't engage in a moral discussion (I already knew those arguments) but rather focused on the consequences. She pointed out that I would have to stay home and take care of the baby and because she worked, she would be tired and not able to help me after work. She very effectively described a very unacceptable lifestyle . . . one without school or any personal freedom. I enjoyed school and the ability to do many things, so the decisions about sexual behavior were easy. I acted proactively to ensure the future I desired.

When I was permitted to date, I quickly learned that there were times when not accepting a date would be awkward. I made an agreement with my mother. Whenever a young man asked her if he could date me, she was to say "No." This was my proactive plan to handle such situations. It worked very well.

My parents made most of the other major decisions (e.g., going to college). I always understood that *not* going to college was not a choice. However, I did select the college (with advice from a guidance counselor) and the major of study. What my parents did not know was that I wanted to be a dancer and did not expect to pursue nursing as a significant career choice. I included a hospital school of nursing among the applications submitted. Ironically, my decision to attend New York University followed an interview at a major diploma school of nursing. When I mentioned New York University, I was counseled not to attend that school, but there was no conflict in my decision because I knew I had made a choice that pleased my family and me. I knew what they valued and wanted.

When I was growing up, people did not move away from their families. Neighborhoods were built by generations of families working and living together. Your cousin lived "down the street" or "around the block." Everyone knew that you were "Mrs. So and So's" niece, granddaughter, sister, etc. I needed a "reason" to leave because of the pressures from the family and people in arenas 2 and 3. I worked as a registered nurse on medical/surgical units for experience while I searched for a reason to leave New York. I found that reason when I was accepted to a 3-month communication training program for members of the helping professions. For my family, education was an acceptable reason for leaving New York, and I also wanted to go to graduate school in California. Being proactive with my family entailed helping them to see the value of my decision from their perception of what was important. In that way, I gained their understanding and support for my decision.

When I finally arrived in California, I did not know anyone. After 1 week, I moved into a house with four other women and a 10-year-old child (the daughter of one of the roommates). It was clear that the group functioned in many ways like a family. We pooled money for meals, took turns cooking, and ate dinner together each night. We even shared the telephone. At the end of the month, we each identified our long distance calls and paid for them and our share of the basic bill. If one of us became ill, we cared for her. Still, most of the decisions I made while living there affected only me.

Before the 3-month internship program ended, I knew I did not want to return home. My decision wasn't whether I would or would not stay in California but how to inform the family that I was not "coming home" to live. I accepted a job offer and returned home on a vacation to inform my family that I was not moving back to New York. Obtaining the job was an acceptable reason to remain in California.

Level 3 — Social Arena (Friends and Colleagues) Decisions

Dealing with decisions that affect the level 3 arena when I was a teenager was not too difficult because most of the students in my class went to college. We had moved to a suburban community where most of the families were upwardly mobile. Only a few students considered vocational alternatives after high school; not surprisingly, these students were mostly minorities who had been programmed to accept less of themselves. Guidance counselors began encouraging the underachievers and minority students to select a vocational track as early as the eighth grade.

As a student who had selected the "college prep track," I belonged to two social groups: a group of "racial minority" friends and a group of "racial majority" friends. Although I received positive responses from my "majority" friends about my decision to attend college, my "minority" friends appeared indifferent about the decision. I kept in touch with a few friends after high school. They all worked and had apartments, cars, and nice clothes. I noted that they were doing the same activities that we had done in high school. Although I did not have many possessions, I had accumulated new experiences and knowledge that I began to appreciate. As the years passed and I continued to face new challenges, I sensed their dissatisfaction with their decisions. My encouragement to them to make changes was met with objections and explanations why they could not. They believed they had no other choices to make. Eventually, our lives became very different, and our friendships waned.

Working brought an entirely different set of social pressures to my decision-making. I often had a difficult time as a registered nurse because of my progressive and empowered vision of nursing practice that I obtained during my nursing education at New York University and by studying with Dr. Martha Rogers (e.g., the advantages of having a baccalaureate prepared and advanced prepared nurse at the bedside). For example, after deciding to take a job in San Jose, I learned that California did not recognize the baccalaureate degree as a credential that determined staff nurse level or salary. They did not seem to understand the additional value of the degree, so I decided to convince them that I should be recognized for my superior preparation and paid accordingly. I explained my educational experiences and obtained transcripts and documentation from the faculty. Eventually, they acknowledged my additional education by increasing the time credited for work experience and, hence, my staff-nurse level. The only criteria they had for establishing wages and staff nurse levels were related to work experience. This is an example of how I had not acted proactively because I had not understood the institution and its policies before accepting the job. I now know there are some aspects of an organization that one can discover as an outsider, whereas other characteristics may only be uncovered as an insider.

Later, I accepted a job with another agency because they based their pay scale on education and experience, but even there my educational preparation was suspect. Most nurses at that time did not have a baccalaureate degree and saw no need to acquire one (imagine what I experienced later when I earned a master's degree and a doctorate). In that and subsequent positions, I learned that if I wanted to make proactive decisions, I needed to know the expectations for nursing preparation of the members of the arena in which I was operating. This situation has been called being "overqualified" for a position. I needed to seek advanced positions, so I became a head nurse. Although I enjoyed being at the bedside, as a head nurse, I was able to role model the kind of care I had been promoting.

One particular experience illustrates the importance of remaining aware of the interactions within arena groups when making a decision. I was the head nurse on a locked psychiatric ward. During each shift, I made rounds and interacted with the patients until a nursing assistant took me aside and told me how nervous I made the staff doing this. She explained that it was not customary for the nurses to interact with the patients. Nurses stayed in the nursing station or administered medication while the nursing assistants interacted with the patients. She said the male staff followed me around to make sure "I was not hurt." Until that discussion, I had not realized how anxious the staff was made by my decisions. This is an example of what happens when one fails to understand the values and expectations within an arena. Here, my decision distracted the staff and impeded their work until I was able to help them redefine the nurse's role.

In another work setting, I learned how important decisions about one's apparel can be to peers and supervisors. I was working as a community nurse educator. Because I encountered a variety of patients each day, I had decided that wearing business attire (dress, skirt, and jacket or a suit) made me feel comfortable and would be less likely to make any patients feel uncomfortable.

I noticed that my supervisor frequently asked me to speak with visitors, often with short notice. One day she explained her behavior. She said that because I always dressed appropriately, she felt comfortable asking me to speak with visitors. She also said she could count on me because I did not alter my style of dressing. I learned that being consistent in my pattern of dress was important in this arena.

In another situation, I became aware of a potential negative consequence from consistency. I learned that sometimes you are offered or not offered opportunities because of others' misperceptions. Once I was asked if I would be interested in applying for a job as a program director. I was excited about the chance to make a change. The person later explained that he had been reluctant to ask me to apply for the position because I seemed so satisfied with my present position. I explained to him that although I was satisfied, I also did not want to miss a new opportunity.

Looking satisfied and doing a good job can be a dilemma if you do not also display a desire for advancement. I have always believed I should perform at my best even if I was unhappy in the position. I also considered it inappropriate to make colleagues nervous because they thought I had unbridled ambition. So how could I do a good job and still show interest in advancement? Networking became the most effective method of letting others know I was interested in job advancement. This did not mean that I had decided to resign and leave my current job; it only meant that I let my network know that I was available if the right opportunity arrived. I could do a good job and not fear missing an opportunity, and my colleagues could be assured that my departure was not eminent.

I have also made what I believe is a proactive decision about performing non-nursing tasks at work. For example, when faced with a "dirty" bed after a patient has been discharged and a new patient is waiting to be admitted, some nurses will offer to wash the bed rather then wait for housekeeping staff to do it. Instead, I would call housekeeping and tell them we had a patient waiting in the emergency department and needed the bed cleaned. In most cases, they would have the bed cleaned and ready for the patient before she or he arrived from the emergency department. It has always been my hope that the staff would try this approach.

I think nurses perform some tasks because they think they lack an alternative or because the obvious alternative is not attractive. If the nurse expects the housekeepers to complain about coming to the unit to clean the bed, she or he might do the task to avoid an unpleasant confrontation. Some colleagues explain their behavior in terms of expediency or as a way to prevent the patient from waiting once on the nursing unit. I have exercised the choice of asking the emergency department staff to keep the patient until the room was ready. The point here is that in light of nurses' other responsibilities, it would be detrimental to clean the beds. In this cost-containing climate, cleaning beds after a patient's discharge could become an assignment for nurses. If that happened, reversing the "new" bed-cleaning policy would be harder than keeping the roles clear proactively. This is another example of how a personal decision made by one nurse can have an impact on how the work of many nurses is defined. Clearly, the nurse must consider all arenas when making a decision; there are no small decisions, not even those about who makes the patient's bed.

The following example about ordering medications demonstrates how a personal decision can affect others. I worked in a hospital where the pharmacy staff delivered medications that were missing from the patient's bin if the information was faxed to them. However, instead of faxing the information, I noted that many nurses used the medications from other patients' bins or requested "floor stock" of frequently used medications. Having observed this nonfunctional behavior, I sought an explanation and decided that the real problem might have been that the nurses did not know how to use the fax machine and were unwilling to say so.

Using the technique of leading by example, I checked each of my patient's bins at the beginning of the shift and made a list of the missing doses. Then I completed the "missing doses" information sheet and faxed it to the pharmacy. After doing this for a couple of weeks I noted that some other nurses were following my example and others asked questions of me about the fax machine. In no time at all, my proactive approach eliminated what had been a problem.

I think the next example of how a proactive decision can affect others is important because I believe every nurse has the responsibility to welcome and help new nurses into the profession. In a hospital where I once worked, I encountered several newly licensed registered nurses who were employed as nursing assistants. When I asked why they were still working as nursing assistants, in each case, I was informed that they were waiting for a nursing position to become available in the hospital. I explained that it was my understanding that at that hospital, all registered nurse positions required at least 6 months of registered nurse experience, which meant experience as a registered nurse and not as a nursing assistant. Because they were not performing registered nurse tasks in their role as nursing assistants, they would never be eligible for a registered nurse position in that institution unless a new graduate program was offered. A discussion with the nursing office indicated there were no plans for a new graduate program, so I counseled the new graduates to get some registered nurse experience at another hospital. Because they did not want to give up their current jobs, I suggested they seek part-time jobs as registered nurses at other hospitals and keep their current positions. I know that at least two registered nurses took my advice. One continued to work at the hospital while working as a registered nurse at another hospital until a position opened on the unit where she was a nurse assistant. Another accepted a job at a different hospital and enjoys the environment there.

Level 4 — Community/Cultural Arena Decisions

As an African American, I am constantly faced with the influence of crucial community/cultural issues when I am making decisions. I am often viewed as a representative of African Americans by both European and African Americans. Today, with greater numbers of immigrants in the United States, this focus has become a greater issue because many people believe African Americans are like those depicted on television and in the movies, which of course is not true.

Generally speaking, most successful African Americans are overachievers. We have to be because higher qualifications are always expected when we apply for a job. We are always placed under a microscope to determine whether we are qualified, contrary to popular opinion. Unfortunately, the American general public remains initially suspicious of African Americans who have not been introduced or recommended by a trusted person. Knowing this, I have sought a recommendation from a European American when seeking a new position at an institution where this was an issue. This decision has always been made in light of how the arena participants accept or reject African Americans.

In most institutions where I have worked, the majority of "employees of color" are in the dietary and housekeeping departments or work as nursing assistants or ward clerks. On a regular basis, I have been accosted by "testy" employees (physician, laboratory technician, or other health professional) who think I have not responded to their requests. Some people have an annoying habit of "barking out" requests and expecting responses. Because I am not in a job category of the persons who usually respond to those requests (e.g., clerical or housekeeping staff), I often do not hear them. When I do hear the demand, my decision to respond or not is not based on the assumption that the person requesting the help should expect an answer from me; it is based on my decision to provide assistance or information.

For example, I was charting at the nursing station when a European American laboratory technician very loudly complained about the pneumatic tube transport system. She said it was not working properly because she had seen exiting and arriving tubes collide. She based her decision on the fact that in the few minutes since she had observed this collision, the system had not permitted another tube to exit. After listening to her repeat her complaint three times, I asked her what message was flashing in the system display. She replied, "Accepted." I said, "Then it will be sent. This happens when the system is busy." I continued charting. More time passed and she made another comment about the system and the fact that she needed to send specimens to the laboratory. Because we were the only two persons in the nurses' station, I suggested she call operations if she was still concerned. She responded, "Well, if you do not care about getting your unit's specimens to the lab . . . ." I replied, "You could speak to the charge nurse to make other arrangements." By this time, I had decided she thought I was the unit clerk and that she wanted me to take on the task and the associated worry. Because she had drawn the blood specimens, I knew that it was her responsibility to get them to the laboratory, not mine, so I walked off to complete a task. When I returned, I noted she was still there, now holding the pneumatic tube. She walked toward me with the tube, and as she got closer, she read my name badge, looked surprised, and said, "Oh, you are an RN, not a clerk." I said, "Yes." She apologized. I could have reprimanded her about assuming I was a clerk, I could have ignored her and turned away hurt, or I could have brushed off the incident as an insensitive error. I chose to smile and go about my business and hope that she would be more sensitive in the future.

As an African American, every day and in many situations I have to decide how to manage these affronts. In each instance, I must make choices while keeping in mind that I am functioning not only in the level 1 personal arena but also in the level 4 arena. My decisions may not only affect me but also impinge on fellow community/cultural participants, and I have a duty to do what is best for them.

This next example started as a level 3 decision. I was working in a hospital at a university medical center. The decision was to get management to give us more clerical coverage so our clerk could attend computer-training classes. As a research unit, we had a database to maintain. The special funding that had provided a staff member to perform this task was no longer available. The hospital, however, had refused the initial request for assistance. At the time, we thought our only options were to keep approaching hospital management with more evidence, hoping we would be able to convince them to change their decision; to get the nurses to perform the task; or to seek another outside funding source. The first option was futile; the second, I did not want to support because it was not a nursing function; and the third was a possibility, but it would take time to identify a new funding source.

One day, I overheard two people talking about the volunteer service at the medical center; they were looking for places to assign volunteers. I scheduled a meeting with the director and learned how the department worked. I explained that we needed someone with computer skills for data entry. By working with them, we were able to find another option, which we selected. As a result, we discovered we were now interacting with the larger university campus. Students and spouses seeking unique experiences or with "time on their hands" contacted the volunteer department. In addition, people from the surrounding communities volunteered at the medical center. We were now part of a larger community need and part of the solution. Over time, we accepted numerous volunteers. We sent our ward clerk to computer classes when we were assigned a volunteer who had been a secretary. Each summer, a local high school sent students to the university for an enrichment experience. One summer, the volunteer service contacted us about a student who was interested in research. The student worked on our unit for 10 weeks. During that time, he learned about the research process and designed and implemented a research study about sleep, using his peers as subjects. He was very excited about his experience and wrote us after he returned to school.

I was proud of our involvement in the larger community. We were able to participate because we were flexible. We accepted whatever amount of time volunteers could provide and were creative in finding tasks they could perform. Taking time to adequately train the volunteers was critical. We gave them frequent praise and thanked them for their efforts. This experience taught me about how much people want to contribute and how to creatively support that goal.

To fully understand level 4 and its impact on other arena decisions, I want to share another experience. It happened several years ago. I attended a health fair where I met a woman who described a product that she wanted to make available to nurses. At that time, I was a nurse manager and interested in ways to increase my staff's enthusiasm for the nursing research process. I met her partners, and we decided we could all benefit if the nursing staff agreed to participate in a marketing study of their product. The nurses were asked to use the product daily and complete a questionnaire about the experience. As a result, the staff learned about the research process, and several of them got involved in existing research or started their own research. The information obtained about the product was incorporated in the marketing plan, and the company's market share increased. The decision to be part of this study benefited my staff, a nurse entrepreneur and her partners, and other nurses because the nurse entrepreneur decided to market the product to new nurses. In addition, I wanted to support this nurse entrepreneur because she used some of the profits from this venture to improve and expand cultural understanding between common citizens of the United States and the former Soviet Union.

Recently, I met one of the staff nurses who had participated in the marketing study. She informed me that she had completed a research project on blood-drawing methods. Her study had compared two methods for obtaining blood samples and the end quality of the samples. She found no difference between the two methods as long as the correct technique was followed. Hearing this success story 10 years later was very rewarding and further validated the decision to get involved in the market study.

Level 5 — Global/International Arena

There is an overlap between the cultural/community arena (level 4) and the global/international arena (level 5). For instance, for 3 years my family participated in a student exchange program so we could learn more about other cultures and so other cultures could learn more about the United States. We hosted young women and men from Europe and South America. Each one commented on how different life in the United States was compared with the image acquired from the movies and television. One student even went as far as trying to find a host family like the one he had seen in a U.S.-produced television program. His own parents were separated, and he wanted to experience living as a family with the parents and the children together.

Earlier, I described a project in which a nurse entrepreneur and her partners were working on improving international relations between the United States and Russia. Through my involvement with this group, I was invited to participate in an international conference of women leaders in Leningrad (now St. Petersburg) and Moscow in 1986. There were 52 women at the conference from the United States. We met with women who had comparable roles and discussed the differences and similarities in our lives. I believe this experience helped us gain a better understanding of each others' cultures and countries. I would not have been invited if I had not decided to get involved in the earlier project.

I also learned later that the entrepreneur group introduced the first Alcoholics Anonymous representatives to Russia and helped develop a group there. I believe by helping this company to succeed, I was able to make an impact on the health of citizens in another part of the world. Although I did not know my participation would have such far-reaching results, this experience demonstrates that decisions made in one arena often affect other arenas, highlighting the importance of considering the impact on all arenas when making even what appear to be small decisions.

Impact of Proactive Decision-Making

Awareness of the influence of arenas on decision-making can help one remain proactive. Keeping in touch with changes or shifts in attitudes or values within the arenas (e.g., information about key people, timing, and presentation) improves the information that is used to implement the decision within the arenas.

In nursing, the role of the nurse practitioner has gained much attention in the past 10 years. When I first learned about physician's assistants and the difference between them and nurse practitioners, I was intrigued and wanted to know more. I talked with nurse practitioners, and I read about their scope of practice in numerous professional journals. I also discovered that there were several nurses in the agency who were certified nurse practitioners but who worked as staff registered nurses because there was no category for nurse practitioners. Seeing an opportunity, I decided to find out what was required to hire a nurse practitioner on our unit. Because I had the money available in the budget, funding a nurse practitioner was not an issue. Rather, as nurse manager, I had to write a job description for a nurse practitioner that would be acceptable to the hospital administration, department of nursing, and school of medicine. Recognizing that this goal extended beyond the nursing department, I began identifying the other members of the organization whose support I needed.

My research was useful because I had to understand the level 3 social arena (colleagues) to implement my decision. Knowledge of physician assistants and their role helped me when I had discussions with physicians. Knowing the position of the American Nurses Association and the California Board of Nursing helped me when I made my proposal to the nursing department. Knowledge about the numbers of nurse practitioners already working as staff helped in getting the position approved because the administration was less hesitant about shifting a registered nurse from one unit to another than in bringing in an "outsider." This story demonstrates how important it is do your homework. This is an excellent example of proactive decision-making using the context as part of your considerations.

Another example that illustrates the impact of proactive decision-making occurred in a hospital where I worked as a nurse manager. Nursing staff members were not allowed to display their academic degrees on their nametags. However, I noted that the physicians' tags did include MD and PhD, so I decided to find out how I could include academic degree designations after the nurses' names on their nametags.

During my planning process of how to accomplish this task, I learned that the nametag design was patient based and was decided by the patient relations department. Patients had complained about being unable to identify who was caring for them. Because the patient population was mostly elderly, it was decided they just needed to know whether the caregiver was a nurse or a physician and that the name needed to be visually prominent.

I knew who were the decision-makers and how they held the power within the hospital. I also knew that my manager and a few of her colleagues did not agree with the practice of eliminating the degree initials from the tags but did not want a political encounter with those who had established the policy. I was sure that if I ordered the nametags through the usual channels, my request would be rejected. To avoid that, I learned where the nametags were made, ordered them for all of my staff, and paid for them myself.

Two things happened when the staff appeared with their new nametags. Managers saw them and never asked that we stop wearing them, and the patients and the staff had discussions about what the different initials meant. It became an excellent opportunity for nurses to educate the patients about the education of nurses. Even though I was ready for any discussions or complaints, they never occurred. A point to remember is that being prepared and proactive allowed me to make a change that many believed impossible. Proactive decision-making can be powerful!

Although I have given examples of successful situations, I do not want to imply that my plans always work out the way I expect or want. With unsuccessful situations, I assume that I have probably missed some information about an arena. I am not discouraged because I analyze them for what I did learn and will therefore be better prepared the next time. The important things are to keep observing the arena, to not be afraid to ask questions, and to keep focused on being proactive.

SUMMARY

There are many lessons to be learned from my experiences and many ways that nurses can use these lessons to improve their decision-making skills and remain proactive. Keeping the following thoughts in mind when faced with a decision will help the nurse stay proactive and ready for the impact of a decision no matter what arena is affected.

1. There are always choices; even undesirable ones may become good options. Be creative.
2. Focusing on choices produces proactive decisions rather than reactive ones.
3. When a decision is to be made, decide on the "what" and then on the "how."
   a. Decide what you want to happen (the desired outcome). Determine what arenas will be affected and what you know about each (i.e., their values, expectations, and goals). Watch for shifts or changes. A change in key personnel often signals a change in values and expectations.
   b. Then determine how you want to get to the desired outcome.
4. Learn as much as possible about each arena. Although this may take time, there are a lot of ways to learn that are fun. The following are some ways to learn more about the arenas:
   a. Read, read, and read! I read as many of the agency public relations pieces that I can, in addition to what they provide to the staff. I look for the meta-message. What is it the agency wants us to know and believe? I then look for differences between what is said and what is done. I also read many different newspapers and journals. I read business as well as nursing journals and then read what the critics had to say. Read futurist literature, like the writings of Toffler, Maynard, Mehrten, Bezold, Slaughter, and Rogers.

b. Embrace patient and staff complaints. I ask the staff and patients to tell me how things would look if they could change them.
c. Ask questions. You will not always get answers, and yes, sometimes you may irritate others, so be careful. Never ask potentially embarrassing questions of management in a big group; instead, pose sensitive questions in a hypothetical manner. When the issue is personal, I ask the questions during a one-on-one discussion.
d. Listen to the radio and watch the television newscasts. Everything is related to everything else, so what happens in Washington, D.C., will affect what happens everywhere else. Note the major issues in the United States and abroad and follow them.
e. Listen to those around you on the bus, the train, in the street, in the stores, and in the parks, gas stations, and so on. You learn a lot about people by just listening.
f. Play the "devil's advocate." It is nice to have a friend or coworker with whom you can engage in lively debates without the other person getting angry. Being able to take the contrary position or defending a position can be instructive and open new approaches to old problems.

In conclusion, the information presented in this chapter about being proactive in decision-making and how my experiences were applied can best be summarized by the following quote:

All that you do and all that you learn prepares you for that which someday you must face (Barrett, 1971, p. 237).

REFERENCES

Barrett, W. E. (1971). *A woman in the house.* New York: Doubleday.

Cohen, M. D., March, J. P., & Olsen, J. P. (1972). A garbage can model of organizational choice. *Administrative Science Quarterly, 17,* 1–25.

Cyvert, R. M., & March, J. G. (1963). *A behavioral theory of the firm.* Englewood Cliffs, N.J.: Prentice Hall.

Drucker, P. F. (1986). *The frontiers of management: Where tomorrow's decisions are being shaped today.* New York: Truman Tally Books.

Higgins, J. M. (1991). *The management challenge: An introduction to management.* New York: McMillan.

Janis, I. L., & Mann, L. (1977). *Decision making: Psychological analysis of conflict, choice, and commitment.* New York: Free Press.

Jones, G. R. (1993). *Organizational theory: Text and cases* (2nd Ed.). Reading, Mass.: Addison-Wesley.

Keiser, S., & Sproull, L. (1982). Managerial response to changing environments: Perspectives on sensing from social cognition. *Administrative Science Quarterly, 27,* 548–570.

Larkey, P. D., & Sproull, L. S. (1984). *Advances in information processing in organizations.* Vol. 1 (pp. 1–8). Greenwich, Conn.: JAI Press.

Mintzberg, H., Raisinghani, D., & Theoret, A. (1976). The structure of unstructured decision making. *Administrative Science Quarterly, 21,* 246–275.

Oxford University Press. (1996). *The Oxford dictionary and thesaurus: American edition.* New York.

Purtilo, R. (1993). *Ethical dimensions in the health professions* (2nd ed.). Philadelphia: W. B. Saunders.

Robbins, S. P., & Coulter, M. (1996). *Management* (5th ed.). Englewood Cliffs, N.J.: Prentice Hall.

Simon, H. A. (1960). *The new science of management decision.* New York: Harper and Row.

Chapter 10

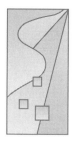

Communicating Effectively

Nancy Dickenson-Hazard
Jane A. Root

Millions of words have been written about communication, and thousands of people have attended communications skills programs—yet we continue to search for ways to communicate more effectively. For decades, researchers have attempted to determine the characteristics of competent leaders. Most studies conclude that "the total effectiveness of leaders rises and falls in direct proportion to their ability to communicate with meaning, their interpersonal insights and actions, their willingness to enthusiastically share their goals and vision and their willingness to be active, positive listeners" (Matusak, 1997, p. 80). To be effective, leaders must achieve shared meaning and understanding in their communications so that all participants reach a common understanding and the subsequent interaction is productive and satisfying.

We all believe we are effective communicators—it is the people around us who cannot communicate. To achieve and maintain a shared understanding, a leader must possess a clarity of purpose and an orientation to service and must be a value-driven person (Matusak, 1997). These basic tools combined with other communication strategies enable any person to be an effective communicator.

Communication, like leadership, is relational. It is a process that requires exchange and is constantly in process. There is no perfect communication, interaction, skill, or technique; there is only openness or better understanding and a shared focus. Over the past decades, computerized information systems have increased the volume of information and rate of exchange of that information. But have we learned to use them effectively, and have they improved the quality of our communications? Senge et al. (1994) discuss the need for 21st century companies to "engage in conversation that isn't polite" (p. 14). Information received is too fast and too much, resulting in a need for a response that is often too abrupt. Before we can engage in only impolite conversation, we first need to understand when we use the term "communication" that we may not be very clear about the use of this term.

In the context of this chapter on communication and leadership, *communication* is defined as the sending and receipt of messages and a shared social experience between two or more people, each of whom has his or her own expectations, experiences, and intentions (Coyle, 1993); it can include exchanges that are

- Verbal and nonverbal
- Interpersonal
- Organizationally focused
- Symbolic
- Culturally focused

Because the menu of options for discussing communication is so exhaustive, we have chosen to provide an overview of the communication considerations that leaders at all levels must understand.

Nurses face special challenges as communicators because their work brings them into contact with many individuals and cultures, all with subtle communication differences. Nurses must be sure that patients and their families have both heard and understood the technical language of health care. Furthermore, the nurse is challenged to create a climate for therapeutic nurse-patient communication that requires excellent listening skills, openness to information, and questions from the client. The nurse must also match what is heard with what is done for each patient's needs. Arnold and Boggs (1995) contend that

> Communication is a basic tool used in the helping relationship. It is recognized as an essential component of the theory and practice of nursing . . . The quality of the communication process, to a large extent, determines the caliber of the relationship . . . Nurses use communication skills to provide new information, correct misinformation, promote understanding of client responses to health problems, explore options for care, assist in decision-making, and facilitate the well being of clients (p. 15).

In addition, the culture determines how individuals inside the organization communicate (Thayer and Barnette, 1994). People want to work in organizations in which they feel free to speak up, but the often-unspoken rules about communication in an organization inhibit truly effective communication from occurring. This creates challenges for nurses in the room of the patient, the workroom, and the boardroom. Nurses who empower and enable themselves and those they serve to communicate effectively within these diverse organizational cultures are leaders. Those who do not still have the potential to be leaders. Booker (1994) suggests communication is a life-or-death matter. If it is practiced effectively, it breathes life into the interaction, creating shared meaning and understanding; if it is practiced poorly, it is certain to kill meaning and understanding.

The first half of this chapter provides a theoretical framework for effective communication that includes three areas:

- Characteristics of effective communication
- How the culture of an organization affects communication
- Importance of feedback

The second part of the chapter focuses on case studies of effective communication in an organization as experienced by a nurse leader.

THEORETICAL FRAMEWORK FOR EFFECTIVE COMMUNICATION

Characteristics of Effective Communication

Research on the characteristics of effective communication indicates that there are three critical factors in effective communication: effective language patterns, the ability to actively listen, and the ability to establish and retain rapport. The absence of any of these factors can create a problem in communication; conversely, the inclusion of these factors should create for the nurse effective ways to communicate with patients and their families, peers, other health care workers, and friends.

■ Language Patterns

Most individuals talk in ways that make it a challenge for their listeners to fully comprehend their meaning; this is because language patterns tend to be unique to individuals. There are four language patterns that prevent us from understanding each other: (1) deletion, (2) distortion, (3) use of vague pronouns and verbs, and (4) nominalization.

Deletion refers to information or material that is completely left out of the communication of the sender. The receiver thus is required to make assumptions about the sender's intent and to "fill in the vacancies." For example, when someone says, "I'm excited," the receiver may either assume understanding of the context of the excitement (perhaps on the basis of what the receiver is experiencing) or, better still, ask for more information ("About what?").

Distortion in communication occurs as a result of distortions in the way the world is being experienced. Distortion comes from our personal prejudices and beliefs that tend to twist our perceptions of how the world works and, therefore, affect our interactions in and with the world. Distortion can take several forms, including distortions in our thinking about *cause and effect* ("something about your behavior causes me to behave in a certain way and I have no choice about it"), *mind reading* (one person knows what others are thinking without direct communication), and *presuppositions* (if the first part of a statement is true, the second part also is true). For example,

■ The Speaker Says	■ The Effective Listener Might Respond
Cause and Effect	
Studying for this examination is giving me a headache.	How is studying for the examination giving you a headache?
It makes me so angry when she's late.	What is it about her being late that bothers you?
You expect too much from me.	What do you think I'm expecting from you?
Mind Reading	
I don't think Mary likes me.	What is it about Mary's behavior that makes you think this?

| My employees know the kind of performance I expect of them. | How do you know that they know what you want? |
| I think she's upset about what I said. | What gives you the impression she's upset with you? |

Presuppositions

I'm really sick, and I'll need an appointment immediately.	What are the symptoms you are experiencing that are causing you to think you need to come in right away?
If you really cared about our relationship, you'd pay more attention to me.	In what ways does it appear that I'm not paying attention to you?
She's not much of a supervisor, and her employees resent it.	What does she do that gives you the impression that she's a poor supervisor?

Note that the effective listener is attempting to gather more information to gain a better understanding of the statement made by the speaker. In doing so, the effective listener avoids asking questions that begin with "why." "Why" questions tend to challenge the speaker and may even be perceived as challenging the speaker's values and beliefs, therefore appearing to be confrontational.

"What" questions tend to be questions that gather information. For example, is there a difference in these exchanges?

■ The Speaker Says	■ The Effective Listener Might Respond
I don't think Mary likes me.	Why do you think so?
	or
	What is it about Mary's behavior that makes you think this?
It makes me so angry when she's late.	Why do you let it bother you?
	or
	What is it about her being late that bothers you?

Vague language, especially the use of pronouns and verbs, creates confusion and misinterpretation. What we say tends to be clear in our own minds because we have the context for our verbal statements, but such comments can lack clarity for a listener. The more specific we are in our language, the greater the chance we will be understood and mistakes in communication will be avoided. The following are examples of vague language:

■ The Speaker Says	■ The Effective Listener Might Respond
It's confusing.	What is confusing?
I learned a lot last year.	About what? In what subject areas? From whom?
I really like working with people.	What kinds of people do you especially like working with?
That lecture was really interesting.	What, specifically, did you find interesting about it?

| Things just seem to be going wrong today! | Specifically, what's going wrong for you? |

Nominalizations occur when we use language that appears to be precise but is not. Words such as "overworked," "problems," and "relationship" provide us with little in the way of concrete information. Without additional information, McKay et al. (1995) suggest you can identify nominalizations because they are too abstract to visualize. For example:

■ The Speaker Says	■ The Effective Listener Might Respond
I think she disapproves of me.	In what ways is she showing her disapproval?
I think we need to make a decision about meetings.	Let's decide how often we need to meet.
This week has been full of problems.	What kinds of problems have you been having?
I don't see any solutions.	What solutions have you already considered?
She's always been so successful.	In what ways do you see that she's been a success?
I thought everything about it was boring.	Everything? Specifically, what did you find boring?
If I'm going to do this project, I'm going to need some help.	What kinds of help do you think you'll need?
I was disappointed in the way the meeting ended.	What was it about the ending that disappointed you?
I really like working with people.	What is it about working with people that you enjoy?
I think that patient is going to need more attention.	What do we need to attend to?

The statements above by the speaker are examples of the way we talk. The responses are provided as examples of ways effective communicators use clarifying questions to gain additional information so they have a better understanding of what is being said. Thus, the sender is responsible for speaking more precisely; if not, the receiver has a responsibility for clarifying what was said if communication is to be meaningful and understood by both parties of the interchange.

There is an old story about a sculptor who worked in stone. He was working on a large piece, using a hammer and a chisel to carefully shape the stone. Suddenly, the hammer slipped, and the chisel hit his hand and badly cut it. He rushed to a hospital, where surgery that saved his hand was performed; however, the man was angry that the accident had occurred, and he melted down the blade of the chisel and broke the handle of the hammer into pieces of kindling. It wasn't long before he realized that he had destroyed the tools he used to express his artistic gifts and to make a living, so he purchased new tools and began to work again.

Language, like the hammer and chisel, is a tool for our use. Like the sculptor's tools, it must be used precisely and with care; used carelessly it can confuse others, can misrepresent us, and may even do harm. Unlike the sculptor, we cannot simply dispense with language. The sculptor discovered that destroying his tools would not solve his problems; no more will refusing to communicate with others resolve our problems as communicators. Improving our "aim," sharpening our communication tools, and understanding that errors in communication are the feedback we need to improve as communicators will all contribute to high-quality communication.

■ Active Listening

Not only is listening a critical part of the communication process, it also is an activity that consumes many of our waking hours, even when we are not in an active communication mode. We listen to music, to the news on the radio or television, to lectures in classes, and to the sermon in church. Listening is not the same as hearing. Hearing is the physiological process of receiving vibrations on our eardrums, making hearing a passive process, whereas listening is an active process that involves interpretation. According to Devito (1995), listening requires five processes:

1. *Receiving a message from a speaker.* A message can be verbal, nonverbal (gestures or facial expressions), or both. Receiving seems simple enough but becomes complicated by our tendency to shift to thinking about what our response will be. Receiving, therefore, requires focused attention on the speaker.
2. *Striving to learn the meaning of the speaker's verbal and nonverbal messages.* We do this through our understanding of the message's context—what we already know about the speaker and his/her perspective—as well as the content and by asking clarifying questions and rephrasing the speaker's words to determine if we understand.
3. *Using understanding to help us in remembering.* The challenge of this activity is that we tend to remember not what was said but what we think was said. We are helped to remember by focusing on the central ideas presented.
4. *Evaluating the speaker's message, judging intentions or motives.* We may be analyzing the message against our own criteria, prejudices, opinions, and beliefs.
5. *Responding.* We may give responses during the speaker's message, both verbal (e.g., "I see . . .", "Yes . . .") and nonverbal (e.g., such as nodding or smiling). Responses after the message is complete may include several dimensions of communication including agreeing, emphasizing, or questioning.

To actively listen to another person is both a commitment and a gift. We all violate these five processes at times and create blocks to effective listening, as when we judge, filter what is being heard, or half listen. McKay et al. (1995) suggest six behaviors that will communicate to others that you are listening:

1. Maintaining good eye contact
2. Leaning slightly forward when listening

3. Reinforcing the speaker by nodding or paraphrasing
4. Asking clarifying questions
5. Staying free of distractions that prevent you from giving your entire self to the speaker
6. Making a commitment to try to understand what is being said

The importance of increasing your skills as a listener cannot be overemphasized. One study of 68 adults in different occupations found that on the average, 9% of the adults spent their time writing, 16% of their time reading, 30% of their time talking, and 55% of their time listening (Barbara, 1971). For health care providers, poor listening can be hazardous to the patient's health.

■ Rapport

The third characteristic of effective communication is the ability to gain rapport with the person to whom you are talking. Rapport occurs when you tune your body language, verbal language, and tone to match those of the other person. Rapport creates a common ground. This happens through the unconscious or conscious matching of behaviors with those of the other person, such as

- Matching voice tempo—accelerating or slowing the speed of your speech
- Matching voice tone—becoming louder or softer
- Matching breathing rate
- Matching body posture

This matching of body postures must be done with subtlety, or it will appear to be mimicry or the person will think you are making fun of him or her. As Laborde (1983) explains,

> Maintaining rapport is a way to synchronize the different experiences, values, and meanings of human beings. External matching accentuates similarities and lays down differences so that understanding and rapport between people seems to increase (p. 36).

Gaining rapport through the external synchronization of our behaviors and physiological responses provides us with a way to emphasize the similarities between us. Establishing rapport increases the trust between speaker and listener, allowing for more open and honest communication, communication that is viewed as supportive and not hostile or negative. When we have rapport with others, the trust between us increases and we do not have to "watch our words."

As with many aspects of life, being an effective communicator takes skill and practice. If you want to learn a new skill, such as how to tell patients not to do something because it is harmful to them, you are encouraged to practice the skill until doing it becomes natural to you. However, many of us do not carry this simple principle over into our communication. Practice the skill by externally synchronizing (matching) your voice tempo and tone, breathing rate, and body posture in your communication with others for 2 weeks and then evaluate whether you think these changes have improved your ability to gain rapport with others.

A basic rule of communication is that communication is the response you get. The response received is feedback about whether the message was understood. Our tendency is to blame the listener for our missent message rather than understanding it as feedback. What we intend to communicate may not be what is received. For example, if you are in a restaurant and you ask the server for a glass of water and he brings you a cup coffee, what does this mean? Let's analyze this error in communication; what do we need to ask ourselves about what happened here?

- Were there physical barriers to the server's ability to hear me, such as noise from other diners or from the kitchen or clattering of dishes?
- Did I speak too softly and the server did not hear the request?
- And, taken to the absurd level, does the server know the difference between water and coffee? For example, do I need to specify that water is the clear liquid served in a glass, not the hot, brown liquid served in a cup?
- Or do I assume that the server has an "attitude" and isn't interested in responding appropriately to the request?

As silly as this example is, how often do we assume that the listener understands our meaning even when we have not provided sufficient "cues" and "clues" to assist the listener? And what do we say to ourselves when the communication we send is not responded to as we predicted?

If you do not receive the response you anticipated, this may mean that the listener does not understand you. Your task then is to change your communication approach until your intended response occurs. For example, if you ask one or more clarifying questions but you observe that the questions are creating defensiveness instead of clarity, you are not getting the communication outcome you sought. Your ability to adapt and be flexible will increase the likelihood of getting the desired outcome.

We do not believe that individuals get up in the morning and say to themselves, "I think I'll do all I can to miscommunicate with others today." Errors in communication occur for a reason, and part of becoming an effective communicator is to reduce the variables that cause communication errors. This is accomplished by practicing clarity in communication, assuming positive intent on the part of those responding to our communication, and understanding that errors in communication are feedback for us about our communication skill level.

Communication in Organizations: Understanding the Culture

Perhaps the most significant factor influencing communication in organizations is the organizational culture. Schein (1985) defines culture as "a pattern of basic assumptions invented, discovered, or developed by a given group as it learns to cope with its problems of external adaptation and internal integration, that has worked well enough to be considered valued and, therefore, to be taught to new members as the correct way to perceive, think, and feel in relation to those problems" (p. 7). A less complex definition is that culture "is the way we do things around here" (Deal and Kennedy, 1982, p. 4). Culture can also be thought of as the rules of the game (Nelson, 1997, p. 64).

These rules dictate how members of the organization communicate with each other and the content of the communication. For example, Nelson (1997) suggests the following questions to assist in an understanding of how an organization approaches communication.

> Is information treated as a scarce good, or does it flow freely? Do communication practices and norms support a sense of professionalism, mutual respect, and decorum? Do norms exclude from discussion personal concerns unrelated to the performance of the organization? Do people feel reasonably comfortable about communicating negative information to superiors? Is honesty in the admission of mistakes interpreted as a sign of strength and professionalism? Do norms encourage ample and honest communication with clients? (p. 65).

He further suggests other areas where there may be communication rules, such as communication about money and performance and what happens to individuals who are the bearers of bad news to the organization. Ryan et al. (1996) write in their book *The Courageous Messenger* that learning how to speak up builds more positive work environments and dynamics. And there is a growing trend in organizations for everything that goes on in the organization to be fair game for discussion and that "disclosure is healthy and restraint is unhealthy" (Nelson, 1997, p. 64). However, Nelson also notes

> The bigger the problem the stronger the propensity toward denial, so people and organizations with more problems tend to deny more. The denial process sucks up large amounts of mental and physical resources, leaving us less energy to deal with problems and thereby exacerbating our difficulties further. Additional difficulties call for the further denial, and so on. Logically, then, the less our rules restrict the subject matter and delivery of communication, the less denial and better health our organization will have (p. 64).

Errors in communication have not disappeared with the addition of complex communication technology such as electronic mail; however, they may change the rules about communication. Communication technology has been credited with increasing the efficiency of communication in organizations, improving the work environment, and "democratizing" the flow of information, thereby reducing the hierarchies that develop in many organizations about both the quantity and quality of information that is shared at various levels. Some organizations have discovered that electronic mail allows for less formal, shorter written messages (Taylor, 1981). Although these trends can be highly positive, e-mail places a greater responsibility on the sender to write clearly.

Similar challenges exist with voice mail, in which a lack of direct feedback, which is usually a part of telephone communication, may create additional confusion about the message. "Face to face communication is the richest communication medium because it allows immediate feedback, has the capacity to provide multiple cues, communicates in natural language, and can be highly personal. A message can be adjusted, clarified, and reinforced instantly" (Trevino et al., 1990, pp. 75–76).

One of the challenges in discussing communication in organizations according to Jablin et al. (1994) is separating interpersonal communication competence from communication competence at the organizational level. The latter usually includes management information systems, communication media and organizational history, and the competencies of those members of the organizations who are responsible for representing and presenting the organization to the internal and external audiences.

At the interpersonal and organizational levels, we assume a rationality in the communication. As Pearson and Daniels (1988) note, "in many day-to-day episodes of communication, people may well 'know' what kinds of behaviors will be both appropriate and effective, yet act in ways that deviate considerably from the behavior that their knowledge would seem to prescribe" (p. 99).

Importance of Feedback

Perhaps the most challenging aspect of organizational communication is giving and receiving feedback. Hathaway (1990) observes that we tend to think of most feedback as negative, but in reality, feedback can be a resource for achieving positive results, a mechanism for improving our work and our relationships with others. In the final analysis, we can accept or reject the feedback we receive from others.

Giving and receiving feedback—telling the truth as you perceive it to be—can strengthen a relationship, increase trust between individuals, and create new solutions to problems. "To tell the truth, you build a bridge. It's a bridge of words. One end of the bridge is anchored by your reason for telling the truth in the first place. The other end is anchored by the needs the person you're telling the truth to will have in hearing your truth and in giving you what you need in response" (Foster, 1997, p. 271).

■ Giving Feedback

Hathaway (1990) states there are three steps in giving unsolicited feedback.

Step 1: Timing feedback. Feedback is more likely to be heard when it is given at a time and place that are free of interruptions and when the receiver of the feedback is not under excessive stress or distracted.

Step 2: Asking permission. Asking the receiver for permission to give feedback increases the likelihood that the feedback will be heard.

Step 3: Being specific. Providing specific examples of the behavior you have observed, explaining your reaction to and your preferences for an alternative that would be satisfactory to you and to the receiver of the feedback, improve the quality of the feedback. If appropriate, benefits that will result from a change in behavior should be included ("I believe our patients will be better served").

Many times, feedback is poorly received because planning of the feedback session was haphazard and ill-conceived. A fourth step (and actually the first in this progression of steps) is to prepare to give feedback. Activities that should be considered before giving feedback include

- Rehearsing what you want to say
- Anticipating the responses of the receiver
- Getting clear about the behavior you observe and the behavior you believe is more desirable
- Reflecting on how you can offer your support for change

It is probably apparent by now that the critical skills for those who lead are competence in interpersonal communication and the ability to handle "people problems." Many nurses feel much more comfortable with the "technical" aspects of nursing, such as budget decisions, giving assignments, and providing nursing expertise to staff and patients that will improve the patients' health status. Some nurses actually perceive dealing with people problems as an illegitimate use of their time. Providing clear and useful feedback or giving instructions, for example, can sometimes be viewed as activities that take up valuable time rather than as critical functions that are part of any nurse's job.

■ Receiving Feedback

Research on the development of successful executives tells us that a significant component of their development includes increasing their self-understanding by actively seeking feedback about themselves.

> Most people believe they do know themselves, but there is overwhelming evidence from psychological research that a lot of energy is expended protecting our self-image. As easy as it sounds, it can be incredibly difficult to accept knowledge of personal limits, to accept responsibility for mistakes, or to recognize skill deficiencies (McCall et al., 1997, pp. 136–137).

What if you receive feedback that you have not solicited? Feedback can be a major opportunity for learning. Weisinger (1981) believes we should ask questions when reflecting on feedback that is unsolicited. Hathaway (1990) suggests we ask the following questions of ourselves:

- Do I hear the same feedback from more than one person?
- Does the critic know a great deal about the subject?
- Are the critic's standards known and reasonable?
- Is the critical feedback really about me? Or is the critic merely having a bad day or upset about something else?
- How important is it for me to respond to the critical feedback? (p. 21)

■ Self-Feedback

Finally, although feedback from others is essential, equally important is self-awareness, or what we think of as "self-feedback." When we are truly honest with ourselves, we know when we can and should improve our work performance, communicate more effectively, be more disciplined or dependable, build new skills, and so on. When we are being honest with ourselves, we know when an interpersonal communication has not gone well or when we have not "done our homework" in preparing for a meeting or a work task. Rather than finding a reason outside of ourselves for these errors and deficiencies, we can be honest with ourselves and consider strategies that would prevent them from occurring in the future. McCall et al. (1997) notes that exceptional executives accept responsibility for their shortcomings and for their own learning and make choices to do something about them. Awareness, through introspection, and feedback from others are prerequisites to change and are essential to the development of leadership.

The technological advances in diagnoses and treatment will continue to expand and bring countless benefits to the patients in the health care system. However, effective communication skills continue to be the most important resource nurses have for expanding their knowledge, appreciating the richness of the human experience, and deepening relationships with coworkers, patients, and their families. There is no better way to provide quality care than to be an effective communicator.

Summary

Communication is defined as the sending and receiving of messages between two or more people. Unfortunately, defining communication is easier than actually communicating, because to communicate meaningfully and fully requires both verbal and nonverbal communication, which brings with it the expectations, experiences, and intentions of both the sender and the receiver. Over the past two decades, the complexity of communication has increased due primarily to technology, including both the increased volume of communication and the speed at which it is exchanged through technologies such as e-mail and faxing.

Ironically, the most effective communication tool continues to be face-to-face interchange, although even face-to-face communication can result in "mixed messages" between the sender and the receiver if effective communication methodologies are not observed. These include rapport, effective language patterns, and active listening. The absence of any one of these factors can create a problem in communication; conversely, the inclusion of these factors should create for the nurse effective ways to communicate with patients, their families, and colleagues and in nonwork relationships.

ONE NURSE'S EXPERIENCES AS AN EFFECTIVE COMMUNICATOR

The professional and popular literature has repeatedly stressed the importance of communication to success as a leader. Each leader develops his or her unique style of communicating with colleagues, constituents, and subordinates, but consistent among all leaders are the abilities to establish and maintain rapport, actively listen, and use effective language patterns. Over the past 25 years, we have been privileged to hold a myriad of leadership positions and during the course of these experiences have learned from both successes and failures in communication. What we present here are one nurse's stories of getting it right sometimes and wrong sometimes but always learning and improving.

Know Thyself, or "What You See Is What You Get"

A prerequisite to effective communication in any leadership role, whether it is leading a work team, a patient and family, or a large organization, is to know yourself. Being comfortable with who you are and developing the ability to articulate this as it relates to your work are all-important to receiving and sending clear communications. The congruence between the leader's values and beliefs and those of the organization are paramount. In many ways, the leader and organization become one, making a match mandatory between what the leader believes and what the organization stands for. Without this fit, neither the individual nor the agency can meet their purposes.

On two separate occasions, I found myself before search and screen committees interviewing for leadership positions. The decisions to seek these positions were driven by two factors: a desire to expand my contribution to nursing and health care and a passionate belief in lifelong growth and development in others and myself. My track record as an administrator was decent, and my skill set was relatively comprehensive. I had come to believe firmly in a working environment that values differences in people and their talents; believes in a cause, in service to others above self; provides room and resources to get the job done; celebrates achievements and learns from failures; expects accountability for doing your best; builds openness, creativity, trust, and respect; encourages cooperation and collaboration; and is an environment that is driven by a vision of what can be rather than what is. In both instances, I was looking for such a place in which to plant myself, with the hope that I would bloom. I had reached a plateau in my preceding positions and knew that the climate and culture of those organizations needed something and someone different. Our long-term goals had been met, future ones were established, and strategies were ready for implementation. I, too, needed new challenges and recognized that moving on was appropriate, being content that the organizations and people I served had grown and developed.

In advance of these interviews, I had been provided with questions, and although they were all appropriate, and necessary in order for the decision-makers to determine the best candidate for the positions, I frankly found them a bit daunting. They were questions/statements such as

- Describe three leadership initiatives you have undertaken.
- How would you develop a strategic plan? A business plan?
- Describe how you have done this previously.
- Describe how you would resolve a constituent or staff conflict.
- Discuss your experiences with evaluation of services. Of performance. Of outcomes.
- What makes you uniquely qualified to assume this position?
- What are your strengths and weaknesses?
- What is your leadership style?
- What is your vision for the organization?

What I realized after several days of asking myself "what have I gotten into?" is that the organizations were not only evaluating my skill sets but also assessing my ability to communicate who I was to determine a fit with the missions of the organizations.

My final approach during the interviews, which I did prepare for, was to convey "what you see is what you get." This was not necessarily a display of attitude but more of a truth statement about who I am and what I believe so the agencies and I would know whether a relationship was possible. I answered each of their questions thoughtfully and honestly and made it a point to clearly state my views about such things as leadership style, business plans, conflict resolution, and evaluation. I also asked questions of them: "What does this organization need from its leaders? What is its governing philosophy? How are decisions made? What are the routes of communication?" More importantly, we discussed what it means to be entrusted to lead, what and whom the organization serves, and what was the history of the organization and its relationships, expectations, hopes, and dreams? As the dialogue evolved, evidence of congruence between my beliefs and values and those of the organizations emerged.

The most telling discourse, however, was when the question "What is your vision for the organization?" was posed to me. This is a question I have been asked in every interview for every leadership position I have assumed, and my answer has always been the same—"My vision is that of the organization. We need to arrive at that vision through a shared process using the talents and expertise of all those involved and touched by the organization." This response, although sounding a bit grandiose, reflects my belief that the lead staff member of any organization is present to *share* the governance for that organization, not to control it. It becomes the responsibility of that leader to execute the vision into reality, to make it happen, and to communicate to the stakeholders as action happens. But many people contribute to the crafting of what *can* be for an organization. As this was expressed to my interviewers, it became apparent that knowing myself not only helped to identify common ground but also began to establish a rapport with my future employers and laid the foundation for open communication.

Knowing ourselves is not always an easy lesson. It does require continual learning, self-improvement, and introspection. It also requires a belief in yourself and a passion for the job. I vividly recall accepting an offer to consult with a not-for-profit organization to teach physical assessment to a group of pediatric nurses. Lured by the prestige of the institution and flattered by the offer, I readily agreed to take on the 6-week course, thinking "How hard can this be? I do this every day." In my subsequent planning conversations with the organizers, I soon found out how wrong I was! I had not only failed to hear what the course objectives were, but I had also neglected to examine what I had to offer. Yes, I did possess physical assessment knowledge and skills, but I lacked the teaching skills, prowess, and confidence to convey this to students. Although I had the passion for the content, I did not have the communication talents to teach it. My initial conversations were filled with distortions (i.e., "I can perform physical assessments, therefore I can teach it" versus "Is doing assessments the same skill as teaching?"). There also was vagueness in our conversations (i.e., "They have confidence I can do this" versus "Confidence in what?"). Nominalization was present as well (i.e., "We need you to teach the class" versus "What are the skills needed to meet the course objectives?"). It soon became obvious that these obstacles impeded effective communication regarding my ability to meet their expectations. Our solution was to pair me with an experienced lecturer while I demonstrated. This experience taught me several valuable lessons: (1) it is better to know your strengths and weaknesses and admit them rather than doing something incorrectly; (2) having confidence in your own abilities before sharing them with others is critical because others are relying on you for leadership; (3) self-improvement is continual and takes many, and sometimes, unlikely forms; and (4) effective communication requires a desire to hear what others are saying, as well as carrying a responsibility for ensuring mutual understanding.

The C's of Communication: "Am I Speaking in Foreign Tongues?"

Engaging in communication that is clear, complete, correct, current, and congruent spells success, with success being measured by the response you receive. In essence, are the objectives of your communication being met, or are you speaking in a "foreign tongue"?

Effective communication involves the messages we send, as well as those we receive. It involves what we say, what we hear, and what each party thinks the other said and heard. When all the C's are present, we establish a shared or common meaning and a shared understanding about the subject of discussion. Without them, we generate frustration and, frequently, mistrust.

Using the C's for communications in large organizations is particularly important and effective for a leader. As the size of an organization increases, so do the scope and amount of information. We are all bombarded with print, electronic, verbal, and behavioral communications. The leader in such circumstances is continually challenged to process and pass on the information that is important for those in the environment to achieve the goals of the organization. Much like being in the center of an hourglass, the leader must ensure that what message is sent does not become bogged down in the middle where she or he sits. The leader must maintain a flow that is timely and relevant to the decisions and actions that need to occur. Likewise, the leader must set expectations and nurture similar communication skills in those surrounding him or her. The most effective skills contribute to making communication clear, complete, correct, current, and congruent.

On assuming a leadership role in a large, not-for-profit member-driven organization, I was met with the challenge of maintaining a flow of information among the members, staff, and a board of directors. I recognized that the first communications to each of these groups were important to future success. Although patterns (once a week or once a quarter) and vehicles (print, verbal, electronic) might change, it was essential to initiate and establish an atmosphere of openness. It was also imperative to convey the same message. This message was that the organization existed to serve its membership. To the board of directors, this message conveyed the following:

> As the elected body of the membership, you have been entrusted with overseeing the well being of this organization. You are members who have achieved

one of the highest honors and weightiest responsibilities the organization can bestow. As executive, my role is to serve as your advisor, to provide resources, to implement policies, to keep you apprised of activities and issues and to direct the administration of the organization's work.

The board of directors was equally clear in their expectations of their role: "To be the guardians of the organization; to represent as a whole the membership and to be responsive to the constituents and changing environments." In addition, the board members saw themselves as responsible for the integrity of governance of the organization and for maintaining accountability for all organizational activity. They further expressed their expectations to delegate administrative function to the executive, seek her counsel on matters before them, support the executive in decisions and actions consistent with organizational goals, hold the executive accountable for the direction of the organization, and evaluate the work of the executive.

This open communication created a shared understanding of our collaborative work, as well as clearly defined mutual expectations. A myriad of vehicles and patterns of communication were subsequently established to carry out this shared understanding. Tools such as facilitated retreats, construction of a governance resource manual and board orientation process, establishment of monthly e-mail updates from the executive, institution of a governance continuum process guided by organizational programs of work, development and use of board of directors and executive evaluation tools and processes, and ongoing leadership development readings and exercises were implemented. With each change of the board, these expectations and tools are reviewed, amended, or confirmed to ensure open communication, shared understanding, and accomplishment of organizational goals.

To the staff of the organization, the primary message was similar: "We are here to serve our members." Awareness of the ambivalence associated with a transition in leadership made it important to recognize both the anxiety and the excitement produced by this change while not losing sight of our primary purpose. It was essential to lay out as quickly as possible how this purpose would be accomplished, and it was also imperative to converse with the entire staff at the same time, knowing that what was said would traverse the grapevine with lightening speed.

At the first all-staff meeting, the one priority that was communicated was that staff should provide the highest level of service to our members; it was explained that we had been entrusted to be responsive to member needs and that the expectation was that this would be carried out by each of us in a timely, accurate, and caring manner.

To provide an understanding of my leadership style, it was explained to staff that participation and cooperation were welcomed and encouraged. I expressed my view that working collaboratively achieves greater results and that we would be working individually and collectively on building team skills. As far as direct supervision was concerned, the situation would dictate the approach: sometimes I would hover, sometimes they would be on their own. However, it was conveyed that I would do everything in my power to provide them with whatever help and resources were needed to get the job done. In addition, an open-door policy in terms of problem solving and decision-making was offered. I conveyed that sharing difficulties was not considered a weakness but that asking someone for help was a sign of collaboration and respect. If a mistake was made, it was far better to be accountable for it, vowing to improve next time and learning from it.

In addition, as we were effecting this change, two other behaviors were expected of staff members: loyalty, which meant giving an honest opinion and engaging in debate, but once a decision was made, carrying it out as if it were their own; and being kept informed, which meant no surprises, because I would much rather hear the problem while a difference could be made than after the fact. Finally, I outlined a consensus-building process we would use to build this new team. It was a process involving listening to individuals and groups; envisioning ways to organize ourselves to more efficiently serve the members; and using resources such as focus groups, retreats, staff development activities, and consultation.

The staff was also clear about their own expectations as employees. They expressed a belief in the work of the organization and regarded themselves as being responsible for providing service, resources, and information to the members. They regarded the organization as one of the best places they had worked and expressed a desire to do the best job they possibly could. Their expectations of their leader were equally lucid: to listen, to be fair in interactions and decisions, to be clear in expectations of them, to facilitate and mentor them in team building, to help them deal with change, and to keep them involved and informed.

The open exchange between staff and leader revealed a mutual understanding based on a shared vision of what we were in the business of doing. Communication such as this positions people to better understand the other person's perspective, limits passing of judgments on someone or something, engenders trust, and fosters generosity of spirit—all of which create fertile ground for building a culture rooted in shared meaning.

The message of expectations to and from the members of the organization was the most important of all communications. As the organizational core, the unified message to members from the board of directors, executives, and staff was that we serve to facilitate their advancement in achieving the mission and goals of the organization. It was conveyed that our expectations of ourselves were fourfold:

- To be responsive to member needs and concerns
- To nurture and protect the organization on the members' behalf
- To oversee the administration of the organization's affairs and activities
- To use a membership-based process to implement initiatives

Also communicated was the high regard in which members were held, as well as a deep respect for the trust placed in us to safeguard and direct the organization. Members received the clear message that it was our job to provide resources and opportunities, which enabled them to fulfill the purposes of the organization.

Expectations of members were also conveyed. It was hoped that individually and collectively, members would involve themselves, their talents, and their resources to live the organizational mission. Member commitment to contribute to goal fulfillment was a high expectation. These messages were conveyed via regular periodic communications through multiple print, electronic, and verbal vehicles. They were well received, as indicated by the increased numbers of members, use of resources, and involvement with organizational activities.

Members themselves were also very clear about their expectations of the organization. Through surveys and focus groups, members expressed a belief in the organization's work and a general satisfaction with the service and resources provided them to achieve this work. They conveyed the expectations of timely receipt of services and benefits, maintenance of the prestige and integrity of the organization, provision of quality products and services, expansion of activities for their changing needs, and receipt of regular communication about the organization and its activities.

This open communication using the C's of communication sustained the growth and progress of the organization. When the door is open to information exchange, it generates the chance to initiate new action or to put people in touch with each other. It provides the necessary data on how to respond and to tailor activities to meet member needs. Members in turn respond by becoming more invested in the organization, and the organization prospers. This reciprocal communication between members and leaders was evidenced by reframing existing programs to a changing membership, creating new activities and services as requested, and witnessing increased member participation and active contribution to the organization.

The most valuable lesson to be learned from open communication is that people just want to be asked. Members repeatedly expressed appreciation for the chance to express their expectations. They were equally enthused by seeing tangible change, which fulfilled their needs in advancing the organization's goals. Their enthusiasm played out as a larger investment of themselves in the organization's work, an outcome the leaders found gratifying. The cycle of openly receiving and sending information resulted in shared meaning and understanding, as well as shared action.

Active Listening, or "The Lights Are On but Is Anyone Home?"

Inherent in using the C's of communication is the ability to listen. Becoming an active, positive listener is a skill that is learned and constantly improved. With its effective development, communication is enhanced and trust ensues—what person does not like to know that his or her thoughts are valuable by having another person pay attention? Without active listening, communication is impaired and eventually stifled in a barrage of barriers and inconsistencies.

Many of us learn the value of active, positive listening by overcoming barriers to it. One such barrier—gazing intently but not hearing a word—was brought home for me when I was a participant at an interdisciplinary meeting with an agenda focused on strategies to reduce the stress of change. There were 10 participants, and all had been asked to share their success and failure stories. Discussion ensued after each story. Having completed the telling and discussion of my stories, I was enjoying and contributing to those of others. Or at least I looked attentive and participatory, but my mind had wandered into other irrelevant areas. Then I heard asked of me, "Isn't this a problem similar to the one you experienced?" In a flash I was back to the venue, realizing that I had not really heard what had been said. Not only did I find it embarrassing to point this out to my colleagues, but I managed to impede the progress of discussion. Luckily for me, many of my fellow participants had experienced this same phenomenon, and the facilitator dealt with it in a humorous way, saying "Does anybody else have their lights on but is not at home? Maybe it's time for a break!" But the experience taught me to maintain good eye contact and jot down notes paraphrasing what the speaker was saying or write down questions that I wish to ask for clarification.

Other stumbling blocks to listening include jumping to conclusions ("The answer to your dilemma is obvious"), planning your response instead of listening ("I find your situation and response unacceptable"), formulating an opinion before the message is finished (shaking your head midsentence while saying, "Approaching this problem by a different perspective will achieve a better result"), and listening selectively (showing boredom). Each of these barriers inhibits and sometimes kills the communication process.

Listening itself becomes a clear means of communication. One of the first activities I undertake when assuming a leadership role is to have one-on-one conversations with each staff member. This provides an opportunity to learn and know more about the organization and the people functioning in it. The basic agenda for the conversations is shared in advance and involves my listening as staff members describe their roles as they are, their roles as they would wish they were, their personal goals, and how I or the organization can make this happen. The setting is quiet, removed from activity, and free of barriers between us (such as a table or desk). Experience has proved time and time again that once the initial nervousness and reticence have passed, both creative and critical thoughts flow abundantly. My role in these conversations is to listen, ask clarifying questions, and come to understand each person and his or her perspective. The information received is invaluable to helping people and, subsequently, the organization to achieve the highest potential.

In one particular conversation in which the employee was quite critical of the organization, she expressed a perception of not being respected for her work. When I asked what being respected meant, she said simply, "being given words of praise." For another employee who was generally unhappy with his employment, citing numerous resource deficits, I asked what made it satisfactory enough for him to stay despite all the negative feelings. His answer was that he really believed in the work of the organization and his possibilities within a new paradigm. These clarifying questions told me several things. First, being recognized for a job well done was a compelling need for all, which prompted investigation and subsequently the development of an annual staff recognition event. Second, despite perceived poor circumstances, a belief in something makes things tolerable, at least for a while. Because of one employee's comment, the relocation of equipment and personnel resources to improve the functioning of the department ultimately doubled performance.

Listening throughout these conversations in a positive, attentive manner provided invaluable data. When synthesized, it revealed areas of common concern and common idea themes. Once the synthesis was validated, this information served as a springboard for action. Listening provided the basis for role redefinition, reorganization, reallocation of resources, staff recognition and development programs, redistribution of tasks, creation of work teams, and much more. The tangible results were an increase in morale and productivity. These conversations were so successful that open chat times and regular visits to work areas were established just to listen to what was going on. Listening helps me keep my fingers on the pulse of activities for the organization and is an effective communication tool that serves as a stepping stone to establishing trust and building rapport.

Establishing Rapport, or "Sink or Synchrony"

Engaging in interactions and building relationships that are characterized by harmony promote confidence and demonstrate a willingness to cooperate. Our behavior and words are the tools by which we establish and maintain rapport. Using them in a manner synchronous with those we are relating to is a challenge and requires a conscious effort to maintain flow with the other person. Rapport building requires confidence in self, a certain degree of vulnerability, and a willingness to be open, courageous, purposeful, and patient. In each encounter, we allow ourselves varying degrees of openness, with our behavior being the indicator of our willingness to create unison.

Several years ago, I employed an articulate, intelligent, attractive, and well-qualified young woman to spearhead a major public relations initiative for an organization. In small-group conversations involving the three or four persons in her department, she was relaxed, conversant, open to suggestions and spirited debate, and creative. She was able to create a synergy between herself and those in the small group—so much so that an outside observer would believe she was a long-time colleague and friend of members of the group. However, in the larger management group of 10 to 12 persons or more, her behavior was totally different. Her posture was tense, her arms were crossed, her eyes were diverted around the room or downward, and frequently, she turned her chair away from the group. Her demeanor was detached, and her tone of voice when she did speak was harsh, with her words haughty or even demeaning. The end result of these almost opposite behaviors was that although her immediate work group functioned quite well in an atmosphere of collaboration, her rapport with the larger group was minimal to nonexistent. Eventually, the distrust created by a lack of similarity between her and the other work group managers began to affect performance. Without the rapport among managers, collaboration and cooperative efforts were impossible. She needed clear communication and positive working relationships with the other managers to do her organization-wide public relations work. Without it, she ran into difficulties in securing the information and cooperation she needed to perform her job. In time, she was able to correct this deficit in her repertoire of communication skills through classes, mentoring, and practice, and she became respected and highly regarded in the organization.

For several decades, I have served as the executive of member-driven organizations. The reality of this role is that with every election or appointment cycle, I have a new boss. On a regular basis, I must create common ground with a new president and board. We must synchronize our different experiences, values, and meanings to be effective for the organization. What I have experienced is that truly significant rapport is much more than behavioral and physiological synchrony. It is an investment and giving of self to achieve a greater good. Paramount in this rapport development is a sustained and clear focus on what is best for the organization. The most successful and sustainable rapport I have experienced requires this mission and purpose focus; a generosity of spirit, time, patience; and a positive attitude. So each time this happens, several tactics have been found to be effective in facilitating the development of this synchrony:

- Extensive orientation to the organization and its history, mission, goals, and culture
- Continual leadership development activities
- Getting to know each person personally and professionally, and letting them know me
- Talking regularly with the board and even more frequently with the president
- Asking and listening
- Sending messages and information openly and honestly
- Being sensitive to, valuing, and respecting our differences
- Creating hospitable space
- Continually asking, "Is this in the best interest of the organization?"

The response to these strategies is generally welcomed, and efforts to build a positive rapport are eagerly pursued. The adaptability and flexibility that have been demonstrated by individuals of the leadership team has been extraordinary over the years. Trust, in an atmosphere of amicability, respect, and lasting friendships, has endured past the point of professional responsibility. Most importantly, the work of the organization has been achieved with ease, and its successes have increased. This occurred because the governing body developed relationships that are equal and collegial versus hierarchical and that focused on policy rather than procedure. They have established a rapport that is unique to them as a group yet permits them to act as a single entity in the best interest of the organization. These boards have proved that establishing open rapport is hard work, fun, and rewarding.

Culture, or "Walk the Talk"

Culture, as defined as the way things happen in an organization, is dependent on communication to exist. It is where all elements of the organization come together to achieve the mission and goals, and it is where the totality of communication happens to achieve the desired response—a successful organization. Whatever an organization desires to achieve occurs through its culture, and whatever the culture achieves happens through communications.

As the environment in which organizational mission and goals are lived out, culture is created, built, and maintained by the leader. In many ways, the leader's personality becomes embedded in the culture of the organization. The leader's beliefs, values, and assumptions are transferred to subordinates and colleagues, thereby creating an attitude and a way for things to get done. The creating and building of a culture require a vision of what is preferred for the organization and takes tremendous energy.

Leaders build culture in two distinct ways:

1. By surrounding themselves with subordinates who think and feel the way they do (this is achieved by hiring only people who meet this criteria or by socializing existing people into it)
2. By role modeling behavior that encourages subordinates to internalize and identify with the leader's beliefs, values, and vision

Because organizations are dynamic systems with development cycles of their own, they are constantly evolving. Such changing requires the organization's leader to understand the organization's culture, strengths, and weaknesses and to consolidate elements needed to maintain the organization's ability to function and grow (i.e., adding stability and permanence) while developing new concepts and skills (i.e., creativity and innovation).

Changing the culture frequently means unlearning things that no longer serve the organization well, a process that creates anxiety and resistance. Although no culture shift is free of challenges, leaders are best served by not arbitrarily changing culture through a dramatic elimination of dysfunctional elements or an edict on how things will be from now on. Letting the culture evolve by building on strengths while permitting the dysfunction and weakness to atrophy over time provides a more stabilizing approach. Cultural dynamics are clearly articulated in the patterns of communication, and change begins with understanding these patterns as illustrated in the following scenario.

To gain an understanding of how things were done operationally in a large, not-for-profit service-oriented organization, I conducted individual interviews, as previously described, with each staff member. An analysis of the content of these conversations revealed many common themes and an overall paradox of wanting to function collaboratively but actually functioning in an independent manner. The rules of the culture dictated top-down centralized communications and decision-making and discouraged cross-departmental or employee problem solving and decision-making. Information was closely guarded based on belief that if it was shared, others would use it to their advantage with the boss. Closed, "grapevine" systems of communication were prevalent versus open, honest, complete systems (i.e., if you wanted to know something about a project, you went to the "organization's busybody" rather than to the person in charge of the project). Critical debate and negative information were discouraged, often for fear of retribution. When concerns or "bad news" was communicated, it was often via e-mail or voice mail. Face-to-face communication was an exception rather than a norm.

Although organizational work was completed, there was relatively little appreciation and, often, knowledge of how one's work influenced that of another or facilitated the organization in achieving its goals. A frequent response was "I didn't know" or "It wasn't in my job description," indicating a lack of concern or interest in doing work with someone else or outside the circumscribed area. *Means,* or the steps in a process, were more valued than the *ends,* or serving the client through working together. In essence, this staff depicted an organizational machine that was functioning with independent parts that did not connect or integrate fully to function together and move the machine faster. A communications audit determined that the way they were relating among themselves (or the rules they were following) did not achieve what they wanted—to be better informed, to work together, and to do the best job they could in serving the clients. On the contrary, the existing system limited information flow, gave out inaccurate information, discouraged rapport and collaboration, and prevented them from doing more efficient, higher-quality jobs. The audit also revealed many strengths: a commitment to the organization and a desire to make it succeed, a sincere work ethic, a dedication to and clarity about whom the organization served, a talented experienced pool of employees, respect and trust in the leaders, a strong history of purpose, and fiscal health. These were all strengths to build on while weaknesses changed or atrophied. A change in culture was clearly indicated, and the use of effective communication was to be the key.

The initial strategy for implementing a culture change was to convene the staff and communicate, face to face, the results of the audit. How communication occurred and how it influenced the organization culture were presented, and the dissonance between "what is and what is desired" was painted. Both positives and negatives were outlined, and the message was given that negatives did not mean retribution but rather learning opportunities. This point was clarified for staff when the question "Have you made an error in your work over the past year?" was asked. All raised their hands. This was followed by "Did you learn something about yourself because of this error?" Again, all raised their hands. Last, "Have you made that error again?" was asked. None raised their hands. The point of the exercise was to emphasize that all of us make errors and that in their culture, failure was already regarded as an end (a strength), not as a means of retaliation (weakness).

Staff dispersed into small groups and were asked to (1) define the characteristics of their optimal work environment; (2) validate those weaknesses or strengths presented by individuals, adding others if necessary; and (3) define three strategies for addressing how to shift weaknesses to strengths so that they achieve the optimal environment. Results of the small group work did in fact validate the results of the audit and defined the optimal work environment as having hospitable space to develop and practice flexibility, accountability, initiative, open communication, collaboration, problem solving, efficiency, accurateness, consensus building, decision-making, responsiveness, and generosity of spirit.

My beliefs about organizational culture were shared, as were those about the importance of collaboration and consensus building. Expectations of staff to participate in this collaboration building based on how they wanted to operate (or how the rules of the new paradigm would work) were stated. I also emphasized we had already taken the first step toward open communication. We had established collaboration and consensus by using the simple tools of listening to each other, we had developed rapport with each other, and we had debated the desired culture characteristics as a collaborative unit, reaching consensus about what the culture would look like and what actions were needed to get there. It was time now to "walk the talk."

It is never as simple as saying, "We will all work as a team now," and having it happen without embedding new definitions and mechanisms into the organization's processes and routines. Nor is it necessarily easy or fast. The culture-building process that was undertaken from the staff's list of actions continued over 15 months, and 4 years later, it was continually being revalidated and refined. It was an uneasy process; as one employee put it, "Change sounds like a great adventure, but it is really scary." Talking about it then, individually or within groups, became very important and was encouraged. Because change means giving up or altering something that is safe and comfortable, it is difficult, making conversation about its difficulty essential. The leader's role is to listen, reassure, and cheerlead. Without the energy and belief of the leader, a new paradigm will never occur. Weekly conversations and going around the building to talk with staff, as well as attending their departmental meetings, demonstrated commitment and support as the changes were initiated.

The basic action plan centered around norms of communication, both verbal and nonverbal, and began with getting to know each other. This was accomplished through two initial activities: a retreat on how to function effectively with differing communication and work styles and a comprehensive orientation program focusing on getting to know each other's work. These activities quickly expanded to include other information-sharing opportunities such as organization-wide distribution of department work plans and weekly updates via e-mail; weekly, then monthly, forums to discuss issues and concerns with top managers; and bimonthly all-staff meetings to evaluate the progress. Communication needs eventually expanded and changed. As situations and opportunities to interact became more diverse, so did the need for learning new communication techniques—techniques such as conflict management, communicating during times of stress, building and working in teams, effective clear e-mail use, and listening before speaking.

Of equal importance to the success of the new culture was recognizing the value of open communication and collaboration to the organization. Human and fiscal resources dedicated to staff education and development were instituted, and individual evaluation, compensation, and advancement were linked to team efforts and results. In addition, departmental and organizational recognition was given at special events to individuals or groups for helping and contributing to the work of others.

Gradually, the culture shifted because people were asking, listening, debating, recognizing, and valuing their work in collaboration with others. When the rules of the new culture were violated, such as bypassing appropriate lines of communication or not inviting an important player to a meeting involving an issue for which he or she had responsibility, other staff members were quick to point out this discrepancy or omission and expected it to be rectified. The critical role communication played was evidenced by impromptu brainstorming, interdepartmental teams convening around an organizational issue, active advice and opinion-seeking of coworkers, group decision-making, and an overall improved understanding of each other's contribution to the work of the organization. Productivity increased and individual competitiveness decreased. Efficiency increased, as did accountability, revenue, and programming initiatives. The mental and behavioral model of the culture was being carried and communicated by the staff. They were "walking the talk." Transformation was occurring, and the organization was growing and developing.

The transformation and growth of an organization can also create a major pitfall for communication—namely, complacency, or being lured into a false sense of security. Organizational growth generally means increased workload and the addition of new members to the culture to alleviate this work overload. The assumption that the new members or even existing ones will continue to embrace the communication style required by the culture is not a sure one because patterns and processes, once established, do not necessarily replicate themselves. With change, these patterns and processes are also continually evolving, meaning that communication can never be left unattended! Because the integration of change is variable in each individual, and thus the organizational system, continual assessment of "Do these rules still apply?" is required, as exemplified by the story below.

After the rapid expansion of service and clients in a not-for-profit credentialing organization, I was faced with the need for additional staff and an integrated computer operating system. This decision was reached after months of consultation and collaborative decision-making between staff and the board of directors. The goal was to build a database that permitted interaction between all aspects of operation from finance and programming to psychometric evaluation, examination development, and record keeping. The center of the database was to be the population served. Because no one with the talent to administer the database was employed by the organization, a search was done, and a talented individual was hired.

Excitement and hope were high among staff for this project, as was some anxiety over whether it would work for them in their jobs. Because the rules of our culture dictated open communication and information sharing, weekly update meetings were held to discuss progress and how we were all dealing with the change. However, little attention was given to how the database would affect our functioning in our jobs, despite intensive training in its use. When the time came to "flip the switch," we all eagerly began working with our more efficient, productive system. Or so we thought!

Because of the lack of attention and communication about how this system would affect our jobs, what actually occurred was that each department began developing mini-databases to create comfortable surroundings in which to function. It was also discovered that our talented database administrator was encouraging and helping departments set up their separateness rather than integrate them technologically, to protect her turf. What had been a collaborative, open communication team effort had evolved to a dependent, almost hostagelike situation, where staff members were subservient to the administrator for accessing information they needed to do their work. The culture had shifted because we assumed the administrator was following our rules of open communication, when in fact information was protected and hard to get.

The "neuroses" of this showed itself in many ways. First, snippy, dictatorial e-mails from the database administrator to all the staff about database access and use became regular occurrences. Second, the staff bypassed the administrator with their requests and concerns, going to colleagues to complain or figuring it out on their own, rather than confronting the issue alone, in a group, or with their supervisor's help. And last, productivity and timeliness were greatly diminished in the provision of service because of the inefficiencies. Closer attention to rapport building, monitoring of open communication, and orienting the new staff to the basic rules of the culture would have provided an earlier assessment of her ability or inability to work with the team. In the end, the administrator's ability to communicate and function within the culture was not effective, despite intensive efforts, so a talented person who held similar values replaced her.

Feedback, or "Deliver the Mail to the Right Address"

Aside from the obvious benefits of new ideas and insights, giving and receiving feedback demonstrate a willingness to learn and a desire to serve. Whether positive or negative, it shows an interest in the persons and situation involved. Giving feedback provides the opportunity to say, "I value you enough to give you my honest, best thoughts on an issue." Receiving feedback says, "I respect those thoughts and will take them under consideration." Framing feedback in this valuing mode makes it a learning circumstance.

Whether delivering or receiving good news or bad news, it is always important that it reach the right person and the right address. Whenever staff approach me with an issue, a project, or a problem, my first clarifying question is generally, "Have you discussed this with those involved or affected by this?" If the answer is "no," the focus of our conversation becomes whom to approach and what strategies would communicate openness. If the answer is "yes," the response is generally to bring them into our discussion so we have the opportunity to learn from each other's feedback and design a solution with our best collective thoughts. Many times in my career, situations such as this have occurred, and time and time again, the need to involve all stakeholders of the issue in dialogue has proved to be effective. Ensuring that the right people hear and respond to the message is the best way to produce satisfactory results.

Giving feedback requires the elements of timing, preparedness, permission, and specificity, as exemplified here. Several staff members from a large, service-oriented, member-driven department came to me with concerns about their new director's management style. Despite the fact that a detailed action plan existed for the department, the staff members felt unclear as to their roles in meeting department goals. They related that the director did not give clear directions, that they did not know exactly what was expected of them, and that the plan was seldom reviewed for status reports. Feedback from staff members was infrequently solicited, and when it was, direction did not improve. They further reported having only sporadic departmental meetings that invariably became bogged down in tangents and details. Of most concern was their being held accountable to the director for outcomes, which were unclear. When queried as to whether they had discussed these concerns with director, half of them had, with moderate results.

Securing their permission to discuss this with the director and their commitment to work on it as a team, I made an appointment with the director to review these concerns and to develop a course of action. The context of the appointment discussion was communicated to the director as "I would like to give you feedback on your direction setting for the department as shared by your staff with you and me." The ensuing discussion took place in the familiar surroundings of the director's office. The specific staff concerns and perceptions were reviewed by the director and me. Although the director was aware of some of the difficulties, the extent of the staff's feelings was not known. The director requested assistance in resolving these issues. After our meeting, the director met with her staff and acknowledged their concerns, listening to their needs. Likewise, the staff listened to the director's concerns about their closed personal community and independent functioning. Through the use of a facilitator, the department was able to rebuild rapport and establish a plan for how they would communicate. Each staff member, including the director, also accepted the responsibility to build his or her individual skills. As a result of the feedback, they relearned how to relate to each other. They held weekly meetings, with an agenda set by all. The director became more specific in her directions and related them to the department's goals. They celebrated and acknowledged project completion or progression, and they found humorous ways to remind each other to stay on the subject and to "deliver the mail to right address."

Employees sometimes view giving feedback as a waste of time. One such manager I worked with not only saw no purpose to feedback but also was so threatened by it that he thwarted all attempts by others to engage in it. If colleagues offered suggestions and insights, he became argumentative and defensive. If asked by subordinates how they were performing, his pat answer was "just fine." This type of response became so frustrating for all those around him that eventually no one wanted to work with him. He was quite clear that he had no need for other people's opinion, leading to his supervisor's making it equally as clear that his services were not needed under those circumstances.

Receiving feedback enables each of us to build on our strengths and improve on our shortcomings. To be a useful tool for individuals and organization, feedback has to be valued and exhibited. In one organization of approximately 50 employees in which I once worked, the following feedback mechanisms were implemented. All supervisors completed education in providing feedback to coworkers and subordinates. This initial 2-day training session focused on what is appropriate feedback to give, the appropriate environment for providing it, preparation for presentation, and effective phraseology. Role playing was completed, along with critiquing by other participants and the facilitator. Supervisors were taught how to identify strengths and weaknesses in an employee and to present feedback as it relates to specific job responsibilities. Workshops were also held with the entire staff on the value of feedback, on receiving it with an open mind, and on how to challenge themselves. Further feedback was encouraged through suggestion boxes and as a regular agenda item for all meetings. The value of feedback was communicated by recognizing "idea authors" whose suggestions demonstrated tangible benefit to the organization, by rewarding individual performance that demonstrated duty above and beyond the call, and by acknowledging organization-wide those actively seeking feedback.

Frequently, people actively seek feedback, recognizing its value in learning how to improve their performance in achieving organizational goals. One such woman I worked with was the marketing director for a large health care delivery system. This employee had created institutionalized mechanisms for receiving feedback. Before a service or program was initiated, she asked the consumers of that product what they would want it to be. She shared that information with her project team, who would give her feedback as well. Once the product was launched, she asked them how they liked it and what they would do to improve it. She called this last exercise "dart throwing" because if any part of the project was deflated by feedback (a dart) thrown by a consumer or coworker, she saw it as her job to reinflate it with insight and strength.

Feedback has little relevance, however, if follow-up is not attended to. *Follow-up* means not only checking on the progress of ideas generated by feedback but also ensuring that it produces meaningful, positive change. For example, after a survey asking staff for their suggestion on topics for education, two such programs were held and were positively received. However, months went by, and no further programming was planned or implemented. In the interim, further feedback was requested on another subject before the organization. This time, the feedback response rate was less than 40%, and a lot of grumbling on "Why bother to answer; things never change" was heard. Through further face-to-face conversations, I learned that staff eagerly awaited and enjoyed regular scheduled retreat and education sessions. When further follow-up activities were not planned, this was perceived as lack of interest on management's part to listen and follow through. When it became understood that this was a manpower problem created by a vacancy in the staff position responsible for designing and putting into place staff education, several employees volunteered to spearhead this effort until a replacement was found. Follow-up, which creates positive action resultant of feedback, is vital to the ongoing use and belief in the merit of feedback.

Leaders of today and in the future must consistently and regularly ask for feedback. However, in a world increasingly characterized by more information provided in less time and with less support, challenges exist for leaders to focus on the vital areas for change from each important source of information. For the executive of a large member-driven organization, these information sources are many—the members, the board, committees, staff, other disciplines, organizations, and donors, to name a few. Trying to know it all and managing what everyone does represent a doomed strategy. The organization and I are better served by other tactics, such as

- Prioritizing information
- Maintaining a focus on the organizational mission
- Having frequent and personal interactions with the stakeholders
- Setting clear goals
- Asking for input on whether behavior and activity match the vision
- Recruiting highly competent professionals, and empowering them to perform
- Valuing differences
- Learning positively, and following up efficiently

These approaches require asking, processing, learning, and responding quickly—all areas necessitating constant work on my part. Elementary to this work, as well as that of every employee, is self-feedback.

Self-feedback is the "ah-ha" of life. It is the ability to look critically at yourself and your performance, identifying areas for remediation. In these revelations, we improve our work effectiveness, as exemplified here.

During an updating session, the director of a large programmatic area was outlining progress on all the projects he was managing. The more he talked, the more detailed he became, saying "I completed the content for the program's promotional brochure, selected the color and font and wrote the cover memo." He hesitated for a moment and said, "I am doing too much micromanaging. I should be outlining content and design, but my assistant is perfectly capable of paper color and print font selection, as well as writing the distribution memo." This particular "ah-ha" led to a shift in who completed which tasks, resulting in increased time for the director to develop new ideas and an increased feeling of worth and responsibility on the part of the assistant.

Another example—this time of not experiencing the "ah-ha"—occurred when yet another director of services was discussing the need to explore advanced technology for a membership renewal and accounting system. The person came roaring into the discussion with a recommendation of considerable expenditure without research or rationale. The more she was queried, the more it was apparent she had not done her background work. Finally, instead of saying, "I need to do more work on this and get back to you," she blamed a coworker for inefficiency in not getting a job done—a job for which she was clearly accountable.

For organizational growth and progress to occur, each employee must engage in some degree of inner work or self-feedback. Without it, the organization and individuals stagnate, being stuck and possibly content with the status quo. With it, both organization and person explore and build their capabilities, expanding their horizon. Stakeholders look to leaders to make this happen.

SUMMARY

Leaders must have excellent communication skills to be effective and successful. Numerous studies have validated the positive outcomes for organizations when leaders listen; cultivate language patterns that give clear, congruent messages; develop meaningful interpersonal relationships; advocate feedback and follow-up; and actively support a culture in which the same behaviors are practiced and advanced. Using these principles of effective communication, leaders develop a shared vision and meaning of the work they, their colleagues, and subordinates do, keeping the vision alive in an atmosphere of openness and trust.

Good communication begins and ends with self. Every person, particularly the leader, must have a clear picture of self, of what is valued and believed, and how that blends with the organization served. Building on the basic concept of matching yourself with the organization, setting out to live out this match is greatly enhanced through effective communication skills. The cycle of developing self within the organization ends with asking and then using the insights and ideas to critically appraise performance. Learning about yourself through the eyes of others perpetuates a clearer understanding of who you are in the context of your job and the organization.

Communications delivered using the C's—clarity, completeness, current, correctness, and congruence—have been demonstrated to produce results for organizations. The principles here are

- When the message is clear, the ability to respond is enabled.
- When information flows openly and is complete, current and correct decision-making is carried out using the best data available.
- When the end result of communication is advancement of the same shared goal, an environment of collaboration and trust ensues, feeding the open communication cycle.

The power and importance of listening have been explored. Active listening also builds trust, an essential element of communication. Valuing what another person has to say is validated through listening. Common ground and meaningful action cannot be achieved among communicants if they do not hear the information being shared. Frequent barriers to listening include such behaviors as being distracted, leaping to conclusions, appearing disinterested, making minimal eye contact, not clarifying or responding to what is said, and being judgmental. Active positive listening breaks down these barriers and builds rapport and the willingness to participate in achieving a mutual goal.

In establishing rapport, the leader comes to know the perspective of other stakeholders engaged in the joint endeavor. Valuing and being attentive to others' points of view establishes trust, the basis of good communication. Rapport also permits a freedom to communicate, allowing the dialogue to focus on the subject (i.e., patient, organization, members) rather than on participants being engaged in defending self-interest.

The culture of an organization is the paradigm by which it operates, and the leader sets these rules. Communication, both verbal and nonverbal, demonstrates the culture and is an important tool for adapting culture to meet organizational needs. Because the world of organizations is seldom static, the environment of its operation is also constantly shifting. Effective communication skills empower those in the culture to work more efficiently through collaboration and shared understanding.

Feedback, whether given or received, provides opportunity for validating the effectiveness of communication as well as for learning. It conveys interest and respect in the other persons. Feedback encourages a vested interest for those participating in it and carries the obligation to response or follow-up. Having been entrusted to lead by a group of stakeholders, leaders have a broader responsibility to seek feedback. It is essential for the growth and progress of not only the stakeholder but also the leader.

Leadership, when done well, is like any other state. It is a blend of skills and talents, and it is visualized and demonstrated through the way the leader communicates. Leaders and those they lead realize their fullest potential by investing in a common vision that is lived out through their communications. The choice is that communication supports or obstructs this vision. Successful leaders assertively pursue the former and remove the latter.

REFERENCES

Arnold, E., & Boggs, K. (1995). Interpersonal relationships. In *Professional communication: Skills for nurses.* (2nd Ed.). Philadelphia: W. B. Saunders.

Barbara, D. A. (1971). *How to make people listen to you.* Springfield, Ill.: Charles C Thomas.

Booker, D. (1994). *Communication with confidence.* New York: McGraw-Hill.

Coyle, M. B. (1993). Quality interpersonal communication: Perception or reality? *Manage, 45,* 6–7.

Deal, T. E., & Kennedy, A. A. (1982). *Corporate cultures: The rites and rituals of corporate life.* Reading, Mass.: Addison-Wesley.

Devito, J. A. (1995). *The interpersonal communication book.* New York: Harper-Collins.

Foster, C. (1997). *There's something I have to tell you: How to communicate difficult news in tough situations.* New York: Harmony Books.

Hathaway, P. (1990). *Giving and receiving feedback.* Menlo Park, Calif.: Crisp Publications.

Jablin, F., Cude, R., House, A., Lee, J., & Roth, N. L. (1994). Communication competence in organizations: Conceptualizations and comparisons across multiple levels of analysis. In Thayer, L., & Barnette, G. A. (Eds.). *Organizational communication: Emerging perspectives IV.* Norwood, N.Y.: Ablex Publishing.

Laborde, G. A. (1983). *Influencing with integrity: Management skills for communication and negotiation.* Palo Alto, Calif.: Syntony Publishers.

Matusak, L. K. (1997). *Finding your voice: Learning to lead . . . Anywhere you want to make a difference.* San Francisco, Calif.: Jossey-Bass.

McCall, M. W., Lombardo, M. M., & Morison, A. M. (1988). *The lessons of experience: How successful executives develop on the job.* Lexington, Mass.: Lexington Books.

McKay, M., Davis, M., & Fanning, P. (1995). *Messages: The communications skills book* (2nd Ed.). Oakland, Calif.: New Harbinger Publications.

Nelson, R. W. (1997). *Organizational troubleshooting: Asking the right questions, finding the right answers.* Westport, Conn.: Quorum Books.

Pearson, J. C., & Daniels, T. A. (1988). Oh what a tangled web we weave: Concerns about current conceptions of communication competence. *Communication Reports, 1,* 95–100.

Ryan, K. D., Oestreich, D. K., & Orr, G. A. (1996). *The courageous messenger: How to successfully speak up at work.* San Francisco, Calif.: Jossey-Bass.

Schein, E. H. (1985). *Organizational culture and leadership.* San Francisco, Calif.: Jossey-Bass.

Senge, P. M., Kleiner, A., Roberts, C., Ross, R. B., & Smith, B. J. (1994). *The fifth discipline fieldbook: Strategies and tools for building a learning organization.* New York: Currency Books.

Taylor, J. R. (1981). The office of the future: Weber and Innes revisited. *The Canadian Communication Quarterly, 8,* 4–13.

Thayer, L., & Barnette, G. A. (Eds.) (1994). *Organizational communication: Emerging perspectives IV.* Norwood, N.Y.: Ablex Publishing.

Trevino, L. K., Daft, R. L., & Lengle, R. H. (1990). Understanding managers' media choices: A symbolic interactionist perspective. In Fulk, J., & Steinfield, C. (Eds.). *Organizations and communication technology.* Newbury Park, Calif.: Sage Publications.

Weisinger, H. (1981). *Nobody's perfect.* Beverly Hills, Calif.: Stratford Press.

Chapter 11

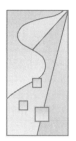

Mentoring
Others

Fay L. Bower

All successful leaders have had mentors and are mentors. They had someone they could confide in, seek advice from, and get help from, and they do the same for others. Being influential and making a difference often are the result of learning leadership skills from others. The skill of gaining recognition and power and the ability to influence others often are learned from those who have recognition, power, and influence. Mentors may have position and title, but they can be without either and still be influential and able to help others.

Mentors are role models and facilitators of career development; they can open doors to opportunity, and they teach by modeling. Being able to find a good mentor and being able to be a successful mentor are two aspects of career development that every leader must have. Furthermore, an important outcome of mentor relationships is that they result in lasting and unique colleague relationships.

Mentors have specific characteristics that allow them to facilitate the development of others. According to Taylor (1992), a mentor is one who takes a personal interest in assisting someone to develop the knowledge and skills needed to meet specific career goals. Williams and Blackburn (1988) believe that a direct working relationship is most beneficial in the development of others. Many (Kanter, 1977; Levinson, 1977; Moore, 1982) believe the best way to mentor someone is to follow the tutorial model, wherein the selection of the protégé is specific, the relationship is close and supervised, and the mentor guides the activities of the protégé. Vance and Olson (1998) believe mentoring is a developmental, empowering, and nurturing relationship that extends over time and in which mutual sharing, learning, and growth occur in an atmosphere of respect, collegiality, and affirmation. The mentoring relationship can even be viewed as a gift-exchange (Gehrke, 1988) and as a collaborative learning experience for both parties (Kaye and Jacobson, 1995).

The characteristics of mentoring relationships vary somewhat; Taylor (1992) claims that a mentor relationship includes valuing the protégé and believing in the individual's potential for success. The mentor is the role model, guide, teacher, coach, or confidant. Hockenberry-Eaton and Kline (1995) believe the characteristics of an effective mentoring environment include (1) providing leadership, (2) showing patience, (3) demonstrating caring, and (4) maintaining loyalty. They point out that building trust in the relationship is an essential

255

component for creating a nurturing environment and that the socialization process experienced during a mentor relationship should be effortless. Levinson (1977) suggests there are several roles that mentors must fill: teacher, sponsor, guidance counselor, and initiator. They also provide moral support and indoctrination into the values and of the outcomes pursued. Vance (1999) states that the mentor guides, models, encourages, and inspires the protégé and that a key role of the mentor is to create an environment that supports the development of both individual and collective mentor relationships.

Ultimately, regardless of the mentor model, the mentor relationship advances from a helping/learning relationship to a cohort relationship. During the mentor relationship, the mentor helps the protégé with career goals that may end in a similar position or one of higher magnitude. Because the mentor's colleague connections can provide the protégé with opportunities beyond those the mentor can provide, it is not uncommon for the protégé to reach heights similar to or beyond those of the mentor.

The impact of mentoring is supported by the literature. In a study by White (1988) in which 300 academic nurse administrators were evaluated, mentors gave their protégés confidence and inspiration and encouraged achievement and intellectual development. Spengler (1982) evaluated 501 mentored doctorally-prepared nurses and found them to have more definite career plans, to be more satisfied with their career progression, and to possess a greater sense of accomplishment. In a study that evaluated mentoring and new graduate nurses, Hamilton et al. (1989) found that new nurses with mentors had increased job satisfaction and leadership behaviors. Clearly, nurses who were mentored have experienced both professional and personal growth (Butts and Wither, 1992; Carey and Campbell, 1994; Martin et al., 1995; Nayak, 1991).

Many benefit from the mentor relationship: the protégé, the organization, the mentor, and others. The protégé is obviously helped as she or he gains help with career advancement. Protégés also learn the value of colleague relationships because of the circle of acquaintances they meet through the mentor. Such colleague systems are the means by which the protégé gains increased access to influence and power. The promise of contacts through the mentor is often crucial for the protégé and helps diffuse some of the emotional tension of the relationship, specifically the tension of taking the next step—to succeed the mentor (Bower, 1993).

Protégés also learn incidental things—how to dress and travel—and important things like the politics of the situation. They learn how to relate to people—especially difficult ones—how to listen, what battles to take on, what issues to avoid, and above all, how to judge a situation. Most protégés learn to look at situations as their mentors would, often asking themselves, "How would the mentor assess this situation?"

Organizations also benefit from mentor relationships. Protégés get things done; they learn and develop while they perform work for the mentor and the organization. The organization benefits by the things that the protégé does under the tutelage of the mentor. If both parties work in the same organization, the mentor also benefits because the things the protégé is doing would have had to be done by the mentor. Because of this help, the mentor can do other things and thus is more productive, which also benefits the organization.

Furthermore, because the protégé often gives credit to the mentor for his or her role in the protégé's activities, the mentor's reputation spreads. The mentor also learns about what works and what does not, so the mentoring can improve. Probably the most wonderful outcome of the mentor relationship is the bond that develops between the mentor and the protégé. The linkage that develops almost always benefits both parties in ways least expected and over a long period of time.

Leaders cannot expect mentoring to occur unless they know what it takes to be a successful mentor and how important it is to have a mentor. The remainder of this chapter is devoted to a presentation of a model for mentoring, followed by the author's experiences with mentors and as a mentor. The specific phases of the mentoring relationship and the many ways one can use the model are described.

MODEL FOR A MENTORING RELATIONSHIP

The mentor relationship model presented here is possible at any level and for any kind of situation, whether it is a one-on-one relationship in an institution or a relationship of two people who are at a distance from one another. Essentially, the mentor relationship model presented here has three elements:

1. A selection process
2. A goal-setting phase
3. A working phase

Normally, these phases occur sequentially, although given the particulars of any situation they may not be exactly as described. If the relationship is established at a distance, the first phase of selection may take longer than when the relationship is between two individuals who see each other daily.

Although it is not necessary for the mentor relationship to be in the same environment, it helps considerably if the individuals have some time together before distance separates them. If separation occurs early in the relationship, there are a number of ways for close and daily contact to occur, such as e-mail, the telephone, and faxing. It also is not unusual for the mentor and protégé to meet at national or regional meetings, where they can assess the protégé's progress. This need for frequent contact (particularly in the early phases of the relationship) is very important if trust is to develop, which is an essential element of the mentor relationship.

Selection Process

The mentor usually selects the protégé; however, there are times when a mentor is selected by a protégé. Persons in high positions have the opportunity to work with many subordinates and therefore have a plentiful supply of potential protégés. Quite frequently, their selection of protégés is by default; that is, they work with assistants who are working their way up and are naturally ready for a mentor. At other times, mentors may purposefully be looking outside their circle of colleagues for protégés for specific reasons. Mentors often want to prepare protégés to carry on their work. It is not uncommon for a mentor to systematically search for a protégé who can complement or add to the work of the mentor or complete a project once the mentor has moved on to something else. Scientists, researchers, and politicians often locate and work with protégés so their work will continue once they are no longer able to do it.

Nursing leaders have always mentored others, but recently, because of the "burnout" of nurses, there has been a new interest in mentoring. Nurse leaders are encouraging other nurse leaders to deliberately seek out students, new graduates, and novice nurses to facilitate their transition into the profession and to assist in their career development (Joel, 1997).

Mentors sometimes find protégés by accident. It is not uncommon for a mentor to find a protégé at a conference, workshop, or national meeting. Mentors often find protégés while talking with participants at these gatherings. They learn about the interests and talents of an individual and how that person could fit into their own plan of work. Sometimes they are intrigued by a person's talents and simply want to help the person reach his or her goal, which often is similar to their own.

Because a mentor relationship often is a socializing experience for the protégé, it is a common experience within professional groups. Physicians, nurses, lawyers, and engineers often have a cadre of protégés who are learning their roles by being mentored by the expert. The expert works closely with the novice and becomes the role model, advisor, sponsor, and teacher. The mentor often selects the protégé because of his or her potential (lawyers often hire associates because of their talents) or agrees to accept a protégé (interns are assigned to specialty physicians) so that the protégé can fulfill certain educational requirements. In nursing, mentors generally select their protégés because they show promise and have established a linkage with the mentor as a professional. The experienced nurse often mentors new graduates while they learn their roles as professional nurses. This kind of mentoring relationship is common in specialty units such as the intensive care unit, critical care unit, and oncology.

Protégés do find their own mentors. Andersen (1999) provides a set of questions that student nurses can use to prepare themselves for a mentor search. Most nurses interested in a career, rather than a job, look for persons who can help them advance in their chosen career pathway. They want someone who knows their area of interest, who is willing to give them time and attention, and who has a network they are willing to share. They want entry to certain activities, and they need to know that the mentor will be willing to offer that opportunity.

Some protégés do not know what they need, but they know they need help with their careers. These protégés need a mentor who knows how to work with novices and who is willing to give an extraordinary amount of time, effort, and expertise. Being close to the mentor is important because there usually is a need for frequent communication. However, protégés can be mentored from a distance if the mentor is willing to use electronic forms of communication.

During the selection of a mentor or a protégé, the mentor and protégé must determine if they are compatible. As they work together, they look for commonalties, areas of difference, ways to communicate effectively, and ways to get the work done efficiently. The protégé may feel this is a "watch time," a time for the protégé to prove his or her worth, but it is actually a time for building trust and commitment by both parties. This phase does not last very long because most mentors see themselves as reasonably good judges of character and talent and know when a relationship is going to work. Protégés also know fairly quickly if a match is not a good one. Problems arise when one party thinks the relationship is not viable and the other believes it is; then, the mentor must resolve the issue because it is the mentor who is the giver and the protégé who is the receiver of the service.

During the selection phase, there are several things that both parties must determine if the relationship is to be successful. First, the mentor must determine whether she or he has the time to devote to the protégé. Some protégés take a lot of time because they are insecure and need support; others need little assistance as they go their way. If the protégé is to be helped from a distance, the mentor must decide whether she or he has the time to keep track of the protégé's activities and can locate the protégé when an opportunity surfaces. Second, it needs to be determined whether the mentor is willing to provide access to his or her circle of colleagues and whether they would be responsive to including the protégé in their activities. Some colleagues do not want their names used or shared with others. Third, the mentor must determine if she or he has the skills needed to help the protégé. Although the mentor and protégé may have a common interest and want to work together, the mentor must be able to advise, teach, counsel, and refer the protégé. Some experts are very anxious to help protégés, but they do not have the patience or ability to advise or teach. They forget what it is like to be uninformed and to need help at a very basic level. Fourth, the mentor must be available when the protégé needs help. If the two are working closely together, then availability usually is not a problem. When the mentor and the protégé are far apart and the protégé needs help, the mentor may be contacted during the evenings and weekends and during travel.

Protégés also must determine if the relationship is a "good fit." Sometimes, the mentor is very demanding or expects too much, so the protégé must determine if this is something that can be negotiated or is not tolerable. There also are mentors who expect the protégé to initiate; if this style of functioning is not acceptable to the protégé, the relationship may need to be terminated. The "fit" of a relationship thus depends on both the mentor's and the protégé's taking the responsibility for determining its viability.

An important aspect of the mentor/protégé relationship is that it ultimately develops into an intimate relationship that must be nurtured, supported, and sustained over time. Having the right pairing of persons will facilitate this process, so the selection of either person is critical. Quite often, two people locate each other and see a common interest, with one having the expertise the other wants. They quickly join together, but without an assessment of the factors described above, the relationship may not develop into one of trust and intimacy. Without trust, the protégé may not get what is sought, and the mentor may not get the satisfaction that is deserved.

Goal-Setting Phase

The second phase of the mentor relationship is when the protégé and the mentor establish goals for the protégé. There are several ways that this phase may progress. The protégé may come into the relationship with a set of goals; the mentor may devise a set of goals for the protégé; or the mentor and the protégé may design the experience together. Some mentor/protégé relationships define goals as the opportunities occur or as the protégé requests them.

For most mentor relationships, there are protégé goals, mentor goals, and mentor relationship goals. Protégés usually want to perform well and advance their careers. Mentors usually want to provide a good experience for the protégé so the protégé can meet his or her own goals. Goals for the relationship usually include the development of a trusting relationship in which both the protégé and the mentor benefit.

Many protégés want to "see the bigger picture," perform at a higher level, make a bigger impact, and develop skills of leadership. They also want to relate to other influential people; to have access to privileged, special, and even secret information; and to be taken into the confidence of those in the "inner circle" of the mentor. Although it may never be said, they also want to make the mentor proud of them and even to succeed the mentor. These goals are not usually stated, but they should be because they help to establish a direction for the relationship and benchmarks for evaluation.

Most mentors want their protégés to meet their own personal goals and to make the mentor proud of them. Although it might not be said, they also know that if they are successful, the protégé will succeed them in their ability to make a difference. Every mentor wants to be part of a successful protégé's career. They also want the experience to be a challenge—one that will allow the protégé to meet his or her goals—but they also know that the experience must not create barriers for the accomplishment of defined goals. Therefore, mentors must be able to judge what the protégé can do so success is the outcome. Nothing is more alarming than to put a protégé into a situation where failure is possible.

The first goal to be reached in the relationship is trust. Because the overall goal of the relationship is to socialize the protégé, the mentor must create an environment in which trust can develop. Successful mentor relationships last a long time even after the protégé no longer needs help and has also become a mentor. This outcome occurs because of the trust that was established and because both mentor and protégé knew from the start that the mentor relationship is the first stage of a lifelong colleague relationship.

Goal setting can be long or short term, or both. Long-term goals are general, whereas short-term goals for the protégé are specific. Most protégés want to advance their careers as the long-term goal. More-specific goals have to do with the nature and level of the position and activity pursued by the protégé as part of the career pathway. For instance, getting appointed to a special committee may be a short-term goal, whereas being part of the decision team for a major change in a hospital may be the long-term goal. Learning to design a business plan may be a short-term goal, but establishing a business may be the long-term goal. Learning leadership skills may be a short-term goal, whereas locating a position as an administrator in a school of nursing may be the long-term goal.

The best way for the mentor to help the protégé meet short-term goals is to have the opportunity to determine how they should be met. Sometimes the protégé knows exactly what is needed, whereas at other times the mentor knows what is best. There also are times when opportunities arise that neither the protégé nor the mentor could have anticipated, so the freedom to determine how a goal can be met often is the mentor's prerogative. This is why frequent communication is necessary. When these unexpected opportunities occur, the mentor will need to contact the protégé quickly before the chance is lost.

Goal setting for the protégé and the mentor occurs at the beginning of and periodically throughout the mentor relationship. A frequent check by the mentor on the progress of the protégé determines when a goal has been met and another is needed. It also lets both parties know when there is stagnation of the protégé's progress or when a better approach should be taken. In some relationships, the protégé assumes the responsibility for letting the mentor know when a goal has been met and seeks advice on the next step. When the mentor and the protégé are working closely together, goal setting and goal checking are easy. Mentoring at a distance means that both the mentor and the protégé must take the initiative for alerting the other about setting and measuring goals. If there is a lull in the communication, the mentor usually contacts the protégé for a progress report. Distance should not be a deterrent to successful goal setting and progress checks.

Working Phase

The working phase of the mentor relationship goes through three stages:

1. Establishing the relationship stage
2. The exchange stage
3. The transition stage

■ Establishing the Relationship Stage

Establishing the relationship begins shortly after both the mentor and the protégé have acknowledged they want a mentor relationship and have identified their goals for it.

During the early phase of the relationship, the mentor and the protégé work together, learning mostly about each other. They learn about each other's work ethics, relationships with others, preferable hours of work (some people do their best work in the evening and some persons function best early in the day), and whether they work alone or spend most of their time in committee work. They also learn about the functions of the role to be developed by the protégé or the activity the protégé wants to pursue; in doing so, they learn about how each other thinks. Some people are deductive thinkers, and others are inductive analyzers. They also learn about what is similar in the way they look at issues and where there are differences. It is truly a time of discovery even when the two have known each other for a long time. For those who do not know each other well, it is a time for gaining a profile of each other's personal and professional lives.

This stage of the working relationship may be long or short depending on the individuals involved. For the mentor to do the best job, the protégé must be willing to tell everything that will help the mentor provide the best experience. This may mean the protégé will outline strengths, share idiosyncrasies, identify fears, tell secrets, reveal deficiencies, and so on. Of course, it is understood the mentor will hold these disclosures in confidence. The mentor may even share some of his or her own mentoring experiences in an attempt to help the protégé see that these issues are not unusual for a protégé.

The boundaries for establishing the relationship vary, depending on the earlier relationship of the mentor and the protégé, the distance between the two, the ability for both to share and learn about each other, and the roles of both. Generally, if the mentor and protégé knew each other before the mentor relationship, the establishment of mentoring is quick with no need to learn the above. If the individuals were strangers before they decided to work together, then the time to establish the relationship will be longer. Distance can also extend the time it takes to establish the relationship; it is much easier to establish a mentor relationship with someone when you can be with him or her on a daily basis.

Being open and sharing will facilitate this aspect of the relationship; however, some people have a hard time sharing personal aspects. The mentor can help the protégé by initiating the sharing. By modeling what the protégé is expected to do, the mentor sets the stage for the protégé to share. How the mentor accepts what is told also affects how open the protégé will be. The mentor must be nonjudgmental and accept what is said without comment or critique.

An important variable to consider during this phase is the status of both the mentor and the protégé. Because the relationship starts out as a parent/child relationship, the mentor must be sensitive to the protégé who has status equal to the mentor's. It is easy for the mentor to create a mentor relationship with a student, a subordinate employee, or a person who is less experienced careerwise. However, there are people who have status but want to shift their activities from one area to another and need a mentor to help them.

Mentor relationships between individuals with equal status usually quickly move into a colleague relationship and have the tendency to be reciprocal—that is, the mentor helps the protégé, and soon the protégé is helping the mentor as they become colleagues.

■ Exchange Stage

The mentor usually determines the activities and referrals for the protégé, but sometime during the relationship the protégé starts to make suggestions and to pose ideas for the mentor to respond to. When this happens, the working phase of the relationship has advanced to what is called the exchange stage. The mentor and the protégé begin working as a team with equal responsibility for the direction and progress of the protégé's development.

One of the critical features of the exchange stage is the mentor's and protégé's ability to give each other negative as well as positive feedback. Mentors need to know when something they have suggested or something they have done did not work or was inappropriate. In trusting relationships, giving negative feedback is not hard. However, if the protégé does not trust the mentor, she or he may withhold important information that would help the mentor make the right connections or provide the best activities. Furthermore, if the mentor does not feel comfortable giving an honest appraisal, the protégé may be denied important help. Honest exchange about all aspects of the mentor relationship is absolutely essential if the relationship is to be productive, effective, or worthwhile.

Exchange between the mentor and the protégé must also be based on realistic expectations. For instance, the mentor must be realistic in the appraisal of the protégé's performance. It may take several experiences before the protégé can master a skill, and the protégé must be realistic about his or her expectations of what the mentor can accomplish for the protégé. Some areas of the protégé's development may take more time to set up than was originally predicted. However, if the mentor and the protégé have shared adequately with each other and have learned to be open in their communication, then disappointments, delays, and repeated performance should not be hard to handle.

The exchange of proposed experiences, of the outcomes of these experiences, and of the quality of mentor's and the protégé's contributions continues throughout the mentor relationship. However, over time, this exchange often becomes less frequent. This reduction in exchange could mean that the protégé has begun to take on more responsibility for the initiation and evaluation of her or his own activities and does not need the mentor. It could also mean the mentor is satisfied with the protégé's progress and is comfortable with less-frequent communication. Frequently, it means that the relationship is entering the transition stage.

■ Transition Stage

The transition from being mentored to being a colleague is subtle and can happen at any time during the mentoring experience. It is also quite possible to be mentored *and* be a colleague. However, most people move from the mentoring relationship into a colleague relationship, particularly if the protégé moves into a position of equal status with the mentor. For instance, nurses who have faculty positions often move into administration, so when a dean is mentoring a faculty member and the faculty member becomes a dean, the two start to relate more as colleagues than as mentor to protégé. However, some would say the mentoring process is never really over, and sometimes a transition occurs and the mentoring relationship is resumed later.

One of the factors that initiates a transition, other than the fact that the career of the protégé is well on its way, is that the protégé starts to take on her or his own protégés. Another factor that moves the relationship into transition is when the protégé has assumed responsibility for the career; however, the relationship may remain as is for as long as the participants want. Many mentor relationships continue for as long as the individuals have a need for each other.

Sometimes the mentor relationship goes dormant—that is, the mentor and the protégé do not converse or keep in contact. This lull does not necessarily mean the relationship has changed or is in transition. A great characteristic of mentor relationships is that they can be operative or inoperative and then be reinstituted when the protégé wants help, support, or advice. However, a sudden stop in dialogue between the mentor and the protégé could mean there is trouble, so it is recommended that the mentor check with the protégé periodically when there is no action. Silence could mean nothing is wrong, or it could mean that the protégé is in need and cannot ask for help.

Periodic lulls in communication usually do not occur early in the relationship but are common during transition. These quiet times are like testing times when the protégé determines his or her ability to "fly alone." Inactivity is usually not discussed but just occurs, so it is best to check to determine the real reason for the lack of communication, particularly if the relationship occurs at a distance.

MENTORING AND BEING MENTORED: AN APPLICATION OF THE MENTOR RELATIONSHIP MODEL

There are many stories I can tell about mentoring, both as the protégé and as the mentor, because I have been involved in both kinds of relationships. Without these experiences, I would not have accomplished what I did, nor would I feel I had made the impact I did. And I know from personal experience how important it can be to have a good mentor. I also know the rewards you get from being a mentor and seeing your protégé advance and be successful. The following stories are about my experiences as a protégé and a mentor, and they are offered to those who want to be both and want to see how the phases of the mentoring relationship can vary.

Being Mentored

I had several mentors during my career in nursing. Most of my mentors were men because there were few women administrators in the higher positions in universities when I was starting my career as an academic administrator. They were not very good role models, but they gave good advice, helped me make the right connections, and moved me into important positions. I learned a lot about what not to do by watching them do the wrong things, and I learned a lot about what to do from those with whom they put me in contact.

I had five mentors who were women. They all were nurses: two were clinicians, and three were professors of nursing. I learned a lot from them about being a professional nurse and later about being a faculty member. They were excellent role models and also gave great advice about what I should and should not do. They could not, in those days, help me make connections or open opportunities for me as my male mentors did, but they gave me the start I needed as a nurse and as a faculty member.

When I was a new registered nurse, a gruff old nurse of whom I was scared mentored me. Even though she was a terror and had everyone on edge, I learned a lot from her. She taught me to think first and to act next, to put my patient first over all other considerations, and to be respectful to all people regardless of how they treated me. Later in my career, another nurse took me under her wing. She was an excellent clinician who helped me learn to be an intensive care nurse and then a head nurse. She also was the one who urged me to go to college, a decision I probably would never have made otherwise.

As an adult undergraduate student, I was privileged to have three professors who took an interest in me and helped me deal with being in school while rearing four children and working. They encouraged me to try new things and to test my limits. I was always into something new when I worked with them. Later, when I became a faculty member, they were there to help me learn that role, too. They had great faith in my leadership potential and were always there to cheer me on. They all became my colleagues, yet I still consider them my mentors.

The stories I want to tell about my being mentored focus on the selection, goal-setting, and working phases of the mentor relationship. Examples of the selection and transition phases of the mentor relationship are discussed from my perspective as a mentor.

Being Mentored as a Student and a Faculty Member

Having a mentor when you are a student is absolutely essential for survival. One of my first experiences as a student with a mentor, who later became my colleague, was when I had to register for senior classes in a large metropolitan university. The day before registration, I was unable to get to the college because I was in the hospital in labor with our fourth child. My husband went in my place, stood in the long line, and probably would still be there if the faculty person had not recognized him and took care of the registration. That event was the beginning of a 40-year relationship. She was the person who listened to my concerns when I was hassled by another professor because I wanted more time to complete an assignment. In fact, she was the only person who understood how hard it was to go to school, care for four children (one teenager, two preteens, and an infant) and a husband, and work. This understanding was very important to me because she was single and did not marry until very much later; even so, she was sensitive to my situation, to how hard it was for me, and to how determined I was to get a degree.

Frequently, her assistance was nothing more than listening to me or pointing me in the right direction for a reference. On the clinical unit, she was tough on us all and did not let me do anything less than the others, but she also did not expect me to do more just because I was a registered nurse, as did some of the other faculty. She did, however, find experiences for me that were enriching and not repetitive because I had been the head nurse of an intensive care unit before I enrolled in her leadership course (which was required of all students). She assigned me to the director of nursing, who became my preceptor; with her, I learned a lot about the politics of the hospital. I followed the director from meeting to meeting and did projects for her that helped me understand the operations of the units that reported to her. I prepared a long-range plan for the nursing division and presented it to the hospital board, an activity I would repeat many times again but with different groups and in several different universities.

My relationship with my mentor in the bachelor's program did not end when I graduated. She was always there when I needed her during my master's program even though I was at a different university. She read the papers I wrote and gave me an honest, sometimes scathing, appraisal of the content and style of my writing. She offered suggestions for improvement and urged me later in life to coauthor a book with her.

After the master's program, my first work in curriculum and consultation was with this mentor; by then I was a faculty member and the associate director of a federally funded project she had written. We worked together in the college from which I had graduated 1 year earlier with a bachelor's degree. She taught me how to write behavioral objectives, to do a concept analysis, and to map concepts across the curriculum. Together, we led the faculty through a major curriculum change, and later I went on visits with her to other schools as a consultant. All during this time we were colleagues, but I always thought of her as my mentor. It wasn't until I became an administrator that our mentor relationship terminated and I sought the help of others in that field. To this day I keep in touch with her, although infrequently, because so much of what I can do and have done is because of her. She was a major contributor to my development, and I am eternally grateful to her for helping me grow and succeed.

My second mentor in college was at the graduate level. She also gave a lot of time to my development. Her contributions, however, were very different than those of my first faculty mentor. I am a very good editor thanks to the lessons I learned from her. She proofread what I wrote and forced me to seek additional resources to back up my statements. She was a stickler for accuracy and a perfectionist when it came to APA format. She also had an interest in leadership, and it was because of her urging that I accepted an invitation to join the Sigma Theta Tau International (STTI) Honor Society of Nursing. I also agreed to run for the presidency of the charter chapter because she convinced me I could provide the leadership the new chapter needed. When there was something I did not know or could not do, she told me where to find information about it. She never told or showed me how to do anything; thus, she helped me learn to be a resourceful investigator, something I am proud I can do today.

She also became a colleague when I joined the faculty, and it wasn't long before I replaced her as coordinator of the graduate program when she became associate dean of the school. It was her nomination of me for professor of the year that provided my first significant acknowledgment on the campus as an outstanding academician. Ultimately, I became the chair of the department because she had urged the dean to make the appointment. Her contributions to my career were to insist I perform in an outstanding way, to take on positions and assignments that were a challenge, and to prepare myself for the future. I was 48 years old when I received my doctoral degree, and it was because she had urged the dean to appoint me as chair that I returned to college. A faculty member with a doctorate had to serve in that capacity. In retrospect, I think it was her way of getting me back to school.

One other professor in graduate school made a big contribution to my career. She taught curriculum and instruction and had just received her doctorate when the fall semester began. She had developed a conceptual framework for curriculum development as her dissertation, and we all had to learn how to use it. Fortunately, this was a wise and useful skill for me to learn because in later years, I traveled all over the country teaching others how to use a conceptual framework to organize a curriculum. After I graduated, she, I, and three other nurses formed a consultant firm; in the 1970s, we provided assistance to more than 250 colleges or universities in the United States and Canada. She introduced me to her network of colleagues, which helped me establish a reputation as a curriculum expert and consultant.

These women were wonderful mentors and are to this day my colleagues. I owe them much for their modeling, teaching, selection of me as their protégé, and support when I needed it.

Being Mentored as an Administrator

The first male mentor I had was the dean who appointed me as chair of the nursing department at the university in 1978. He gave me my first chance to be an administrator. Later, after he left the university and became the president of an osteopathy school in San Francisco, he wanted me to be his vice president. That same year, I was offered the position of dean at another university, where I met my second male mentor, who was the vice president of academic affairs and my boss. I did not take the vice president position at the osteopathy school because I wanted to be a dean of nursing and I thought it would open more doors for me in the future. In fact, all of my nurse mentors urged me to take the dean position. It proved to be the right choice because the osteopathy school was later sold to a national firm and moved out of San Francisco.

Both of these men were very good to me. They helped me understand the politics of the institutions and how important it was to be connected to a power base, even though neither of them succeeded in surrounding themselves with those in power. They assigned me to important committees and asked me to chair critical task forces. I went to many regional and national meetings as a representative of the universities because they knew I would make contacts there. In fact, both of them set up meetings for me at these conferences so I could build a network. They even told me whom to contact and whom to avoid. Both of them believed I would make a good college president, so their advice and actions were always the basis for their recommendations and work with me. Although they never met one another and were by nature very different, they both promoted my career in the same way: they helped me get connected so I could build a network, and they placed me in positions that were challenging but highlighted my talents.

The third male mentor was a priest who was the president of the university. When my boss, the vice president of academic affairs, suddenly retired, he recommended that I serve as the interim vice president while a search was conducted. I agreed and served in that capacity for one and one-half years. I worked closely with the president and learned a lot about the Jesuits and how to be a fund-raiser. The time I was in that role and the year that followed when I was the university planner and institutional director of research were critical for my next position as the president of a small college. In those roles, I learned about planning, the importance of providing a vision, and the value of a team approach to running a university. Although he was not a particularly good role model, he was good at helping me learn more about university governance and union negotiations. He appointed me to head major committees; he also gave me the freedom to create a planning office, and he supported my efforts at institutional planning—something that had never been done on the campus. We tried a lot of things—some that failed and some that succeeded. With his encouragement, I revamped the budget and the process used to develop it; I also successfully brought the university through accreditations of the business school, the nursing school, and the total university. I failed at revamping one of the colleges but learned later that the seeds I planted came to fruition after I left. I appreciate the support he gave me, the opportunities he provided, and the way he let me try new approaches. Mentors who can let their protégés stretch are hard to find. He also believed I should be a college or university president, so much of his help was provided with that in mind.

One other man played a major role in my career. He was the chair of the board of directors of the college where I was president. He actually was the reason I left the West Coast and dragged my husband to the Midwest. His biggest contributions to my career were having faith in my judgments and always being there to support me. I had difficult tasks to accomplish, and I knew I could do what was needed because he was there as buffer and confidant. He helped me prioritize our options, to get connected in the city, and to get support for the college from the community.

All of these men selected me as their protégé and helped me by supporting me, placing me in positions of influence, setting goals (even though they were not always stated), and introducing me to influential people. They are still a part of my life, although they are now much more like friends than mentors. We are all retired except the priest, who is the chancellor of the university and doing what he does best—raising money for the university. Although I never had formal plans or goals with these men, we always knew the direction in which we were heading. In fact, my first male mentor was the one who put the idea of being a college president into my mind; without ever sharing that with the others, they all came to the same conclusion. I am grateful to them for having the vision I did not have and for helping me reach that goal.

Mentoring Others

I have mentored and continue to mentor many nurses. The stories I tell here are about those protégés who exemplify the points I want to make about how the relationship was established, what role I played, and how the relationship changed. The first story is about a protégé whom I have known for 25 years and whom I continue to mentor and about how our mentor relationship was established and progressed.

Our relationship began when she was a faculty member and I was her dean. It developed over time from an informal friendship into a mentoring experience and then into a colleague relationship. The role I played was mostly as role model, teacher, and advisor, yet I do still support her and try to open doors of opportunity for her. She initiated the selection when she came to me one day and formally asked me to help her develop as a faculty member. I accepted the request, and we began by looking at what she could accomplish.

Together we set many goals for her: getting a doctorate, learning to be a good teacher, taking a leadership role, and being a researcher and writer. To meet these goals, I helped by being on her dissertation committee, coteaching with her in the classroom, giving her advice about being the director of a graduate program, doing research with her, and writing several chapters in books with her. Even though we do not live in the same state now, we communicate daily by e-mail and I frequently fax her information, ideas, and projects she has asked me to do or critique.

Over time, we have learned to be honest with each other, which means I frequently tell her what *not* to do or what she has done that was not very smart. Her naïveté still often gets in the way, which can cause me to loose patience, an action not appropriate of the mentor. Her feedback to me helps, as mine does for her. We are very open with each other and have developed a trust relationship that has helped us both during the 25 years.

One of the issues I have had to cope with is my tendency to parent her. Although mentors need to be helpful and supportive, it is not appropriate to parent the protégé. This means I have had to watch my tendency to scold, to not do what is necessary for her to do, and to look carefully at my expectations. I have had to ensure that we did not develop a codependent relationship. Because we know each other very well and want the relationship to grow and thrive, we monitor each other so a codependent relationship does not develop.

At times, I have had to push, challenge, and insist that she try something else. At other times, I have had to urge her to stop, think about, or reconsider something else. This kind of open communication is possible only if the participants of the mentor relationship trust each other and know that the advice is in the best interest of the protégé. I have also had to learn to step back and let her make mistakes when she would not listen to my advice. Letting the protégé make errors is hard but it can also be very growth producing for both persons.

Like my own mentors, I have had a vision for her and have most recently had to revise it. She has surprised me with her newest challenges and how she has met them. A mentor must be careful not to limit the development of the protégé, especially if the relationship has gone on for a long time. I think distance has changed our relationship and has allowed her to grow in new ways and encouraged her to assume more responsibility for her professional growth. It has also helped me to see that being geographically close is not necessary for protégé development.

My second story is about a young woman I have mentored since she was an undergraduate student in nursing, when I was the dean. In fact, many of my mentor relationships began when the protégé was a student. It is natural for a professor to be a role model for students because the professor can socialize the student into the profession of nursing. This young woman was often in my office asking for advice, seeking help with coursework, and talking with me about nursing. Professors who are open and accepting will find students in their offices, which is a wonderful opportunity to begin a mentor relationship. Our relationship began because she initiated it and because she was persistent and kept herself within my view. However, it was I who saw the potential and recognized the need for someone to facilitate her career. She kept in touch with me after she graduated and went into the army, and she involved me in her graduate study after she fulfilled her military commitment. She wrote letters to me apprising me of her progress in the army and sought my advice about opportunities when they arose. When I made trips to Washington, D.C., I would visit with her and get an update on her career. During her graduate study, I listened to her concerns, read and critiqued her papers, and counseled her about the best way to proceed in the program. Sometimes she followed my advice, and sometimes she did not.

When she was a student, I acted as teacher, confidant, and supporter. When she was ready to apply to graduate school, I wrote her a reference letter; I did the same when she recently applied for a new position. I also reviewed her resume and helped her think through the interview process. In each of these instances, she initiated the exchange; however, I have called her with ideas, have suggested different options available to her, and keep her in mind when I hear about vacancies and opportunities in nursing. She now lives in a city far from me, so we, too, communicate by e-mail, fax, and telephone. Currently, we are more like colleagues, but I still often mentor her when some new opportunity arises in her life.

I have one protégé who is currently in doctoral study who also initiated our relationship, but her story is different. We worked together in 1996 when she was an extern at STTI and was assigned to me. We were planning the ARISTA II conference, which was a summit meeting of high-level individuals in health. Nurses, physicians, insurance executives, academic officers, writers, entrepreneurs, public servants, and hospital administrators were brought to Indianapolis to the headquarters of STTI to discuss the future of nursing. I was chair of the leadership institute that sponsored the event, and my protégé was there to help me. She was a faculty member at a university in the south and was doing the externship as a way to learn about leadership. We were in a meeting; the discussion was exciting and stimulating, and we needed someone to record it and lead the discussion. I looked at her and pointed to the blackboard, indicating that I thought she should volunteer to do the job. She shook her head, indicating "no." I said as I looked at her, "You can be the facilitator, help us out." Shocked, she got up and did the best job anyone could have done. I was proud of her, and later she told me she was glad that I had insisted she do it. Sometimes, the mentor needs to push the protégé to do things; the trick is to push them into activities you know they can do well.

Our relationship is fairly new and began as an assignment; however, it grew in ways we had not expected. At her request, I wrote a letter of reference for her when she decided to go back to school to get a doctoral degree. I had been urging her to do so, and then one day, I got a telephone call, and she told me she had decided to apply. The day she was accepted, she called me again, and I felt as happy as she did about the acceptance. I have not heard from her in a long time, but I know that when she is ready, we will resume our relationship. A lack of communication does not necessarily mean the relationship is over. I know that she is very busy teaching and going to school, so I have not bothered her; I will when I know that she is less busy.

I have another nurse protégé who is a young man in academia. I hired him for his first faculty position in California in 1980. I met him at a national convention in Houston, Texas, and knew after the interview that he had great potential and would fit the position for which we were recruiting. I have followed his career with interest and have helped when he wanted me to. Recently, he decided it was time for him to move on, so we began a review of the positions available in the United States and Canada. I nominated him to positions, wrote recommendations for him, and called some of my colleagues to find out about some of the places where he wanted to apply. For about 3 months, we worked closely together, searching, analyzing, and picking the places he would apply or where I would nominate him. He called after each interview, and we analyzed his reactions. When it came time for his decision (he had two offers and a third possible one), I helped him look at the advantages and drawbacks of each. I also went to his going-away party at the university, where he was serving as associate dean. I am proud of his accomplishments and that I could be part of his pursuit of a new position in his career. Like me, he wants to be a college president, so I imagine I will be called into service for him again in 5 years when he decides to reach for a vice president position.

Our relationship has spanned that 18 years, but for about 8 of those we were not in touch. I knew that when he was ready and needed mentoring, he would let me know. I monitored his career from a distance; that is, I kept track of him through others who worked with him. Sometimes, the mentor knows more about the protégé by asking others. You get a different perspective and one that is more holistic when you consult those who have a working relationship with the protégé.

As you can tell, my role with him was mostly as advisor. I have never been his teacher or direct role model; however, I know that I have been a role model for him because I hear from others what he says about me. Mentors must always remember that what they do speaks a lot louder than what they say and that news spreads very quickly, especially if one is in a position of high visibility. When I was president of STTI I had high visibility, and those who knew me were quick to know what I was doing. It was also in this role that I gained many more protégés because young professionals are always looking for someone to help them with their careers.

One of my protégés started as a colleague and then became a protégé. She and I met when I moved to the Midwest and became president of a college. We worked together because she was on the alumni board. She was also a director on the kidney transplant unit in the hospital adjacent to the college. Our graduate students were precepted by her, and I heard a lot about her from them. I immediately noted that she was highly motivated and a quick learner and that she got things done. As time passed, we became good friends, and when she was terminated from the hospital during a cutback, she turned up in my office for support. That was the beginning of our mentor/protégé relationship.

For a period of about 3 months, I was her confidant and advisor while she considered her next step. I urged her to take time (she received a nice settlement from the hospital and did not have to rush into anything) to consider what she wanted to do next. I did not know until later that she was having difficulty deciding what to do because she could not envision herself doing anything different.

To reinforce her worth during this difficult time, I gave her several important tasks to do for the alumni association. I have learned that when people are in a transition from one job to another and are frightened about the unknown and the transferability of their abilities, they need to believe they are important and needed. Keeping busy was not the issue, but having something to do that highlighted her worth was my intent.

I remember the day she came in to see me to tell me she had a tremendous offer from a firm that built hospitals; the firm wanted to establish a consultation division for reengineering hospitals and wanted a nurse in that division. It sounded good, and she liked the idea, but she wanted to know what I thought about the job and the salary. It was a good offer, but I knew they needed her because of her experience with reengineering and I thought the salary should be more. I told her to ask for $20,000 more, at which she gasped and nearly fainted. I do not think that I will ever get used to the way nurses do not value their talents; clearly, she was worth more than they had offered. She was afraid they would not give her what I suggested, and I said, "So .what? Nothing ventured, nothing gained. And you are worth it." In this case, I was trying to boost her image and to help her learn how to negotiate. "If they won't go to that figure, negotiate but do not take what they offered. They need you," I said.

"But I do not know if I can do that job," she said, and I replied, "You know more than you think you do. Go for it."

The next day, she returned all smiles because they had agreed to pay what she asked without any negotiation. She was amazed that it had worked. The next day, I had a big bouquet of silk flowers on my desk as a "thank you" from her. Letting your mentor know that you are thankful for the help is important. And letting the protégé know that you are proud of her or his ability to try something risky is also important. I told her how proud I was and that I knew she could do it. Later, she told me that my faith in her was very reassuring and helped her see her worth at a time when she was unsure of her abilities beyond what she had been doing for the past 17 years.

This mentor relationship has been through many phases. Currently, she is learning to write for publication. She also became the president of a new chapter of STTI, a position that I urged her to assume. She is still very involved with the alumni association and plans on getting more involved with STTI. I am looking for an international committee I can help her get assigned to because I know she is ready for that kind of work. Knowing your protégé's capacity for work and advancement is important so you can make the best recommendations and give the best career advice.

Sometimes, a protégé is selected after a service has been provided in another context. As I said, I did a lot of consultation with schools of nursing in the 1970s. One of those schools I worked with had gone through some pretty horrendous changes in administration, and the new chairperson needed help. A colleague and I met her at a national convention, and we agreed to help her with a curriculum revision. That was the beginning of a relationship that spanned more than 20 years and moved from consultation for the program to a mentorship with her. Although I have continued to be the curriculum consultant for the program, I have also helped her since she became a dean. I had her as an intern at my school, where she spent time with me as part of her doctoral work learning to be an academic administrator, and was a member of her dissertation committee. We have done research together, and I have sponsored her to a leadership fellowship, written letters of recommendations for her, placed her on an international ballot for office on the board of a national organization, and been available for personal professional advice.

This story about being a mentor is a little different because it is an example of how a mentor relationship can evolve from a different activity. Of note is that it was after we had known each other for a long time that the personal need overtook the program need; this was probably because we had time to develop a personal relationship as well as a programmatic one.

There are times when I thought I had not been a good mentor and had not been able to help the protégé only to find out later that I had. Early in my career, when I was a neonatal intensive care nurse, I worked with a young nurse who was very good at what she did but had no idea where she wanted to go with her career. I talked a lot about going to school and the advantages of an education. We worked nights together, so I know that I must have driven her crazy with my talk about the value of an education. Nearly every night I urged her to go to school and to think about nursing as a career.

I left that job when I became an assistant professor at the university, and I lost contact with her. It wasn't until a couple of years ago when a woman came up to me at a regional conference and said "Thank you" that I realized I was talking to that same nurse from the intensive care unit. She was thanking me for the advice of long ago and wanted to let me know that she had recently received her doctorate and was a professor of nursing in a university in the east. She also told me that she had been watching my career and had gained a lot of help as she saw me as her role model. This story suggests that you can be mentoring some one and not even know it.

The last protégé I want to introduce is one I selected because I saw a potential for success and a need for assistance many years after our first encounter. This protégé was also a student when I was dean. She appeared to be on her way and very capable and did not need a mentor. In school, she was the president of the student nurse association, active in class activities, and very involved at her church. She is beautiful, articulate, and smart. I remember giving her the diploma at graduation and wishing her success. That was in 1985. I had not seen her since then until 2 months ago, when she called to say hello.

I had seen her aunt at my 50-year high school reunion and asked about her, telling her aunt that I would like to hear from her. I was interested in knowing what she had done. When her call came, I arranged to have lunch with her. It was at this meeting that we established the mentor relationship and I promised to help her. She had recently married and moved back to the San Francisco Bay area; she was looking for a position in a hospital and wanted someone to talk to about her career. The other day, I received a letter from her, so we will meet again. She clearly needs dialogue and direction even though she has acquired a new position. People often need mentors in the prime of their careers simply because they are looking to the future and know that having someone with a network is important.

SUMMARY

Being mentored and having a mentor are very satisfying experiences. The roles I played in both positions were different, yet being mentored by a good mentor helps you become a good mentor in turn. I know that I am a good mentor because I know what a poor one is like. But even my poorest mentor was a big boost to my career and me, so in that sense I guess that there are no bad mentors if you know what to look for and what kinds of experiences are possible. I think that I have learned as much as those I have mentored and have gained as much as they did. This fits the model presented by Kaye and Jacobson (1995), who believe mentors will increasingly view themselves as learning partners.

Overall, there are several aspects about my mentoring experiences that I want to highlight:

- Mentors often do not have to search out protégés. If they are open and available, a protégé will find them.
- Having high visibility attracts protégés. Without any effort, high-visibility nurses will accrue protégés.
- Distance can help a mentor relationship, particularly if the relationship is of long standing.

- It is possible to learn from a mentor who is a poor role model. Because the mentor can offer a variety of services, being a poor role model does not make one a poor mentor.
- Connecting protégés to others is an important activity, but the mentor must know whether the person the protégé is referred to is willing to take the protégé.
- Mentoring takes time, effort, and commitment. Do not take on the job if you cannot meet these requirements.
- Mentor relationships can go dormant and still be viable. When you least expect it, the relationship will resume.
- Protégés do not always take your advice. This does not mean it was bad advice or that the protégé is disrespectful; it means the protégé may see things differently and may need to test his or her own judgment.
- Mentors and protégés do not have to be of the same gender, nor do they have to be in the same business, but they must have common goals.
- Keeping the mentor relationship from becoming a codependent one is a full-time job and the responsibility of both the mentor and the protégé.
- Mentorships arise from a variety of experiences; sometimes they are part of a colleague relationship or begin at a conference or a workshop, or they are arranged as an assignment. Staying flexible helps facilitate the possibility of the development of mentor relationship.
- Mentors may think they are not doing it right, but it is the protégé who is the best judge of the mentor's impact.
- Mentoring relationships serve many purposes for both the mentor and the protégé and provide several advantages for both persons. Listed below are just a few of the advantages and benefits.

For the mentor, the relationship is a way to

- Help the next generation of nurses get prepared for leadership roles
- Extend one's self through the work and role of the protégé
- Help another professional
- Grow and develop one's own skills as a teacher, counselor, advisor, and role model
- Extend the network of colleagues

For the protégé, the relationship is a way to

- Learn and develop new skills
- Advance one's career
- Become part of a network of colleagues
- Learn how to be a mentor

The mentor relationship is as old as time. Socrates was a mentor, and so was Martin Luther King, Jr. Throughout history, mentors have been helping protégés. Nurses have mentored others but have done so mostly as role models. More recently, they have begun to see the true value of mentoring and know that it is an essential element of any leader's repertoire of behaviors and that it includes helping protégés advance their careers. Leaders have a responsibility to see that the next generation of nurses is prepared for the role of leader. What better way is there to do this than to learn from the successful leader as a protégé? I think this chapter can be summed up by a quote:

Come to the edge.
It's too high.
Come to the edge.
We might fall.
Come to the edge.
And they came. And he pushed them. And they flew. (Source unknown)

REFERENCES

Andersen, C. A. F. (1999). Mentoring and networking—The student's perspective. In C. A. F. Andersen (Ed.). *Nursing student to nursing leader.* Albany, N.Y.: Delmar.

Bower, F. (1993). Women and mentoring in higher education administration. In P. T. Mitchell (Ed.). *Cracking the wall.* Washington, D.C.: College and University Personnel Association.

Butts, B. J., & Wither, D. M. (1992). New graduates: What does my manager expect? *Nursing Management, 23*(8), 46–48.

Carey, S. J., & Campbell, S. T. (1994). Preceptor, mentor, and sponsor roles: Creative strategies for nurse retention. *Journal of Nursing Administration, 24*(12), 39–48.

Gehrke, N. (1988). Toward a definition of mentoring. *Theory into Practice, 27*(3), 190–194.

Hamilton, E. M., Murray, M. K., Lindholm, L. H., & Myers, R. E. (1989). Effects of mentoring on job satisfaction, leadership behaviors, and job retention of new graduate nurses. *Journal of Staff Development, 5*, 159–165.

Hockenberry-Eaton, M., & Kline, N. E. (1995). Who is mentoring the nurse practitioner? *Journal of Pediatric Health Care, 9*(2), 94–95.

Joel, L. A. (1997). Charged to mentor. *American Journal of Nursing, 97*(2), 7.

Kanter, R. M. (1977). *Men and women of the corporation.* New York: Basic Books.

Kaye, B., & Jacobson, B. (1995). Mentoring: A group guide. *Training and Development,* 23–27.

Levinson, D. (1977). *The season's of a man's life.* New York: Alfred A. Knopf.

Martin, M. L., Tolleson, J., Lakey, K. I., & Moeller, E. (1995). VALOR students: A creative type of perceptorship. *Federal Practitioner, 12*(4), 47–50.

Moore, K. M. (1982). The role of mentors in developing leaders for academe. *Educational Record, 63*, 22–28.

Nayak, S. (1991). Strategies to support the new nurse in practice. *Journal of Nursing Staff Development, 7*(39), 64–66.

Spengler, C. D. (1982). Mentor-protégé relationships: A study of career development among female nurse doctorates (doctoral dissertation, University of Missouri—Columbia, 1992). *Dissertation Abstracts International, 44*, 213B.

Taylor, L. J. (1992). A survey of mentor-protégé relationships in academe. *Journal of Professional Nursing, 8*, 48–55.

Vance, C. (1999). Mentoring—The nursing leader and mentor's perspective. In C. F. Andersen (Ed.). *Nursing student to nursing leader.* Albany, N.Y.: Delmar.

Vance, C., & Olson, R. (1998). *The mentor connection in nursing.* New York: Springer.

White, J. F. (1988). The perceived role of mentoring in the career development and success of academic nurse administrators. *Journal of Professional Nursing, 4*, 178–185.

Williams, R., & Blackburn, R. (1988). Mentoring and junior faculty productivity. *Journal of Nursing Education, 27*(5), 204–209.

Chapter 12

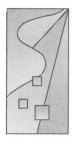

Letting Go and Taking On

Linda Arnold

Health care reforms in the 1990s have triggered incredible changes in the environments in which nurses work. No matter what is encountered in these new environments, it is how the nurse responds that counts. Their responses will, in part, be based on their psychological reactions and on how rapidly they can shed outdated thinking and behaviors. Those who assume leadership during times of change will be the ones who (1) can best understand themselves, (2) can recognize when they are stuck, and (3) are able to let go of ways of working that are not functional and assume ways of doing things that fit the demands of the new work setting.

This chapter is about letting go of ideas, behaviors, philosophies, and existing points of view that do not fit anymore and taking on new perspectives that are consistent with the changes occurring. *Letting go and taking on* is an ongoing process of giving up some ideas and taking on others or assigning someone new to a task previously performed by a licensed person. For instance, it could mean giving up the idea that care for patients must be given only by a professional nurse or that there is only one right way to accomplish a goal. It could mean evaluating the skills of the unlicensed person and letting him or her provide the aspects of care that match those skills. It could mean leaving one job and seeking another that fits one's existing point of view about patient care or that brings more joy to the caregiver. Thus, letting go involves both attitudes and actions and can be partial or complete.

Nurses have not been very good at delegating care and have stated it was because they were concerned about the quality of the care. "Healthcare organizations [have] created roles and relationships to meet the challenges of providing quality, cost-effective care. New care providers are being introduced into healthcare environments with the expectation that licensed staff will provide oversight. Professional nurses are concerned about the implications for their professional practice" (Person, 1997, p. 12). It seems that nurses are worried about whether the delegate will provide correct care and wonder whether they can delegate tasks without compromising their roles as professionals, so rather than delegate, they perform the tasks themselves. Pollack (1996) explains this lack of delegation by saying, "Sometimes the person, who can accept on an intellectual level about not delegating as much as he or she should, cannot change the approach because the real problem is emotional" (p. 21). Thus successful delegation depends, in part, on the nurses' abilities to observe and *understand* their abilities to let go.

Interestingly, the struggles in learning to delegate are those of letting go of anything and have a lot to do with control. Although most of us intellectually understand that we have control over very little in our lives, we do have the ability to make change and to adjust to change. Even knowing this makes us uncomfortable, so when letting go is necessary, we tend to hold on to what we know works and what we believe should be in order to control the world around us. However, this attempt to control can lead to problems if the need to let go is greater and more appropriate than our need to hang on to ideas, values, or behaviors.

Letting go takes many forms. For instance, the nurse can accept a new idea while dropping an old view or while taking on new responsibilities. It can be something as simple as asking someone to do what you have usually done. The hardest part about this process is the range of emotions that accompany these changes. Person (1997) says letting go is hard because most behaviors not only have become comfortable and habitual but also fit one's vision of how things should be. Nurses often take on new responsibilities without letting go of others until they find themselves overworked and stressed. Some nurses have not learned to take on and let go at the same time.

A common response to holding on is stress. *Stress* can be defined as the feeling one gets when existing points of view and ways of functioning no longer fit or work but are continued. Existing points of view are the beliefs, values, or opinions that constantly influence our behaviors and thus our communications. Sometimes, they lead to difficulty when they do not fit the environment in which they are acted out. For example, imagine the nurse who believes her method for doing a certain procedure is correct and the only way to do it. Her point of view is probably that she knows best because she has experience and knows what works; therefore, everyone should do as she does. Obviously, holding to this point of view will lead to tension and stress for the nurse and for others who may want to do the procedure differently. It can be said that letting go of "should" is a good way to allow for differences in practice and to avoid stress.

Letting go of outdated points of view is hard and often the reason for tension in work environments. The effort expended and the resultant conflict between what is needed and what is done that does not work become so great the person feels anxious, fatigued, and sometimes angry. Typically, the person blames others for these feelings because there is a lack of awareness of the root of the problem. Alternately, the individual does understand the problem and wants the world to return to the way it was so that the existing point of view that underlies the behavior can remain untouched. Clearly, this attempt to hold on to an ideal that can no longer be implemented in the new world of health care is one of the sources of stress for some nurses.

Letting go for some nurses seems like giving up or not caring when it often is nothing more than changing the method for reaching the same goal. In the current managed care environment, there is a different staff mix and often fewer resources than before. Coming from the old point of view, some say they cannot provide care in this way. Once one decides that something is impossible because it should be the way it was, the opportunities for creative thinking and problem solving are greatly reduced. Letting go of the old point of view and accepting a new one would bring these nurses to the same goal but in a different way. Moving away from the absolute and "should" frees one to accomplish the best outcome that is consistent with the circumstances.

One of the more difficult aspects of this process of letting go is identify what is being held on to. Every nurse, regardless of the specialty or level oi practice, will have to ask several questions: Do I like what I am doing? Am I stressed and unhappy? Do I blame everyone else for how miserable I feel? Have I retired while on the job? Am I doing anything about my situation? Will I be able to find the energy and creativity to have an impact on the system in which I work? Although the answers to these questions will be different for each nurse, if the answers to most of these questions were "yes," then the next step is to let go of something. There simply is not enough energy and creativity to deal with today's challenges if the old identities and ways of thinking do not work anymore. The nurses who discard the old ways and old ideas will take the lead and have the greatest impact on their practice and on the profession as a whole.

This chapter presents a model for *letting go* and *taking on*. It provides (1) a way to examine yourself and your attitudes, behaviors, and points of view and (2) strategies for letting go of things that no longer work. Every leader, regardless of the level, must be able to let go and take on to be effective.

TRANSITIONS: A MODEL FOR LETTING GO AND TAKING ON

A transition model developed by William Bridges is an excellent way to look at ways to let go. Before change can take place, says Bridges (1991), "One must understand that it isn't the changes that do you in, it's the transitions" (p. 3). He emphasizes the importance of the emotional component, the internal process that occurs during change. Before Bridges, the focus of attention during change was on getting the external pieces in place and ignoring the struggle people might have with the change. The nurse was expected to adjust to fewer professional staff and more inexperienced and less-skilled personnel. If the nurse resisted these changes, she or he was labeled a troublemaker. Bridges (1991) points out that "psychological transition depends on letting go of the old reality and the old identity you had before the change took place" (p. 4). Thus, before the nurse can adjust to change, she or he must make the psychological transition, and this takes time. In other words, without transition, change will not occur.

Phases of Transition

Bridges' transition model has three phases: the ending phase, the neutral zone phase, and the new beginnings phase. People going through change have to go through these three phases before any change really occurs; if there is a delay in any phase, the change is delayed.

■ Phase 1: The Ending Phase

In the initial phase of a transition, there are endings and losses. Even when the change is positive, one has to let go and say good-bye to the old way. Even when one gets a promotion, a raise, a higher faculty appointment, or an opportunity to have an impact on the system by placement on an important committee, there is a loss and a letting go. How could these rewards be considered a loss? Imagine the letting go that might be needed with these new opportunities. You are no longer in the old position with those you have worked with for some time, at the earlier salary with all of its tax advantages, in the previous faculty position with its lesser responsibilities, or in a place where you weren't expected to provide new ideas. The new opportunities undoubtedly bring new expectations and more responsibilities. There will be more demands on your time, which could interfere with your personal time and probably create more stress. If the change and transitions are by choice, one can rank the loss and letting go against the positives of the change. When the change and accompanying transitions are not within your control, there is more stress from the unexpected losses and endings. Bridges (1991) states that one must understand "failure to identify and be ready for the endings and the losses that change produces is the largest single problem that people and organizations in transition encounter" (p. 5). This is also true if the change and ensuing transition occur in one's personal life.

■ Phase 2: The Neutral Zone

Bridges describes the next phase of the transition model as the neutral zone. This is when the old is gone and the new has not yet been totally accepted or identified. This phase offers both risk and opportunity, and although its length is variable, it usually lasts longer than the external change. During this time, the nurse may be looking for a familiar method or marker to hold on to. This is why we commonly hear "But we always have done it this way" during this phase.

The recent external changes in the health care delivery system have included the downsizing of staff and the additional loss of familiar team members. These losses of the valued aspects of health care delivery are the reason the length of this phase has been long and uncomfortable for the staff. Nurses need time for grieving and adjusting to the new.

Because of the discomfort felt by those in the neutral zone phase, there are a number of predictable pitfalls. The most common mistake nurses make is to do a "geographic"; this means there is a tendency for nurses to leave their present jobs because of the changes and the unknown outcomes of the changes. As organizational turnover increases, so does the tendency for nurses to start looking elsewhere for employment that they think will offer more security. Sadly, today's health care environment does not provide stability, so nurses who have sought it have found that within 1 year after changing jobs, they are back looking for stability again. Bridges (1991) comments, "painful though it often is, the neutral zone is the individual's and the organization's best chance for creativity, renewal, and development" (p. 6).

The most beneficial approach during this phase is to remain in place and to use the time to see what direction the organization will take and what opportunities arise because of the change. There is no doubt this phase will include a struggle; however, because all of life can be a struggle even in the happiest and most successful times, the task is to avoid having the struggle become suffering.

Suffering includes the development of victim behaviors that are manifested by blaming, feeling sorry for one's self, being paralyzed and resentful, and being at risk of making poor decisions. Peters (1994) states that "blame obscures the true nature of problems. As long as you're holding someone or (something) else responsible for your failures, you're casting yourself in the role of victim, powerless to act except in response to the actions of others" (p. 126). Thus, the victim role leaves one consistently in a reactive, as opposed to a proactive, mode.

If one allows the victim mentality to continue, the next step can be a move into resentment. Resentment can pervade the organizational and personal neutral zone. Nothing drains creativity and energy more rapidly than the impotent feeling that accompanies resentment. Dalrymple (1998) discusses the outcomes of resentment and says, "If the world is unjustly stacked against us, any effort on our part to improve the situation is futile" (p. 32). In today's health care climate, it is not surprising to find a struggle; however, the key for leaders at all levels is to recognize the difference between struggle and suffering and to help those in transition move through the struggle without suffering.

Persons in the neutral zone may be in various stages of transition. It can be difficult for the nurse who has let go of the old format and is taking hold of a new one to deal with those who have decided to suffer. It is not uncommon to hear nurses who are suffering say "no" or "yes, but" to every suggestion made for establishing new routines. However, the negative attitudes of coworkers must not be allowed to interfere with the positive attitudes displayed by those moving forward. Although passing through this phase may be difficult, it is not impossible if one does not expect everyone to let go at the same pace. The key for those making the transition is to identify those who are also moving forward and to join them for support.

■ Phase 3: New Beginnings

The final phase of the transition model, according to Bridges, is "new beginnings." He says, "starts take place on a schedule as a result of decisions. Starts involve new situations. Beginnings involve new understandings, new values, new attitudes, and most of all, new identities" (Bridges, 1991, p. 50). During this phase, there is a need for lots of communication. Because of the anxiety and turmoil of the neutral zone, people do not listen or hear as well as they usually do, so an extra effort on the part of leaders must be expended to provide information and more information and then more information. It cannot be assumed that saying anything once is enough. There also must be a willingness to be patient and to continue working with those who are having a hard time. It is very important to avoid blaming and labeling those who are slow to let go.

As each person searches for a new beginning, it is crucial to remember that new beginnings rarely occur overnight or with great intensity. Usually, it is a slow and steady process forward, with one step at a time. Bridges (1991) says, "We forget how indirect and unimpressive beginnings really are, and we imagine instead some clear and conscious steps that we ought to be taking" (p. 135). The key, however, is to remain alert and energetic and to recognize each opportunity as it emerges.

As nurses struggle with the changes evolving in the health care system, there often is a lament that this current system is not the vision of nursing practice that drew them to the profession. They note that these changes do not fit the model that they had imagined or had actually been part of until recently. However, Levine (1982), who writes about the process of death and dying, said, "I have seen how much suffering is created by our models and resistance to the givens of the present. A kind of mental cramping develops from holding to the models of who we think we are and how the world is supposed to be" (p. 54). Thus, acknowledging that the system in which you work is no longer the one you entered is the first step into the new beginnings zone. Nurses who are able to do this are on their way to looking for a new role, new working relationships, and a new attitude. Those who have decided to hold on to what is familiar regardless of its fit are on the road to suffering. Others may chose to let go of the current job and to search for a model of practice that fits the present circumstances. This could include looking for a different setting, a new role, new working relationships, or even a new attitude.

There is another way of letting go that occurs quite frequently during change; this is when doing the job using the old ways during change becomes so unbearable that the worker gets physically sick and is thus forced to let go. As the health care system changed and nurses have been expected to take on more responsibility, some nurses have continued to use the old ways to cope. Instead of saying "this is more than I can handle," they continue to act on their existing point of view by trying to do everything even though there was never enough time and they felt stressed and like failures. Eventually, they became sick. Illness created a letting go that would not have happened on its own. The physical self did the job when the emotional self would not let go. Understanding and using Bridges' transition model represent a way to avoid letting go by becoming sick.

Summary

Being an effective leader includes the ability to let go of ideas, values, and behaviors that no longer work during change or to let go of activities that others can do. Bridges suggests that it is the transition, not the change, that is difficult. He also points out that it is our inability to let go of our existing points of view that blocks our ability to move through the three phases of transition (ending, being neutral, and new beginnings).

The inability to let go often is the inability to give up control and involves a self-evaluation of one's existing points of view and how they fit with the changing world in which we live. The story that follows is about one nurse's use of Bridges' transition model when she was confronted with change in her career.

TRANSITION THROUGH CHANGE BY ONE NURSE USING BRIDGES' MODEL

To this day, my mother does not know I was fired, yet the events of that Friday afternoon are still a vivid memory to me. Strangely, I can still remember exactly what I was wearing and how my boss wouldn't look me in the eye. He said it was either him or me, so it had to be me. One of my department managers stopped me in the hall to see what was wrong, and with disbelief in my voice, I told her, "I've been fired." She started to cry, but I walked dry-eyed to my office and called my husband. That critical meeting was the starting point of my personal story of letting go and taking on.

Entering the First Phase of the Transition Model

Bridges' (1980) comments on endings describe my own ending as a nurse administrator. "Considering that we have to deal with endings all our lives, most of us handle them badly. We take them too seriously by confusing them with finality—that it's all over, never more, finished. We see them as something without sequel, forgetting the fact that they are the first phase of the transition process and a pre-condition of self-renewal" (p. 90). At the time of that meeting, I do not believe Bridges himself could have convinced me that my job loss was going to be the best thing that happened to my career; I was in shock.

There had never been a time in my life when I was not working, including all of the years I was in school. Nor had I ever experienced what could be called a failure. I asked myself: How could one be fired and not be seen as unsuccessful, as a failure? I could not picture what was ahead for me, and that was terrifying. I was in the ending phase of transition and did not know it.

That feeling of not knowing the future was not new to me. It had been with me for a long time because many aspects of my position were not satisfying; in fact, they were often extremely stressful. I had considered returning to school but only as an escape and because there did not seem to be anything else I could do. Because many of my peers had similar complaints about their positions, it was easy to believe these feelings were to be expected. It really did not cross my mind that my unhappiness had to do with my job's not being the right one for me.

In addition to my sense of discomfort, it was a time of tremendous turmoil within the organization, and I naively ignored the political implications for someone in my position. I believed that as long as the nursing department was running smoothly and I was working hard, any problems that arose could be solved. Although there were lots of stories from my colleagues about nurse administrators being sacrificed during organizational struggles, I never thought that it would happen to me. I can see now that it was my lack of political savvy that left me vulnerable to termination.

Obviously, the emotional aftermath of this forced letting go was very painful and reinforced my concerns about my professional future. Even more disturbing was acknowledging that I might have continued doing something that I did not enjoy because I was unable to let go. I was holding on to something that didn't work; I was stubbornly denying the benefits and the need for a change.

Why did I hold on to something that was not working? In hindsight, I think it was because it is human to not like change and to stick to familiar patterns even if they are painful. Holding on felt like control even though I knew I had little control over things. I held on to what I was doing even though I knew it was not healthy for me. Holding on seemed to protect me from experiencing an ending. Bridges (1980) says, "Endings are experiences of dying. They are ordeals, sometimes they challenge so basically our sense of who we are that we believe it will be the end of us" (p. 100).

We seem to hold on to what is not working and is not healthy for us because we have a model of ourselves in a certain role and can identify our successes only within that context. We can't see ourselves doing something else. This was the struggle for me. From the time of my entrance into nursing school, I wanted to be a nurse leader, a nurse administrator. My evaluations in nursing school emphasized my potential as a manager, and I never really considered any other position. All of my education was directed toward that goal. Levine (1982) reminds us that "Models create such expectation by preconceiving, like any philosophy or idea, a sort of tunnel vision" (p. 54). My identity became merged with the model of administrator, so it was very hard to let it go.

Sometimes, our identity becomes tied to the idea that we can manage many roles at the same time. At one of my workshops, a participant asked for suggestions on how she could handle her time more efficiently. She was a single mother with three children who was working full-time and attending school part-time. She wanted to know how to manage her time so she had more time with her children. My suggestion that she consider letting go of some of her activities to make room for more time with the children was not acceptable to her. She had promised herself that she would go back to school without affecting the rest of her life. She admitted she was feeling stressed and was having sleep disturbances but felt that better management of time would overcome these problems. No amount of advice from me or the rest of the audience could influence her to let go of her model. A health problem or something happening to her children will probably trigger letting go for her. It could occur sooner if she would consider the transition model.

The process of holding on can lead to many different outcomes depending on the situation and the intensity of the stress. Holding on created erosion of my self-acceptance and self-worth. I began to believe more and more strongly that it was a deficiency within me that was the problem. I believed the situation would get better if I worked harder, longer, and more creatively. Many of the nurses who attend my workshops have had the same experience with holding on.

Driving yourself to do better works for a short time, but rarely does it work over a long period of time. Another recent situation supports this statement. A nurse leader I know developed a program for providing quality care to certain groups of low-income patients. She wrote the grants, did the fund raising, created the marketing plan, and then did the marketing on her own with some financial and material support from the sponsoring institution. In addition, she provided some of the patient care. The program was very successful, but as the health care climate became more financially demanding, the clinic was adversely affected. With each new problem, the nurse took more and more on herself in an attempt to keep costs and personnel needs to a minimum. By the time we met, she was severely stressed and depressed and barely able to get up in the morning. However, the biggest problem was her image of herself. Although she realized the health care industry was different, she believed she should have been able to overcome the changes so the project could have survived. I understand that statement because it was just like the one I held on to for a long time after I was fired. That word "should" got in our way of letting go.

Another nurse at a transition workshop I conducted shared a similar story. The hospital where she worked was downsizing, so she decided to join every committee she could and to take on new projects as a guarantee against being laid off. She was feeling overwhelmed with all of the work and jokingly hoped she would be removed from her job so she could get a rest. Later, I found out that she did lose her job; while deciding what to do next, she took a part-time job. After being forced to let go, she took her time looking at other options. She was into the neutral zone.

After listening to many stories about forced letting go and remembering my own, I find a common theme. Every one of us felt relief after letting go. I remember sitting at my desk in my office shocked and hurt as I had never been before in my life but very aware of feeling a huge sense of relief. At least I did not have to come to work the next day. At the time it did not make sense, but now I understand more about the stress I was feeling and how much I needed to let go of the job. It is also an example of the duality of feelings that can occur during an ending. In the months that followed, it was reassuring to remember how relieved I was, especially during those times of doubt in the neutral zone phase.

Maneuvering Through the Neutral Zone

It has always seemed strange to me that Bridges calls the second phase of a transition the neutral zone because in my experience, it is far from neutral. For me, it was a time of shock and numbness alternating with fear and panic. At first, it was wonderful to sleep late, to have time to read the newspaper, and to enjoy a leisurely cup of coffee. However, it was also much like other aspects of life—reality finally set in, and I had many immediate responsibilities to complete that were not very attractive.

Because of my position and responsibility for a large department, I scheduled a meeting for the first Monday after I was terminated to officially say good-bye. I had already started to dissociate and cannot remember much of what I said, but I do remember the feelings, the honesty, and the support in that room. There was sadness, shock, and disbelief, but there was also a lot of love and caring. This was the first time I had shared how stressed I had been in the job. I had not meant to do this, but the mood was just right, and before I knew it, I was telling them things I had never before shared.

That meeting sparked the beginning of a most difficult time for me as I entered the neutral zone. I found I was no longer comfortable with the people I had worked with for many years. I received calls from those I had supervised, peers from other departments, and colleagues from other hospitals; they wanted to comfort and support me and often asked me to lunch and other events. I found myself saying "no" and not wanting to answer their calls. The irony of this situation is that previously I never had time to see friends outside of work, and now that there was time, each telephone call or lunch invitation triggered sadness and more pain. My coworkers were well intentioned and sympathetic, but being with them was too distressing for me; it was more painful being with people than being alone. My feelings were similar to those grieving the loss of a family member, but the death in my life was the loss of the image I had of myself as a leader. For a number of months, I was in this stage of grief before I realized I had something I could do.

Another aspect of my life that made this time in the neutral zone difficult for me was my position as secretary and member of the board of directors of a state nurse administrator's group. The high visibility of this position made it impossible for me to avoid telling my story again and again. Although my peers were sympathetic and supportive, I felt like a person with a contagious disease. I did not fit anywhere, and those around me did not relate to me as they had. I had heard about others losing their jobs, but I never thought it would happen to me or that I would feel like such a failure. Looking back, I realize now that I was in a daze and "on automatic pilot" while performing my assigned duties, which included participation in an annual conference. Bridges (1980) describes this period of the neutral zone by saying,

> People in transition are often still involved in activities and relationships that continue to bombard them with cues that are irrelevant to their emerging needs. Because a person is likely to feel lonely in such a situation, the temptation is to seek more and better contact with others, but the real need is for a genuine sort of aloneness in which inner signals can make themselves heard (p. 121).

Although I found it hard to be alone during this time, I was not drawn to others and thus was able to hear the signals when they came.

The turning point came one night at the administrator's conference. It had been a long and difficult day, and I could not sleep or even relax. It seemed like everybody else was happy and successful and I was the only loser at the meeting. This was my only episode of "victim thinking," and it did not last long. A friend from the board was staying across the hall from me, so I asked her to come to my room, where I started talking about how I felt. I started to focus on me as the person and not as the administrator who needed to be successful. After that meeting, I began seeing a counselor and started to explore the direction my career could take.

This episode triggered my second "letting go." This time I needed to let go of seeing myself in a negative way and of needing to hide how hurt I was. The process of letting go is ongoing and continues clear through the transition. Bridges (1991) explains those first few weeks with this message: "One of the most difficult aspects of the neutral zone for most people is that they don't understand it. They expect to be able to move straight from the old to the new. But this isn't a trip from one side of the street to the other. It's a journey from one identity to the other, and that takes time" (p. 37).

It wasn't long before I began to receive telephone calls from headhunters about available administrative positions. A couple of them were sure that I could be placed within weeks. This amazed me. Who would want me? I had been fired, and were there still employers who might want to hire me? It sounds naive, but never having been fired in my life, I had this idea that you had only one chance and if that one didn't work out, you were through for life. I found out there are many, many opportunities if you look and wait.

As the numbness and shock subsided, I started to consider whether management was for me. This questioning process was difficult because it was hard to turn off the negative self-talk that included many "shoulds" and "if onlys." I learned later that this negative chatter in our heads is one of the dangers of the neutral zone. If you have a tendency to place high expectations on yourself, as I did, the discomfort and empty feelings during this phase can create a type of paralysis and a loss of confidence in self. The counseling sessions I was pursuing were effective in helping me stay out of this self-depreciation. It was a struggle to stay in a positive frame of mind and to accept a "wait and see" posture, but I did.

One of the exercises I pursued in counseling was to list all the different tasks, duties, behaviors, and requirements of my administrative job and to assign a value based on my enjoyment of doing each one. The list was quite lengthy, but there were few on that list that received high values. Telephone calls, meetings of all kinds, and communications with physicians received low values. Those that were rated with high values were counseling, teaching classes, and motivating staff at all levels. I realized that most of my time was spent doing the former as opposed to the latter, so it quickly became apparent that I needed to change my career goals.

This assessment of my administrative duties helped me look at what had happened at the hospital with a less-judgmental attitude. I discovered my boss was under attack from the physicians and they were leveraging our institution against one nearby. He also had been meeting with the former nurse administrator in secret on the weekends to discuss the nursing department. He had not taken me into his confidence about the politics of the institution, nor were we working together to solve the problems. He believed in sharing on a "need to know" basis. All of the administrative staff were under tremendous stress because it was "every man for himself." I had had no experience at this level to know how to protect myself, nor was there anyone I could go to for advice. I cannot believe how trusting I was. I did know that my boss was not communicating with me, and when I questioned this, he gave me an indirect answer, which I did not question for a more specific response. I know now that I was already in a daze at work and in a survival mode. In part, learning this explained my tremendous feelings of relief as opposed to anger when I was fired. I was glad to be out of there and did not know it. In some way, I had already said good-bye but could not let go on my own.

Looking back, I now realize that my lack of experience in a large organization and my inability to see the big picture contributed to my termination. I had concentrated my efforts on the nursing department and had not balanced my attention by gaining a broader view and building a political base (see Chapter 4 for a discussion on seeing the big picture).

Some of my colleagues urged me to fight my termination by filing an unfair labor suit, but because of the public exposure, I decided not to pursue any legal action. More importantly, I realized I was not happy in the position, that management was not where I wanted to be anymore, and that I had been holding on when I should have let go. In the seminars that I conduct now, I often share my experience with the audience and point out that it took a jolt (like being hit on the head with a 2 × 4) to get me to let go and that there are better ways to do it.

There is an emotional element to address in the neutral zone, and for me it centered on my feelings toward my boss. This is a more painful process and takes more time to resolve than any other aspect of letting go. I was angry at my boss and the previous nurse administrator, both whom had betrayed me by meeting in secret to discuss problems with the nursing department. I knew this kind of thing occurred all of the time in many organizations, but until it happened to me, I had no idea how difficult it is to handle feelings of abandonment and betrayal.

The most important aspect of the neutral zone for me, however, was the time and space I gave myself to determine my next action. I had received a severance package, so I could take my time finding a job. I was finally able to be alone, to read, and to assess my strengths. I looked at my talents and found I had two important skills: counseling and speaking. My master's degree in psychiatric nursing had provided me with excellent counseling skills that I had infrequently used to help the nursing staff with their job stress. I had planned on doing staff counseling more frequently, but with my other administrative duties, I never had the time I needed. However, no matter how busy I was, I made rounds and talked with many of the staff each day. Frequently, these conversations would turn into informal counseling sessions, although brief and superficial. I enjoyed these sessions and had even considered doing counseling full-time, but I never pursued the idea.

My role with the nurse administrator group offered me many opportunities to speak on various subjects, and the more I spoke, the better I liked it. People told me I was a good speaker. As a result of my self-assessment, I discovered I had two skills I could pursue now. This new awareness gave me hope that I believe helped me get over my anger, fear, and general anxiety. I was experiencing what Bridges (1991) had written about when he said:

> During this apparently uneventful journey through the wilderness, a significant change takes place within people. That change represents a kind of inner process in which old and no longer appropriate habits are discarded and newly appropriate patterns of thought and action are developed (p. 46).

New Beginnings

According to Bridges (1980), "We come to beginnings only at the end. It is when the endings and the time of fallow neutrality are finished that we can launch ourselves anew, changed, and renewed by the destruction of the old life phase and the journey through nowhere" (p. 134). I read that passage many times and finally understood it when I began to consider my new beginnings. I had no awareness of how down I had been until I emerged ready to let go and move ahead. When I was immersed in my job, I believed there were few opportunities ahead. As I entered the new beginnings phase, I saw the choices as unlimited. Of course, there was still some uncertainty, but it was nothing like the hopeless feeling of holding on to beliefs that did not work.

One of those beliefs I held on to that did not work had to do with leadership and what it meant. My education began in a diploma nursing school setting at a time when most of the opportunities for advancement in nursing were in management. Even though there were nurse educators writing about clinical leadership, I believed real leadership was provided in the hospital setting in a line position that provided the salary and prestige all nurses ultimately wanted.

When I was told I had a potential as a leader, it was clear to me where I belonged. As I continued my education, receiving bachelor's and master's degrees, I was clearly moving in the direction that mattered and did not consider the possibility of any other form of leadership. I was so focused that I could not let go of one idea to take hold of another. I think this happens to a lot of nurses who miss opportunity because they are narrowly focused. In Chapter 4, the author discusses the importance of networks and how to develop and nurture them. This process is particularly important during the new beginnings phase of transitions because the network can help when the time for new opportunities arrives. When you have been in a position for a period of time, people do not think of you for other work, nor will they know you have gone through difficulties or when you are ready for new directions unless they are told. Others will not know what phase you are in unless they hear from you. The network can be very helpful during these stressful times.

I was out of touch with my network during the endings and neutral phases, but during the new beginnings phase, I starting contacting them. When I started making telephone calls, I found it difficult to say "Here I am, ready to work," but that was more because I had loss contact than because I was afraid they would not respond.

In the early part of the new beginnings phase, I was still unclear exactly what my direction would be. I was looking for enough work so I could contribute to living expenses. Part-time work seemed appropriate to meet this goal. I highly recommend part-time employment during this phase because it allows you to have space and an openness to new opportunities if they arise. I know that I was fortunate because I could take time off and work only part-time, but even if there are financial pressures, I suggest accepting a cutback in lifestyle to postpone full-time employment if you are still unsure of what you want your work to be.

When I was finally ready to seek something new, I called the members of my nurse administrator group and let them know that I was looking for consultation work. Then I had a business card printed. This may seem like a small step, but for me it was a major one. I did not know what to put on the card or what to call myself. I was afraid people would laugh when they saw it. It was at this point that I retreated to some of the self-doubt I felt in the neutral zone. To cope with this self-doubt, I called some of my business friends and asked their advice. I also acquired a few sample cards from the printer. With both inputs, I was finally ready to design my own business card. Clearly, the network helped me when I wavered with doubt.

I learned one very important lesson during this time. Many calls can be made, but it takes only one return call to open a new door. That one call came to me from a nurse administrator who was new to the area and looking for someone with administrative experience to help her reorganize her department by upgrading the policies and procedures in preparation for a Joint Commission on Accreditation of Healthcare Organizations (JCAHO) visit.

This consultation visit in preparation for JCAHO review was perfect for me, but I still wanted to pursue opportunities in psychiatric nursing. That opportunity came to me in a circuitous way. I was serving as a clinical faculty member at a nearby university and was at a meeting when I met a nurse administrator who was looking for a psychiatric clinical specialist to work part-time. This position would allow me to explore something I had always wanted to do and to be in a setting where I could learn more about the true meaning of leadership. At about the same time, a colleague from my previous job called and asked if she could talk to me about a personal problem. We met in an office in my home, and I knew right from the start that counseling was going to be part of my future. What started out as no work had now developed into three different projects. Still lurking in my head was an interest in private practice, but because of these three new opportunities, I postponed immediate action about that interest.

The position of clinical specialist was a powerful way to begin anew. The stability and hours of the job were helpful, but the most valuable experience was working with leaders at all levels. It was my first chance to function in a staff position with informal authority as opposed to the formal authority designated by a management position. I was surprised to find that I was more at ease in this format. I valued the chance to work with the other clinical specialists and admired their knowledge, competence, and commitment to quality patient care. The total experience was one of the most positive experiences of my career.

My part-time job and the consultations I provided allowed me to move toward my goal of private practice because I had the time needed to learn more about establishing a business. I began reading books about starting a business; the first thing I learned is that you need a business plan. At first, I was afraid that if I put an idea on paper and it did not work I would end up with another loss. I learned this was another example of how my confidence was still fragile. However, I seized the opportunity and outlined some initial goals I wanted to pursue. Fortunately, the house my husband and I had recently purchased had a room that I could convert into an office. The next step was to alert the network about what I was doing and to ask for their help with referrals. I never used the word "entrepreneur," although according to *Random House Webster's College Dictionary* (1991), an entrepreneur is a "person who organizes and manages an enterprise, especially a business usually with initiative and risk" (p. 447), and that's what I did. I also joined an organization of nurses in business; that contact helped me with the details and logistics of establishing a business. Additionally, I had to work my way through the paperwork of certification and conforming to regulations. All of this was time-consuming but necessary. Starting a business is truly a work in progress, and it remains so to this day.

There are many different details to handle when you are in business for yourself; just when you think there couldn't be anything else, another issue surfaces. I never thought about the lack of revenue when sickness occurred or a vacation was taken. I never would have taken a position without benefits, but here I was starting a business without them. I also had never had to do much paperwork or record keeping for tax purposes, and I had never before paid estimated taxes. Tough as these new experiences were, they were the easier activities.

I also needed to establish structures for dealing with patient care issues. I had to find someone to be available for my patients when I was away, and I needed a psychiatrist for medication referral and for my own consultation. I was glad that I had not listed everything I needed to do and have in the beginning because I might not have started into the business at all. However, I was able to take care of all of these issues easily because I had found the work that was right for me. None of this work seemed too much, even though I worked long hours seeing private clients after working at my clinical specialist job.

As my business became more demanding and I was traveling to make presentations, I began to feel overwhelmed by the amount of work I had assumed. I was still working as a clinical specialist, and it was evident that I had to let go of that phase of my career. This time I was holding on because I loved the work and because I enjoyed and valued my colleagues. In retrospect, I probably held on too long, but I had learned my lesson, so I resigned my part-time position and experienced another ending.

Another interesting transition occurred when I moved from working with many professionals and the stimulation of a large hospital setting into a solo practice environment. On some days, the only contacts I had were with my clients. I missed the quick consultations in the halls and the ease with which I could arrange a lunch with my coworkers. In my new position, it was more complicated and usually took a lot of calendar juggling to arrange a simple luncheon with a colleague. Access by telephone, e-mail, and faxing is available to most of us, but there is nothing like having people within talking distance. The neutral zone of this transition was less distressful than the previous one, and I learned to schedule at least some contact with a colleague on a weekly basis. I learned to schedule my clients so that I had enough time for coffee breaks and luncheons and to be out of the office on a regular basis.

In the short period of 8 months, change, transition, and a new direction occurred in my life. I was fired from a position, became a consultant and a clinical nurse specialist, and then established my own business. I followed the transition outlined by Bridges and worked through some difficult feelings and experiences. The outcome is incredibly satisfying and probably wouldn't have occurred if I had not been required to let go. Bridges (1980) summarizes this experience when he says transitions are "endings and beginnings with emptiness and germination in between. That is the shape of the transition period in our lives and these times come far more frequently in adulthood and cut far more deeply into it than most of us imagined that they would" (p. 150).

Delegation

Delegation is another form of letting go; it means passing a task from yourself to another, and it involves the three phases of transition. The new managed care environment of the current health care system requires that nurses make better use of their time and skills. In many instances, this means they must delegate to others, who often are unlicensed and less skilled. Delegation of this kind is a major change in our model of nursing and therefore sweeps every nurse and the profession into a transition process. Because transitions are psychological processes people go through to make the changes, the transition is internal and the change is external. Thus, all nurses will go through endings, the neutral zone, and new beginnings and do so in their own individual ways. However, it is important to remember that this particular transition, like any other, offers opportunities for nurses to take the lead in the establishment of a cost-effective and safe way of delivering nursing care. The success of delegation is to let go of an old idea, accept a new one, and work through the feelings and fears that accompany the change.

■ Endings

As difficult as it is to accept, many aspects of health care, as we have known them, have ended. We are now into a managed care model in which payment for care is prepaid by third-party payers for a defined population rather than being paid to individuals after the service has been provided. The first step in the endings phase is to let go of the fee-for-service model. This is not easy because it is the only one that we have ever known, but just as I struggled with letting go of the nurse administrator role, nurses must let of the idea that fee for service is the only way to accomplish reimbursement.

Letting go of the fee-for-service model is essential, for it is the reason there is an increase in unlicensed personnel in hospitals. Prepaid reimbursement means the hospital must live with the prepaid amount available for those covered by third-party payers (the government via Medicare or insurance companies) who will receive care, and if the institution expends more than it received, it must take the loss. To manage this new reimbursement model, hospitals have chosen to keep employment costs at a minimum. Because 90% of their total costs are for personnel, more unlicensed personnel have been hired because they cost less than professional staff.

At the seminars I present, I have frequently expressed my support for letting go of the old way of delivering nursing care and often have been faced with opposition. There seems to be the belief that if we do not violently fight against this new model, we are traitors to the cause of good patient care. I believe that we as professionals must not polarize on this subject with only two views when historically we have delivered care in a variety of models, some not unlike this present one. During my years as a nurse, I have worked where care was provided by an all-professional staff, by a team consisting of one registered nurse and a number of nurse assistants, or by persons with different skill mixes. Because there has never been a perfect way, the best way is the way that fits the present situation. I believe there will continue to be changes and more opportunities for nurses if they can say good-bye to what no longer fits and work hard to devise ways to deliver quality care in the model that prevails.

■ Neutral Zone

Obviously, many nurses are in the neutral zone when it comes to delegation. The old way of delivering care is gone, and nurses are still trying to find a new way to use the personnel available when assigning care. There are many delegation models being tried, but there seems to be plenty of room for new designs if innovators are willing to pursue their ideas.

In this phase of the transition where new options are considered, it is also a time when people can become trapped by neutral zone hazards. Many of the audiences I address contain nurses who are falling into the "victim mentality," which is disturbing because it is not only demoralizing but also de-energizing. Victims by definition are powerless and thus are not able to move forward. No institution wants workers who are stuck and feel like victims.

There is a big difference between having sadness and anger with the changes and being a victim. A normal part of any transition is the feelings associated with loss, and these reactions will usually pass with time. However, being a victim requires a lot of energy to sustain and takes a huge toll on the affected person. Feeling victimized makes it nearly impossible to think positively and creatively, and if allowed to spread and grow, it breeds personalizing, blame, and ultimately apathy. Statements such as "This is not fair. How can we be held responsible for the care and ask others less skilled to provide it?" indicate that the nurses are personalizing the change and have not resolved their feelings about doing something different. Although there may be real issues that need to be discussed, nursing has always used delegation in some form when care was provided. The issue is not delegation so much as it is one of change and the transition needed for the change to occur.

A nurse at one of my workshops shared the following scenario that illustrates the impact victim behavior can have on change. This nurse was a member of a committee selected to review work redesign models for implementation on her unit as a pilot study. Many hours were spent educating and training the staff in a new model. There were a few staff nurses who were unable to accept the changes and a number who did not like them but were willing to try; thus, there were nurses who were stuck in the endings stage and some in the neutral zone. A couple of nurses with years of seniority started to complain and framed their comments as victims. They wanted to know "Why are they doing this to us, and why are we always the ones who have to work the hardest?" The nurses taking the lead with the project were patient and tried to help the complaining nurses make the transition, but the victim complaints continued and escalated. Soon it was apparent that this unit was not going to be useful as a research site, so another unit was selected for the implementation of the new model. The negative environment of this unit lasted a long time, and many of the nurses who were making the transition transferred to other units. Ultimately, those who remained drove off anyone who had a new idea or was willing to change. This is a good example of how some people react during the neutral phase when they are unable to resolve their feelings. For them, change was not possible. Sadly, it is these nurses who are removed or who stay in the job and make it miserable for everyone else.

The most productive way to move through the neutral zone is to know about Bridges' model and to be aware of the hazards of the neutral zone so they can be avoided.

It is unfortunate that Bridges' model was not part of the education of the nurses in the story told at my seminar. I am frequently asked to provide a workshop on change to angry and apathetic nurses after they have reached these barriers in the neutral zone. I wish that I had been contacted earlier, but I try to help the participants understand what is happening to them and to provide ways for them to resolve their feelings.

The following list of recommendations is offered for those who are being asked to work with more unlicensed personnel and to delegate and are having difficulty in the neutral zone.

- Beware of the pitfalls of the neutral zone, such as personalizing the experience and the development of victim feelings.
- Remember that each person proceeds through this phase at his or her own pace.

- Be supportive of those who are unable to resolve their feelings, but do not get caught up in their negative rhetoric.
- Keep attuned to your own feelings, and contact your network for support.
- Remember that there have been a variety of delivery models used in nursing to provide care, and delegation is not a new one but it is being used in a different context. Changing the delivery model is not the problem; learning to make the transition of feelings about the change is the issue.

■ New Beginnings

According to Bridges (1991), "New beginnings often abort because they were not preceded by well managed endings and successful neutral zone transition. While new beginnings cannot be forced they can be encouraged, supported, and reinforced. There are four specific ways to help someone develop skill as a delegator:

- Explain the basic purpose behind the outcome you seek. People need to understand the logic underlying delegation before they can put their minds to work on it.
- Paint a picture of how the outcome will look and feel. People need to experience delegation imaginatively before they can give their heart to it.
- Lay out a step-by-step plan for phasing in the outcome. People need a clear idea of how they can get to where they need to be as delegators.
- Give each person a part to play in both the plan and the outcome itself. People need a tangible way to participate in the development of their own delegation skills" (p. 52).

Summary

Looking back on that difficult time in my career highlights the many lessons to be learned about change and transition. Without question, it is important to assess those stressful times when change is bound to happen and to do it in a nonjudgmental manner. We usually respond to stress by immediately criticizing ourselves or blaming others and seldom use the time and energy for a simple analysis of what is actually happening. Evaluation is also made more complicated because we tend to wait until we are at a breaking point before noticing that there is something wrong. I wish that I had been able to take the time to evaluate what was happening to me at the time it was happening. Since then, I have learned that using a scale of 1 to 10 is a helpful way to measure one's stress level. If the rating is 5 or higher, it is time to ask whether there is a point of view or way of working that is making the situation more difficult. It is also important to identify what you are holding on to and what is keeping you from letting go.

I have also learned that there are two questions that must be answered before new responsibilities are accepted: Who am I doing this for? and What toll will it take on me? Of course, taking on tasks and responsibilities to help others is understandable, but the effect of this "taking on" on one's ability to function professionally and personally must be evaluated. I found out that there is little or no use in assisting others if you are barely able to work because of the pressures on you.

Another important lesson I learned was that my point of view about what leadership encompassed had prevented me from pursuing other career alternatives. Once I let go of the idea that management was the only way to be a leader, I was able to enter a leadership role of a different kind and, in fact, to influence many more nurses and the profession as a whole. I am particularly thankful to the clinical specialists I met and worked with because through their practice, they demonstrated what it truly means to be a leader.

Another lesson I learned was that the environment of work influences productivity and personal growth. It's one thing to know about the work, but it is equally important to know under what conditions you will thrive. At the beginning of my career, all my experience was within an organizational structure, and that seemed right at the time. Now that I have experienced private practice and managing my own professional speaking career, I value the freedom and do not miss the politics. In my administrative position, I was dependent on how others were performing and how others presented me to my boss and the physicians, who had the power at the hospital. However, my boss gave me up in a minute when the crisis occurred. I swore that I would never be in a position like that again. I wanted to be judged on my performance and by those people to whom I provided direct service.

From the responses in my workshops, many nurses are intimidated by the idea of entrepreneurship and seem to lack the confidence to take the risk. That is a common response and was mine, also. I never considered establishing my own business until I was forced to let go of my old models. A review of how quickly the number of nurse entrepreneurs has grown in the past 10 years illustrates the importance of erasing any doubts about what nurses can accomplish. I am very successful and thankful that I was forced to let go of what did not work anymore. Others can learn from my experience and let go on their own.

The last lesson I learned involves the concept of "willing." This idea is important in every change and transition in our lives. Being *willing* means allowing yourself to consider different options. It means listening to the ideas of others in a way that you may have resisted in the past. If one is willing, it's easier to be patient in the neutral zone and to savor the accomplishments of the "new beginnings." Being willing does not necessarily mean accepting any idea or plan that is proposed, but it means participating in the debate and working toward a compromise. If ever there was a time when nurses needed to be willing, it is now. If nurses are not willing to let go of the points of view that no longer work and become part of the creation of new models of nursing care, they will be left out of important changes. If they are not willing to let go of points of view about themselves, they are risking spending careers surviving as opposed to thriving.

My experience is a wake-up call to all nurses, particularly if nurses are to take the lead. It is an example of how letting go makes a difference in a nurse's life, but it should also act as a model for other kinds of letting go and not be confined to career choices. There are plenty of times in the daily activities of nurses when letting go is the best action to take. To hang on to ideas, activities, values, and attitudes when clearly something different is needed is to limit options, curtail opportunity, and miss a greater role in the delivery of health care. Holding on also places in the hands of others the decisions that will ultimately be made.

I have begun a new life as a nurse, and I thank those who pushed me into it. I have joined a large group of nurses who have established their own businesses and are successfully serving the public. We are leaders in a new and exciting trend and have shown by example that the nurse has the ability and the skills to take the lead. I am sure that letting go will be necessary throughout my career, and I know that I will not be caught unaware of my talents again and will be able to examine my points of view much earlier and more effectively.

REFERENCES

Bridges, W. (1980). *Transitions.* Reading, Mass.: Addison-Wesley.

Bridges, W. (1991). *Managing transitions.* Reading, Mass.: Addison-Wesley.

Costello, R. (Ed.). (1991). *Random House Webster's college dictionary.* New York: Random House.

Dalrymple, T. (1998). The uses of resentment. *Psychology Today, 28*(2), 30–33.

Levine, S. (1982). *Who dies?* New York: Anchor Books.

Person, C. (1997). Delegation: Risk management implications for nurses. *Creative Nursing, 3*(1), 12–15.

Peters, L. (1994). It's your fault! *Redbook, 183*(5), 126–129.

Pollock, T. (1996). Mind your own business. *Supervision, 57*(3), 21–24.

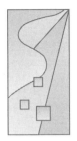

Chapter 13

Keeping
Informed

Terry W. Miller

Keeping informed is an essential skill of effective leaders. Keeping informed not only provides the leader with information but also keeps the leader from being caught unaware or out of touch when important decisions must be made. Keeping informed is often equated with being current, with being smart, and with being ahead of the pack. Keeping informed is a powerful way for leaders to accomplish their task of leading, for those who have information are the best prepared for decision-making and action.

Having information is like having a life preserver when the ship is going down. It is the backup for whatever may happen because being uninformed is a risk no leader can afford. Persons with information are ready for action, whereas the uninformed must delay until they have more information. Being informed is clearly an asset, and being without information is a liability. Being informed is a preventive strategy as well as a proactive one.

Keeping informed is a strategy anyone can learn. It is not difficult to learn how to locate information, how to recognize valid sources of information, or what to do with information once it is available. However, it is clearly a skill that not everyone has but that leaders must acquire. Even the most inexperienced persons can succeed if they are informed and use the information they have strategically. Considering the empowerment one gains with information, why are so many people not informed?

This question and many others are answered in this chapter. There also is an in-depth discussion about many facets of information acquisition and use. A multifaceted framework for gathering, analyzing, and synthesizing information is presented, as well as a simple but complete assessment of how to acquire information via the Internet. It also includes a discussion on the significance of the personal and professional contacts needed by an informed leader. As each aspect of being informed is presented, a personal application on how information advances the leader is also presented.

THE SIGNIFICANCE OF INFORMATION TO LEADERS

When skills in argumentation and communication are about equal, it is usually the person with the newest and best information who prevails. This is because the best-informed are less likely to advocate unwise positions (Rieke and Sillars, 1997). Although leaders do not know everything, they typically know more than those around them or know how to use what they know to a better advantage.

People follow leaders for reasons, conscious or not. One reason they follow is because leaders have the conceptual capacity to cope with an increasingly complex level of information that the followers need to comprehend or use (Levinson, 1995). A leader must provide common meaning and understanding of what may seem to be unconnected bits of information or seemingly unrelated events so others can use the information. When leaders fail to connect critical bits of information in work situations and communicate the connection to others, productivity falls and people become frustrated in their work. In a 5-year study by the Jensen Group (1998) at Northern Illinois University, interviewers discovered that more than 60% of the workforce could not find or translate information they needed to make fast and successful decisions.

Although many people may have the potential, they stumble on the path to becoming a leader because of their lack and misuse of information. This has caused them to pursue dead-end paths, wasting resources and alienating any constituency that could be served by their particular expertise. Poor-quality media (information sources that serve a marketing purpose or sensationalism), more than the truth, perpetuate misinformation.

Information and the leader have a symbiotic relationship. Leaders gather and use information. They also create information and often are the source of much speculation by others. Finally, leaders often provide information to others to guide, challenge, mentor, validate, brainstorm, and socialize. It is no wonder that being informed is essential for a leader to be effective, yet how leaders become informed and use information are different from what many people believe.

Research by Mintzberg (1989) and Krass (1997) indicates that leaders are consummate consumers of information and tend to prefer oral media to aggregated information. They rely heavily on personal contacts, informal relationships, and direct observation when possible. Formal sources and processes are often used to document, demonstrate, or substantiate what the leader already knows.

These points are partially illustrated by the answer given by the head nurse of an innovative critical care unit at a national meeting. She was asked why her unit's sophisticated computerized monitoring system was successfully integrated into patient care and subsequently worked so well. She replied, "We started off very conventionally, and read books on planned management for change. We then threw them away and decided to like each other!" (Bryan-Brown and Dracup, 1998, p. 3).

Andy Grove, the Silicon Valley pioneer and long-standing chief executive officer of Intel, states (1997):

> I have to confess that the type of information most useful to me, and I suspect most useful to all managers, comes from quick, often casual conversational exchanges, many of them on the telephone. . . . It's obvious that the quality of your decision-making depends on how well you comprehend the facts and issues in your business. This is why information gathering is so important (pp. 204–205).

Along with interpersonal roles and decisional roles, Mintzberg (1989) and others (Laudon and Laudon, 1997) believe that informational roles are basic to leadership.

> You often do things . . . to influence the things slightly, maybe making a phone call to an associate suggesting that a decision be made in a certain way, or sending a note or a memo that shows how you see a particular situation, or making a comment during an oral presentation. In such instances you may be advocating a preferred course of action, but you are not issuing an instruction or command. Yet you're doing something stronger than merely conveying information. Let's call it nudging . . . For every decision we make, we probably nudge things a dozen times (Grove, 1997, p. 205).

Regardless of the type of leadership style, information plays a critical role. Authoritarian leaders attempt to control information flow. Charismatic leaders provide information in a way that is seductive for many, whereas instrumental leaders are able to provide a sense of stability with the use and synthesis of information. There is great power in information, if one knows how to get it and what to do with it.

WHAT DOES BEING INFORMED MEAN?

Does being informed mean that you can cite obscure facts and statistics without referring to texts? Does being informed mean knowing more information than most people? Or does it mean being the first to know something that others will want or need to know? Consider the sports fan who can cite almost every statistic about his or her favorite team and players. This person knows the rules, watches many games, and consistently reads the sports section in newspapers and magazines, yet it is highly unlikely that this sports fan would be able to be the team's manager or coach. What the fan knows is *trivia*. What this sports fan does not have is the operational knowledge or decision-making ability it takes to lead a professional team.

Have you ever encountered someone in an emergency situation who could not function? Before the situation, this person seemed to know more than anyone, but when it came time to make critical decisions based on the information that the person had, the transformation of thought into action failed. Being informed implies effective use of the possessed information; if the information is not useable, it remains *trivia*.

Have you ever characterized someone by saying, "She can't see the forest for the trees."? This statement implies that the person being described cannot get beyond the details of the situation. It is easy to get overwhelmed by details or so focused on minutiae that one loses the sight of the goal. It is important to frequently step back from a goal or one's work and look around. Understanding what it means to be informed requires you to be able to see both the forest and the trees *and* to understand their relationship and importance to each other.

Leaders recognize that too much information, as well as too little, can affect a decision. If a person gathers only certain types of information, the decisions are likely to be limited from the onset. If a person understands only the big picture, it will be very difficult to convince others to work out the details in such a way that the big picture becomes a reality or is attainable. Leaders need to know how much information to gather and use, as well as to recognize the difference between minutiae and significant information.

Being informed is an ongoing process of gathering information and using it. Being informed basically means you have the ability to collect, process, store, and disseminate information to support or constitute effective decision-making. You discern and seek what is important to your goals. What you do not know, you strive to find out without being paralyzed in the meantime; that is, you can tolerate the uncertainty of not knowing when necessary to proceed with what has to be done.

A FRAMEWORK FOR BEING INFORMED

How do leaders become informed at a level that allows them to make good decisions in a timely manner? Clearly, it does not happen by cramming. It requires a commitment to ongoing learning. An effective leader has the ability to discover what is important information and to use it better than most people. This ability develops by

- Finding good sources of information
- Asking questions
- Listening and analyzing the answers
- Doing something with the information acquired

Throughout these four steps, the leader is gathering, analyzing, and synthesizing information to make decisions and to determine how to transform those decisions into action.

Finding Good Sources of Information

Never in the history of humanity have there been so many sources of information readily available to so many. This rapid expansion of information availability is redefining leadership. There are tremendous pressures on leaders to incorporate the latest technological advances into the way they interact with people, as well as how they make decisions and take action. Leaders are expected to deliver more choices to constituencies and be accessible in person and by mail, telephone, fax, e-mail, and interactive video. People now have the ability to validate or challenge a leader's information within minutes, if not seconds, from around the world. What people know is becoming more important than where they are in the world (Dickenson-Hazard, 1996).

■ Information Resources on the Internet

The Internet and the World Wide Web (WWW) have received much hoopla the past decade for many good reasons. Consider the resources available to patients and their families on the Internet, recognizing that new consumer health care sites are being added to the WWW every day. One can easily get information about a specific condition or disease using one of the many search engines, such as Yahoo!, Alta Vista, Metacrawler, Lycos, or Infoseek.

The federal government's Healthfinder (http://www.healthfinder.gov/default.htm) provides links to databases, publications, reports, other websites, and nonprofit organizations related to consumer health (Federwisch, 1997). Some excellent commercial sites are available free as well, such as MedicineNet (http://www.medicinenet.com/hp.asp?li=MNI). Both care providers and health care leaders are being challenged by the expansion in information accessibility through thousands of websites on the Internet.

One only has to complete a successful information search to understand why the Internet has become the world's largest and most widely used information network. It is a network of thousands of networks around the globe, both commercial and private, that is used 24 hours a day, every day. There are six basic functions inherent to the use of the Internet. Laudon and Laudon (1997) classify and describe them as the following:

1. *Communicate and collaborate*—the ability to send electronic mail messages, as well as transmit documents and data, within seconds
2. *Access information*—the ability to search for documents, databases, and library card catalogs, as well as read electronic brochures, manuals, books, and advertisements
3. *Participate in discussions*—the ability to join interactive discussion groups and conduct primitive voice transmission
4. *Obtain programming or processing information*—the ability to transfer computer files of text, computer software programs, graphics, animation, and videos with sound
5. *Find entertainment*—the ability to play interactive video games, view short video clips, and read illustrated and animated media
6. *Exchange transactions*—the ability to advertise, sell, and purchase goods and services

Simply stated, the Internet is an international network created by connecting thousands of computer networks (called LANs for local-area networks and WANs for wide-area networks) such that any computer network can send information to and receive information from the others. Internet capabilities include e-mail, Usenet newsgroups, chat rooms, Telnet, gophers, Archie, Wide Area Information Servers (WAIS), File Transfer Protocol (FTP), and the WWW (Laudon and Laudon, 1997). The Internet is becoming easier to use but has been difficult to develop because of variations in its three essential components: client/server architecture, graphic-user interfaces, and hypertext languages. Much work has gone into the Internet and its parts, such as the WWW, and much more is to come.

Instead of hunting through catalogs of information by reading them on site one by one, the WWW user can log onto a computer that is linked with the WWW through an Internet service provider (ISP). There are literally thousands of ISPs, including most universities and commercial ones such as America On-Line (AOL) and NetCom. Many ISPs are expensive, so it is wise to shop around.

Regardless of which ISP one uses, the information from the WWW has to be transmitted into the user's computer. This can be done in several ways, with the fastest ISP costing the most. Whether one has access with a telephone line and modem, Ethernet (an ISDN line) microwave transmission via satellite, or a television cable company, one would get basically the same information. What varies is the speed by which one can receive information. Speed is critical with graphic interfaces, large amounts of text, and multiple documents.

Once the information is transmitted to the computer site, the computer or workstation must use software called a Web browser program to make the Internet information understandable or readable. Some ISPs include the software necessary to browse the WWW with their services. Presently, the two biggest and most common programs are Netscape Navigator and Microsoft Internet Explorer. Ultimately, the Web browser you use allows you to download pages, pictures, sounds, and graphics at different websites.

Laudon and Laudon (1997) state, "The value of the Internet lies precisely in its ability to easily and inexpensively connect to many diverse people from many places all over the world. Anyone who has an Internet address can log onto a computer and reach virtually every other computer on the network, regardless of location, computer type, or operating system" (p. 273). Using the Internet, a nurse in Lima, Peru, can cheaply and almost instantly send information to a nurse in Terra Haute, Indiana, as well as receive it. She can also hold on-line discussions over an issue with nurses around the world in a chat room, as well as search for library sources and order books without leaving her computer desk. She can even take courses for college credit and submit articles for publication.

Although many people equate the WWW with the Internet itself, the WWW is one part of the computer networks linked around the world. The WWW is basically a set of standards for storing, retrieving, formatting, and displaying information. These computer-coded standards make information resources stored in computers quickly accessible and readable to other computers. The WWW serves as the graphic interface for the Internet so you can access millions of information sites (called websites) by merely pointing and clicking on its screen location or by keying in its website address.

Two excellent sites for nursing information are maintained by the University of California San Francisco School of Nursing (http://nurseweb.ucsf.edu/www/othnrs.htm) and the University of Buffalo Library (http://ublib.buffalo.edu/libraries/units/hsl/internet/nsgsites.html).

Both of these sites link the user with hundreds of information resources, including professional organizations, specialty sites, college and university schools of nursing, and subject directories.

If the site is in the public domain and access is unlimited, which many are at this time, you only have to do the following:

- Turn on the computer that is connected.
- Boot up one of the search engines that is available through the Internet provider to the computer.
- Type in the words that represent what you are looking for, and voilà—you will usually get multiple websites bearing a relationship to the key words you have typed.

■ Search Tools

At present, there is no complete index to the resources available on the Internet because they change by the minute. The only certain way to find the location of information on the Internet is to know where it exists—its address. An Internet address is basically a code consisting of a mailbox name@host name. For example, my address is millertw@plu.edu. One of the most useful features of the Internet is that you can find addresses of information sources that you do not even know exist by using search tools. Once an address is found, you can very easily save it with what's called a *favorite* or a *bookmark* for future use.

Search tools include Internet directories and search engines. The directories are lists of categories, starting with the most general and going to the most specific. Basically, a search engine is a computer program tool that enables the computer user to locate specific sites for information on the Internet. If you know what you are looking for either as a category or as specific topic, you can enter your inquiry into a search engine and it will find information for you.

Entry into any one of the many search engines (e.g., Yahoo!, Infoseek, Alta Vista, Lycos, Excite, Webcrawler) can be accomplished by typing in key words or a specific address or by pointing the cursor and clicking on the highlighted link. Search engines enable you do this because they are collections of information that are catalogued, indexed, and linked. Search engines look for the words (key terms) that you enter on your computer in all the places those words are indexed. Different search engines work in different ways, so it helps to know how they differ to make the best use of them for information gathering.

I was conducting a search for a legal case and was able to adequately document my position for the defendants so the suit was dropped early in the discovery period, before going to trial or obtaining multiple, expensive depositions. Search tools have enabled the user to shift from merely simple hypertext browsing to content-based searching whereby the user describes a query and the system being used locates the information that best matches the description. Once the user becomes proficient with search tools, access to complex databases is possible.

■ Limitations of the Internet

Anyone with access to the Internet can download information. There are, however, limits to what is available on the Internet, and it is critical for the user to understand the quality issues inherent in relatively unregulated information sources. Some networks are highly protected and therefore not readily available to the common user.

Many commercial websites require users to enter personal data and/or credit card information before the user can gain full access to them. The user has no real assurance that the receiver will not inappropriately use the personal information. Also, personal information sent over the Internet becomes accessible to anyone during transmission unless special security features are used. Fortunately, most browsers contain security encryption that will safeguard most transactions.

Information resources on the Internet are generally structured in one of three ways: file archives, gopher files, or hypertext documents, which correspond to the Internet facilities of ftp, gopher, and WWW. There also is WAIS. Information found by using WAIS has not necessarily been indexed by anyone and often is the best source of obscure information. The tradeoff is that WAIS is harder to use than the three common Internet structures. The WWW presents information in a user-friendly hypertext format, but gopher remains the simplest of all.

The Internet contains many resources that overlap one another because there is no overriding organizational scheme or structure at this time. Other than equipment and on-line service, the user's knowledge of search tools determines the value of the Internet as an information resource. Whether information is not indexed or how and by whom it is indexed will determine how the user can gain access to it with a computer.

The more the user knows about how search tools are actually designed and the specific rules for using them, the better the Internet will serve *some* of that person's information needs. It is important to try out different search tools on a regular basis and to ask others about what they prefer to use when researching a topic and why. Even if a person is already a sophisticated Internet user, it is good practice to periodically experiment with new tools and websites for information retrieval.

The user can be fooled into believing that information on the Internet is comprehensive because of its sheer quantity. Some information is not available on the Internet for a variety of reasons. Some publishing firms and authors do not want to circumvent other media markets. Also, providing information and maintaining access to that information are costly and time-consuming tasks. Anyone who "surfs" the net has encountered "gravesites" that are no longer useable or acceptable. There are literally thousands of old websites that clutter most information directories.

Henderson and Poulin (1998) offer suggestions for using the Internet. Five suggestions that should guide the user while searching for information on the Internet are to

1. Make sure you are in the right place so you spend your time searching for what you need instead of "surfing" all that's out there.
2. When in doubt, doubt, because almost anyone can put up almost anything on the Web.
3. Consider the source to determine what authority or expertise validates it—one way is to check the URL to determine whether the domain is commercial (.com), governmental (.gov), nonprofit (.org), educational (.edu), network (.net), or a two-letter code for country of origin.
4. Identify the purpose of the website.
5. Look at the details for indicators of substantive information beyond the "bells and whistles."

■ Real Power of Information Technology

Having the latest in information technology does not substitute for or equate with being informed, but it helps. The powerful attraction to the novelty of innovation, along with remarkable integrated marketing about the latest technology, plays like sirens to a leader needing solutions, yet one only has to review the many failures of information technology to achieve the results promised or the newly created problems with its implementation to place information technology in a realistic light.

Information technology often fails to meet expectations because purchasers choose something inappropriate for what is needed or the people using the technology are not properly instructed about its capabilities. Even if the information technology is custom-made for the organization or group, users experience the pitfalls of being testers while trying to carry out the usual work assignments.

Leaders who have invested resources into new information technologies must become a part of the adoption along with others in the group. Sometimes leaders fail to learn the capabilities of their workplace's information technology; instead, they continue along the "old" communication lines or obtain information in the "old" way. This creates new work for everyone because subordinates are expected to use the new technology, yet they have to accommodate to the leader's old way.

Many people are uncomfortable with new information technology because of language problems. Each new technological advance adds new language and acronyms to our vocabulary. Just like each generation of teenagers develops its generation's vernacular, technophiles use language in a distinctive way, such that those out of the loop are unable to participate in discussions or become intimidated.

Oddly, some people hide behind a vocabulary because they are neophytes to the field in question or they are insecure with what they know. This posturing is easily overcome by asking people directly to explain what they mean. Those who will be good sources of future information and who are comfortable with their knowledge base usually take the time to explain the technology. Those who do not are eliminated as future references. However, this does not mean that the novice is relieved of the responsibility to study information technology as well.

Regardless of its limitations, "leadership decisions about information technology are critically important to the prosperity and survival of the institutions and organizations in which they work" (Laudon and Laudon, 1997, p. 5). Good leaders are aware that information systems can markedly alter life in an organization or a culture. They recognize that the productivity of people is highly dependent on the quality of the information systems serving them.

E-MAIL

E-mail makes it possible to disseminate information within the office or around the world in a matter of seconds for a minimal cost. Beyond one-to-one communication, e-mail is especially powerful because of mailing list capabilities with *listservs*. The use of listservs, which allow the sending and receiving of messages from more than one person or entity simultaneously, eliminates the drudgery of repeatedly sharing information among more than two people or entities. For example, members of professional organizations can be notified of critical legislation or rallied to write their legislators in a matter of minutes using e-mail.

When a user subscribes to a listserv, he or she automatically receives messages from the source of the listserv, other members on the listserv, or both. If the listserv source is commercial, the intention is to sell *something* to the members on the listserv or to provide a means of subjecting the members of listserv to advertising on the Internet. This is fine as long as the user obtains desirable or valuable information. There are so many listservs that on-line directories are available to assist the e-mail user in selecting the more useful ones. Periodic review of the value of any listserv or on-line service being received is necessary to eliminate nuisances and save time.

The biggest downside to e-mail (just like telephones) for the organization is when people send and receive personal messages that have no value to the organization or work setting. Also, people can waste considerable time reading unsolicited promotional messages and other nuisances from *spammers*, who are people or information sources who take advantage of an e-mail site (address site) by sending unsolicited advertisements or messages to the site.

It is important to learn the simple etiquette of communicating by e-mail. It is easy to mistakenly think that a recipient of a message or piece of information wants it, even though the person did not request or expect anything from the sender. Common courtesy dictates that e-mail users step back from their messages before sending them and ask several questions:

- Why am I sending this message?
- Is the message appropriate for the persons who will receive it?
- Have I properly addressed the recipients of the message?
- Is the level of formality or informality appropriate for the recipients?
- Can my message be misunderstood or harmful to the recipients either directly or indirectly?

It is important to remember that someone else can retrieve every message sent and received. Computers and servers have a history that is retrievable by those people who maintain them. A knowledgeable person can access what e-mail has been sent from a computer site, as well as determine what websites have been accessed. It is foolish to send messages that could be damaging or highly confidential without knowing the risks. Also, the user should not send messages to all members of a listservice when it should go to only one person or a select few.

Leaders must develop ways to effectively prioritize what and when information is gathered, as well as how to use it. Information systems with multiple, interactive databases are constantly being developed to help people make better decisions. The interaction between an information system and the user is influenced by many mediating factors, including the structure of the former and the personality of the latter. Standard operating procedures, politics, culture, the surrounding environment, and management decisions also mediate this interaction.

A massive amount of new information is constantly being generated in health care. Nurses and other health care providers need access to this information to provide the best care, do the best research, effectively manage others, and teach the next generation. Being well informed makes the difference between having a voice and being ignored as a professional.

DATABASES

A *database* is simply a collection of data gathered and stored in a specified format. For example, an address book with the addresses and telephone numbers of people you know is a database. The purpose of a database is to make selected information more retrievable and useable. Databases can be used by computer users to assist them with problem solving and decision-making and even simulate hypothesis testing.

At their best, on-line databases offer very quick, precise, and flexible searches. They can be used for specific pieces of information or for broadly defined exposure to information sources. At the high end (the most sophisticated and usually the most expensive), there are interactive databases that can be used to manipulate information, as well as to gather, store, and disseminate information. Some databases even allow very powerful search strategies, so complex analyses can be accomplished within seconds.

The use of on-line health care databases enables nurses to keep up with the research and to selectively focus on what is available regarding a particular problem or situation in a fast, unobtrusive manner. Collaboration and communication with other experts and sharing of ideas are essential to health care institutions (Laudon and Laudon, 1997). The user needs to know the scope of health care information required and to decide which areas to concentrate on for the task at hand. The advent of managed care with economic incentives to control costs has spawned the growth of new systems designed to closely monitor all aspects of health care.

New concepts such as economic credentialing, by which a provider is evaluated on his or her cost-effectiveness, is now possible with electronic data processing. Refusing to accept this innovation because of its potential for misuse or belief it should not happen is not preventing the data miners from analyzing massive amounts of information to identify cost centers and to synthesize ways to eliminate or reduce those cost centers, down to the individual level. Therefore, it may become critical for professionals or workers who want to have some control over their destiny to understand how the data will support or limit their future, as well as define their work.

Health care transaction systems are data-gathering mechanisms using three types of data: the International Classification of Diseases (ICD), the Physicians' Current Procedural Terminology (CPT), and the National Drug Code (NDC). Together, these systems provide massive databases that give an overview of patient problems and the associated health care utilization; some gross outcome measures are described by these systems as well. None of these databases contain information describing the quality, type, or cost of nursing services (Jones, 1997).

Jacox (1995) believes that nursing as a profession will have to develop better databases. She believes that nursing is invisible or indistinguishable in the present health care–related databases, pointing out that nursing care received by most patients is not independently described or distinguishable from care provided by others. The nursing care provided is not directly reimbursable or appropriately valued when the third-party payers use health care–related databases for reimbursement decisions.

At the individual level, documentation and data collection systems used by nurses have historically been uncoordinated and nonstandardized, varying greatly among practice settings. A series of reports over the past several years has supported the need for a collection of uniform data that can be used to support clinical and managerial decision-making. The Iowa Intervention Project (1997) found that staff nurses who are told about the databases and their uses were eager to participate in documentation efforts that can make possible the inclusion of nursing data at state and national levels.

DATA MINING

Leaders are often confronted with a need for a highly sophisticated information analysis with a defensible level of certainty based on "the numbers." Although they may intuitively know the answer, the decision made always requires numerical or statistical justification. Also, there are times when they need a new perspective on the information they have, but there are too many factors, numbers, or pieces of information to analyze together. Whether there is a need for a quantitative justification or a new outlook for making a decision, the computer can help.

There are many ways a computer program can sift through databases that are analogous to what people do when they analyze information. Five methods commonly used for this sifting are by associations, clusters, sequential patterns, similar time series, and the two-step process of classification followed by regression (Rae-Dupree, 1997). Recognizing associations among many pieces and sources of information is difficult and time-consuming. A computer program can take large amounts of data and identify numerical or statistically significant relationships by creating algorithms for those relationships.

For example, in many health care organizations, nurses are treated as costs, as opposed to revenue generators. If the organization serves thousands of people, there will be far more data regarding those services than an individual can comprehensively analyze. Also, there will be factions competing within the organization for resources. Those who can justify their services best with "hard" statistical data will have an easier political battle to wage than will those who do not. Also, a comprehensive analysis using the data-mining technique will likely produce some surprises that can refocus the problem in more constructive terms.

Personal experience over the years strongly indicates that if nurses do not learn how to do their own data mining, which requires access to databases, they will fall prey to those who do, regardless of what the information will objectively show. This is not a cynical view about information sharing as much as it is an awareness that people will serve those who support them financially over restructuring a system to empower people who do not support them financially. Presently, data miners in health care are the third-party payers, such as insurance companies, the government, and other institutions.

NURSING INFORMATICS

Nursing informatics is developing as a discipline to assist nurses in a variety of practice settings, especially with nursing functions. Some believe that medical informatics adequately address the needs of nursing and therefore can solve informatics problems of nursing. Others have invested heavily in developing and touting the value of nursing having its own informatics system for information gathering, analyzing, and synthesizing (Turley, 1996). It appears that informatics will change the way in which clinicians understand the information available to them.

■ Quality of the Information

The use of the Internet has brought into prominence the need to critically evaluate information sources. There are hundreds of articles addressing the need to evaluate information. To determine the quality of information, regardless of its source, it is useful to consider its scope—that is, how much, how broad, and how deep is the information. Is the information validating what the person already thinks, or does it support a change in the person's position? What are the long-term as well as the short-term implications? Will people need to do something differently by having this information?

Leaders recognize that unreliable information can take on a life of its own if not properly handled at an early stage. Ultimately, the leader uses information by transforming it into action. This is usually done directly but always uses the help of others. To sort through the information that is available every day, the leader must have a direction in mind while gathering information—a focus. This does not mean leaders will not change direction—they often do—but they are often looking for that critical mass of information that solidifies their decision to act in a certain way or commit to a certain project through its completion.

■ Yourself and Others as Sources of Information

Even with all the new telecommunications, the Internet, and e-mail, there remain two primary sources of information: yourself and others. Although we expect information sources to tell us the truth about reality, even the most objectively quantifiable data are affected by human interpretation. How you develop yourself and connect with others will determine how good your sources of information will be.

Let's start with *yourself* as a source of information. The more awareness you have about the world around you, the better you are as a source of information to yourself and others. If you are having difficulty with a problem or a situation and you feel your solutions or approaches are limited, it is likely that you are using only one mode of thought. Gathering more information may not fix the problem because of what you are *not* doing with the information you already have. Wells (1998) aptly states,

> Often information gathering is a barely disguised way of avoiding thinking and decisions. There is more information about the past and the present than we could ever gather and use. There is no information about the future, the terrain of strategy. No matter how much information we gather, we can never completely remove the uncertainty about the future. . . . Thinking requires a knowledge base that depends upon our access to information. Thinking is necessary to arrive at the decisions that lead us to act (p. 30).

When I was a clinical nursing supervisor at a large private medical center, we had a problem with the escalating costs of maintaining supplies on the nursing units. Nurses and physicians often took more materials than needed and carelessly opened sterile packages without reading about the contents. Meetings and inservice programs did not work because costs continued to escalate to the point of a "police model" for correction of the problem being considered.

No one wanted to return to the time-consuming model where everything had to be ordered from a central supply service. It was felt that it would increase paperwork and, more importantly, seriously delay treatments. More information gathering did not help. No matter how often this problem was addressed, the same solutions were proposed, until the problem was redefined from an individual practitioner's perspective as opposed to the institution's perspective.

The solution was simple. We labeled everything in the supply area of each nursing unit with its per-item cost. Every time someone obtained an item, the person was instantly reminded of its costs to the institution and therefore the patient. Within 6 months of labeling supplies with their respective costs, there was a decrease in supply costs of 40%, adjusted for patient census and acuity. What was needed, once the problem of costs was identified, was not a solution to reduce institutional costs of supplies but a solution to reduce the per-item cost, coupled with getting the information directly to the item user.

Using only one mode of thought greatly reduces the probability that the value of any piece of information is recognized or that many sources of information are a source of power. Although there are many ways of thinking about information and its uses, we tend to favor one approach over others. I tend to agree with Mintzberg's (1989) statement:

> Implicit in a good deal of management science, information systems design, and formal planning have long been the assumptions that strategy making is relatively static, orderly process (it is anything but); that discontinuities can be forecast through systematic procedures (there is no support for this whatsoever); that strategic management can be detached from operating management, with the senior managers informed by "hard" (namely computer-generated) data (managers who believe this are ignorant in two ways); and ultimately that the processes of making decisions and developing strategies can be formalized, or programmed, by systems that rely above all on decomposition (p. 69).

If you think of information and its sources in hierarchical terms, you must be aware of what values underlie the criteria for establishing the hierarchy in the first place. Consider a surgical procedure being done on an immunosuppressed patient. A simple omission in aseptic technique can have disastrous results, yet many health care providers do not value hand washing as much as they value other more complicated and seemingly important practices. Also, if the significance of something will be considered only when presented by persons with the highest positional status, their informational biases become the information-filtering system for everything shared.

Some people are very logical thinkers and discount what others describe as an intuitive approach to problem solving. Wells (1998) states, "Logic works best when we need to make extensions in ideas from a known information base. Intuition operates better when we want to make extensions from our experience and when a leap in imagination is necessary" (p. 37). Consider the quote by Sikorsky (1997), who has given us the helicopter:

> I do not pretend to explain the nature of the process of intuitive discovery, but I can give a few examples of how it works. It may be in the form of a fact or information held in the memory for which there is no data or known foundation, but supported by a firm conviction that it is true. . . . I always had a belief, even as a small boy, that I would sometime build and fly large flying machines. Consciously, I did not pay much attention to this idea because for many years I considered it simply impossible, but subconsciously the conviction was always there. Intuition works even when one does not recognize it as such (p. 366).

Regardless of how information is gathered or used, we all need to learn to be creative thinkers. The highly acclaimed visionary in science and technology, James Burke (1998), has eloquently stated

> [All people] are going to have access to the same information that leaders and bureaucrats have had in the past...(and) have access to lots of information that these leaders don't have, because a leader or a bureaucrat only has a certain amount of time to learn what it is they want to do. . . . But at any level, what you are talking about is one and one making three. The process of change, it seems to me, is almost always the juxtaposition of concepts, entities, ideas, people, or whatever, brought together in a way that has never happened before. And the result is that you tend to get something that is more than the sum of its parts (pp. 12–13).

Now let's discuss *other people* as information sources. People are perhaps the most valuable and dangerous sources of information. As leaders gain status and power, it is remarkable how many people will offer information to them on any given topic, yet one of the constant problems for a leader is how to disentangle the cold, hard facts from the rather warm feelings of the people dealing with these facts (Baruch, 1997). It is important to listen to those who you do not favor, as well as those who make you most comfortable.

Many of us often demonstrate the concept of *actor-observer bias* (Kelley and Michela, 1980). The term identifies a judgmental bias whereby people place greater emphasis on situational factors when explaining their own behavior and greater emphasis on dispositional qualities when accounting for similar behavior in others. For instance, when a nurse fails to chart adequately, she or he may attribute the error to a lack of time, whereas when other health professionals fail to chart adequately, the nurse attributes it to their lack of care or competence.

Nothing transmits information faster than personal information networks because information sharing is a normal part of human behavior. Unfortunately, information can be easily distorted or maliciously altered to hurt or damage others. We all have encountered the gossiper who seems to relish rumor mongering. There also are people who share information in such a loaded, proscriptive, or euphemistic way that it is difficult to understand their real opinion about something. Although they may be socially or politically correct, they offer little and thus are not a good source of information.

It is important for leaders to listen carefully to those around them and to expose themselves frequently to those outside their professional circles as well. Wells (1998) states, "Each discipline brings its own valid way of viewing the world, thinking about problems, and understanding information" (p. 7). Much of the trick comes with experience and with developing rapport through trusting relationships with others. Leaders are selective about how they obtain information and quickly learn the differences among sources in terms of importance, timing, and authority.

The importance of an information source is determined by your dependency on it for achieving your goals. If the source of information is in error and you are highly dependent on it, something will have to be done to correct the source or lessen your dependency on it. If you are uncertain of the source and are highly dependent on it, you will have to validate it with other sources of information. Leaders quickly learn that it is risky to depend heavily on one source of information.

Asking Questions

Most people become uncomfortable when they find themselves in conversations that are fraught with uncertainty. They become bored in conversations when clarity is not offered. The quality of a communication is often judged by the amount of new information that is shared coupled with the amount of uncertainly that is left out. Leaders are often approached by people who ask unusual questions or who are intimidated by the situation. Subsequently, effective leaders stop periodically and privately assess whether a conversation is clear and leading to anything new. When nothing new is being shared about ideas, interests, or feelings, they alter the dialogue so it is more productive and satisfying to all involved.

Several techniques can be used to improve information sharing. To make a good impression, effective leaders quickly establish rapport by identifying and sorting out the relevant values of their audiences. This is crucial to their ability to obtain commitments and to build high-level credibility. They recognize that asking questions that improve the exchange of information requires good speaking skills. Tactfulness, self-disclosure, and asking for feedback often leads to better rapport and indicates trust in the other person. Perception checks are necessary to prevent misinterpretation. When people lose sight of the key issues, leaders bring them back. Thus, it is important to be able to determine the status of the discussion at any point in time. In other words, where does one's line of questioning and the information shared stand in relation to making a decision or taking an action?

Asking open-ended questions allows others to respond according to their own boundaries. Asking closed-ended questions focuses others and sets parameters for the information being shared. Asking content questions ensures that there is substance, and asking process questions ensures that something is doable. Regardless of the kind of questions the leader asks, the payoff is information and should show that the leader is interested in what others think and feel about information.

Although it is commonly considered impolite to question or challenge other people's information, it is often necessary to temper what is heard with a degree of skepticism. It is important to determine who are the decision-makers and what are their goals, as well as who wants to be or tries to act as the decision-makers.

Some helpful ways to get better information are

- Stay focused on what you need to know.
- Do not ask questions you do not understand.
- Take time to frame your questions.
- Prepare in advance the questions you want to be answered.
- Do not ask questions that do not deserve an answer.
- Avoiding cueing the person being questioned.

- If a response to your question is evasive, take note, rephrase the question, and try again.
- Be courteous in your tone of voice and the content of the question unless your goal is to fight and not necessarily to obtain information.
- Ask your question, and then listen.
- Allow time for your question to be thoroughly answered.

Stuart Wells (1998) claims, "It is the fear of looking ignorant that inhibits most of us" (p. 15). Leaders, however, recognize that the risk of appearing ignorant is a small investment for the reward you gain over time by asking questions. This is not to say you ask questions to draw attention to yourself or to embarrass others, because to obtain good information, questioning must be genuine and done in a considerate manner. Most people will approach a person with better information when they know they will be asked questions about what they have to say or offer.

Good listening comes from a balanced posture that is neither too confrontational nor too unchallenging. The leader asks questions in a cooperative, critical manner with decision-making in mind. To elicit the most information through questioning, begin by asking yourself what is known, what is not known, and what needs to be known to make the decision. When a conversation or questioning is going nowhere, it is helpful to reframe the interaction to find a common ground.

Ultimately, leaders ask questions of themselves. Their answers are the results of gathering and analyzing information coupled with what and how they think. This process of synthesizing information into a decision is what helps the leader envision new approaches and solutions. There are many questions I ask of myself, knowing that most questions do not have only one answer. I ask until I get to the point of being able to make the necessary decisions to accomplish what I need to do.

Although mathematical calculations and experimental demonstrations are associated with scientific proof, rhetorical evidence for decision-making is more complicated. When inconsistencies exist between sources of information, merely adding new information of an equally unsatisfactory character will not improve the situation. Regardless of the type and degree of evidence to support a decision, some level of uncertainly may always be present.

Listening and Analyzing Answers

Too often I have been guilty of waiting for my turn to speak instead of listening to what is offered by others. Whether it has been to draw attention to myself or to insert my point of view, the result has been that I did not discover what I could have learned. Listening is essential if you are to learn new information, clarify uncertainties, or extend what you know.

To listen is to be with another person is such a way that the person feels that you care and understand what is being conveyed. Listening requires patience and is an active process, yet listening does not mean giving advice, providing solutions, making suggestions, or relating what is being said to your own life until you are sure that that is what the teller wants and expects. Listening means to hear and give attention.

Silence is one of the most obvious signs that a person wants to listen, yet silence can be threatening and make people feel uncomfortable or self-conscious. Also, it is important to listen with one's eyes as well as with one's ears. Good listeners watch for signs of communication in addition to what is being spoken. Facial expressions, gestures, body movement and posturing, or the lack thereof all represent forms of nonverbal communication.

According to Ash (1997), "Listening is an art. And the first tenet of the skill is undivided attention to the other party. When someone enters my office to speak with me, I don't allow anything to distract my attention. If I'm talking to someone in a crowded room, I try to make that person feel as though we're the only ones present. I shut out everything else" (p. 138).

It would be a different world if more of us followed Ash's approach to human interaction. Just think how much better patients and their families would feel if they received more undivided attention. Having consulted in many cases in which health care professionals were sued, I am convinced litigation could have been avoided if the defendant, and sometimes the plaintiffs, listened more and talked less.

Leaders must learn to listen to themselves as well. The relationship between thinking and listening is critical to the leader. In its most powerful form, listening to one's self provides a means to self-knowledge and personal transformation. It is crucial that leaders have time to themselves in which feedback and inputs from other sources can be integrated into the self such that clarity of thought and purpose becomes evident. Only then can the leader pull all the information gathered into something new and parsimonious.

■ Analyzing Information and Its Sources

So how does the leader discern usable information from bad? Here is the information paradox. We should not look or read for *information* as much as for *ways of thinking* about the information. We should not just approach a source by asking "What information can I get out of this?" Rather, we should ask "How does this source work? How does it offer, argue or present information? How does it reach its conclusions? How can I use it to develop my own thoughts, approaches, or solutions?" In other words, the leader learns to analyze information for ways of thinking about the information.

The following are some steps for analyzing information and its source:

• Determine the *central claims* of the information source and the *purpose* of the information.
• Distinguish the *kinds of reasoning* the source uses: Does it appeal to a theory or theories? Are any concepts defined and used? Is any specific methodology laid out? If there is an appeal to a particular concept or theory, how is that concept or theory then used to organize and interpret the data?
• Examine how the information is *organized:* by different disciplines (e.g., nursing, medicine, business, and law) or organized and presented in a different way.

- Evaluate the *kinds of evidence* provided to support the information. Are primary or secondary sources used? Is the evidence statistical? Is it anecdotal? Could evidence be stronger?
- Determine whether there any *gaps, leaps, or inconsistencies* in the information. What are the unargued assumptions? Are they problematic? What other information contradicts or raises issues with this information?
- Evaluate the overall *power or significance* of the information. If it has little or no perceived value to you, what about to others? Internally questioning the significance of something in relation to another person's agenda or purpose helps to put the information into the proper perspective.
- Place the information in *context*. This includes understanding who owns or controls the information. What audience is the information for: just you or everyone, and why?
- Remember that *bad information* helps the leader to make better decisions if he or she can recognize it for what it is.

There is one great fallacy in leadership circles: to decompose is to recombine; in other words, analysis includes synthesis. Ultimately, synthesis is not analysis but rather is rooted in the mysteries of intuition. Analysis and synthesis differ not only in how they work but also in their respective strengths and weaknesses (Mintzberg, 1989). Often, people who can skillfully analyze a situation or problem cannot put together a new approach or offer a different solution. To synthesize, you must take information and construct something different than what existed before. The ability to synthesize requires creativity and vision that the analyst alone often lacks.

The interaction between an information system and the leader is influenced by many mediating factors, including the structure of the former and the personality of the latter. Standard operating procedures, politics, culture, the surrounding environment, and management decisions also mediate the interaction. Leaders should be aware that information systems can markedly alter life in an organization or a culture (Laudon and Laudon, 1997). Leaders can also kill the spirit of an organization with too much information.

■ Information Overload

People are exposed to more information than ever before. In short, people receive and are expected to produce more information than what was believed to be possible only a few years ago, much less reasonable. It is no wonder that information overload has become part of the modern world. Research by Lewis (1996) has indicated that two thirds of the managers at all levels report tension with work colleagues and loss of job satisfaction because of stress associated with information overload. As many managers also report that their personal relationships suffer as a result of information overload.

The accessibility of information through telecommunications, publications, and the WWW has exponentially expanded the markets for both the producers of information and the users. Certainly, there is more information generated and disseminated in 1 second than any one person can possibly absorb. It is the leader's approach to information management that prevents information over-load, and the approach changes with time, technology, and context.

Information management involves controlling the amount of information people receive and send. Inherently, it involves interrelated issues of quantity, quality, timing, and format. The quantity is dependent on what is available and how much the person or organization can afford, as well as on what people need to know. How much information people receive and send greatly affects their stress level and, subsequently, their productivity. Quality can also become an issue because people often do not initially recognize the value of some information, or they overestimate the value of it. The quality of information is closely linked to timing. Timing is a critical factor in information use because if information is not received or used in a timely manner, it loses value. The format in which information is received, stored, and sent affects its timing and therefore its value. Creating a sustainable format by which information is received in the simplest and most direct manner in a timely way, by those who need it, is an essential goal of good information management. Good information management greatly reduces the likelihood of information overload.

Doing Something With the Information You Have

Effective leaders have developed ways in which they can effectively prioritize what, when, and how they gather information, as well as how they use it. They are often able to see relationships among pieces of information that most people ignore or do not understand. In other words, doing something with the information you have is more about comprehension, relevance, and association than about the quantity of information possessed in any given context. To illustrate this point, I want to share a personal story about making the most out of limited information.

My father had a new tractor that stripped a gear. He took apart the gear case, piece by piece, and laid each piece out on a light-colored blanket in the exact order he took it off. He did not know the names or even the purpose of many of the parts because he had never seen them before this disassembly. When he came to the part that was clearly broken, he examined it carefully and found a small serial number engraved on its side. He then telephoned a tractor distributor of that tractor brand and ordered the part using the serial number. When the part arrived in the mail, he went back to the blanket with the tractor parts and put them back together in the exact reverse order, using the new part instead of the broken one. Although my father did not attend college, read with difficulty, and had never worked on the gears of a tractor before, he was able to solve his problem using limited information.

My father intuitively knew what was wrong with the tractor because of his experiences with automobiles. He was able to correctly analyze the situation based on what he observed and experienced while running the tractor after the gear broke. He strategically planned the disassembly in a manner that would prevent confusion and minimize what he would have to remember. His framework for fixing the tractor relied on what information he had readily available to him.

■ Your Comfort Level With Uncertainty

Many people knowing as much or more than my father did would not have attempted to fix the tractor. They would not have been comfortable with the degree of uncertainty he had. Leaders have to tolerate a level of uncertainty that is often unknown to those who hold others accountable for the decisions being made. In other words, leaders have to make decisions and take action based on those decisions without knowing for certain that they are correct. They are risk takers.

If leaders must have tolerance for uncertainty that exceeds most people's comfort level, how do they develop this level of comfort to be such risk takers? The answer flows from four philosophical constructs that apply to information systems (Rieke and Sillars, 1997):

- Uncertainty is pervasive.
- Information is inherently ambiguous.
- The attraction of certainty is powerful.
- Timing is everything.

UNCERTAINTY IS PERVASIVE

Have you ever encountered people who appeared confident and comfortable about a particular subject or about trying something, who later revealed that they were really uncertain about it? Uncertainty is all around us, yet most of us are still able to get things done with what information we have. At other times, we find ourselves unable to make decisions or act because we are too uncomfortable with the uncertainty of the situation. In these situations, we usually are choosing not to decide or act because we want more information.

The leader's ability to make good decisions with limited information is often what distinguishes him or her as a leader. It seems that leaders have a comfort level with the pervasiveness of uncertainty that most of us do not possess, yet they do not make rash or impulsive decisions. Instead, leaders develop the best rationales or justifications for their decisions as possible, subject them to the best criticism possible, and then proceed, even though they are not absolutely certain it is the best thing to do. It is the power of justification and critique that allows them to proceed even when there is uncertainty.

INFORMATION IS INHERENTLY AMBIGUOUS

Have you ever listened to a lecture, watched a movie, or read the same book as a very close friend and discovered that you interpreted what you heard, saw, or read differently? Language and information are inherently ambiguous. Leaders understand this and take time to operationally define what they are thinking and clarify what they hear from others.

Information will always be filtered through the norms of the culture and through the individual who is gathering, analyzing, and synthesizing it. Cultural differences contribute to the ambiguity of information because what is deemed important by each culture varies. It is important for leaders to recognize cultural differences and to disseminate information carefully, using a process that clarifies both the value and the meaning of the information being shared.

I have worked in two major health care centers. Throughout my tenure at both institutions, I participated in a significant number of "codes." During these resuscitation attempts, I soon realized that the code leaders set a tone and established a process beyond any written protocol. Those who calmly and deliberately stated each step seemed to have better patient outcomes. Regardless of whether a controlled study would bear this out, I know the participants felt more secure about the extremely demanding, intense situation in which a life had to be saved when a calm, deliberate approach was used to direct the code.

My experiences with mentally ill patients on a locked adolescent psychiatric unit taught me even more about how the delivery of information can be used to incite as well as to calm. Some of the teenagers were very adept at manipulating their less-knowledgeable peers. They accomplished this in a variety of ways: sharing half-truths or partial information, picking an inappropriate time for sharing information, selectively exaggerating or downplaying certain information, and so forth.

People provide and receive information with a certain mental orientation that varies greatly from person to person. It is the way an individual perceives, understands, and interprets the information that matters. Any marketing director knows how the presentation of information plays on the mental orientation of the receiver to promote buying. There is a need to recognize that different techniques can be used to persuade people, including themselves, to value something more that they normally do.

Some people are more likely to believe information when it is supported by testimonials. Others are more likely to believe information that is delivered by an attractive person of the opposite sex. It is also easy to "jump on a bandwagon," mistakenly believing that consensus represents the truth. Because there are so many techniques of persuasion, it is always important for leaders to differentiate between what is mere persuasiveness and what is valuable information.

One way to orient yourself to the way information is being presented is by asking the following:

- Does the person or source seem logical or intuitive?
- Is the informant synthesizing an opinion or analyzing what has been presented?
- Is the information divergent from the norm or unifying in scope?
- Is a holistic picture or pieces of a puzzle presented?
- Do I get the information in a sequential, simultaneous, or disjointed manner?
- Does the information source sort out the information in a hierarchical—top-down or bottom-up—manner, or does everything seem to have equal weight or value?

These questions can also be extremely helpful during a group discussion because they provide a way of aligning the direction of information being presented and often reduce conflict. Differences of opinion may remain, but it will be easier to gain insight as to why and take from each opinion something of value for future decision-making.

In addition to having a certain mental orientation in any given situation, people tend to favor certain senses over others. Ask yourself whether you prefer to read information, see information, hear information, taste information, or feel information. Most of us have come to be visual and aural to the point of not even considering the other ways of gathering information except in limited contexts, such as eating. The best clinicians have developed their ability to smell, taste, and feel information, as well as to read and hear information.

■ The Attraction of Certainty

The history of philosophy illustrates how much effort has gone into removing uncertainty from our decisions and actions. In theory development, we classify prescriptive theory as the highest form of theory because of the perceived control it offers for decision-making. One of the main reasons that commercial franchises, such as McDonald's, succeed is their appeal to those valuing reliability and predictability over surprise and uncertainty. Rieke and Sillars (1997) claim, "The attraction of certainty seems stronger than ever today. Many of the most important debates are predicated on the presumption of self-evident and absolute rights. . . . Issues of abortion, genetic engineering, in vitro fertilization, welfare . . . euthanasia . . . and many more are frequently approached in such absolute terms" (p. 7).

Leaders enjoy the perceptible comforts of certainty as much as anyone. They strive to minimize risk and find certainty in their decisions. However, leaders must recognize that valuing certainty will not provide the stability one might anticipate with such predictability. Overvaluing certainty promotes ritualistic behavior. Consider nurses who consistently have defined nursing more as fulfilling time-consuming tasks than as achieving positive patient outcomes. Not demonstrating the connection of nursing care rituals with real outcomes defines the value of nursing only from the caregiver's perspective. To prevent managing the present to the detriment of the future (Wells, 1998), leaders must balance the desire for certainty with the need for change. The degree of change versus the degree of certainty is a matter of politics and timing.

■ The Politics and Timing of Information

It is an incredibly misguided belief that politics and the timing of information can be ignored. This is because people and organizations are often competing for resources. One way to guide one's pursuit of information is to determine who is making the decisions related to an issue or a problem and when the decisions will be made. People debating each other without knowing who will ultimately make the decision or after the decision has already been made expend considerable energy and often fail to change anything.

How, what, when, where, and with whom information is shared make up the politics of information. Consider the politics of drug addiction. Whether it is a disease or a criminal act depends on who provides the information. If the person becomes addicted at age 8 versus at age 21, is it his or her fault, someone else's fault, or nobody's fault? How much federal research money should be allocated for the treatment of addicts versus the incarceration of addicts? Should law enforcement officers be required to share information about drug users with health care providers, or the other way around? The answers to any of these questions are continually redefined because of politics and the timing of information.

Leaders must know how to strategically gain and use information because the importance of information is affected, if not determined, by its timing. Consider when nurses at a large health care institution are negotiating a new contract and the press is filled with stories regarding the rising costs of health care. If the negotiations stall and a nurse strike is eminent, public support will be determined by how the public understands the issue in terms of personal costs and their own health care. If the public has the overall impression that meeting the nurses' demands will do nothing more than drive up health care costs, the nurses will find minimal public support.

In addition to understanding how to strategically use information to advance an agenda, the leader will often have to respond to damaging information. This is called *damage control*. Damaging information occurs for a variety of reasons; most often, it is due to a lack of understanding or misperceptions about a problem or an issue. Sometimes, it happens because someone wants to sabotage a project. Regardless of whether damaging information has a basis in fact, the leader must respond to it in a way that will maintain his or her support base.

Often, the value of information goes unrecognized for a long period of time. Consider that the physics for magnetic resonance imaging was developed and available for decades before imaging was used in clinical practice for diagnostic purposes. Without political support, it is difficult, if not impossible, to bring major projects to fruition. Leaders quickly learn that political support greatly enhances financial support.

■ Privacy and Information

To complicate matters, people in leadership positions are sometimes unable to share information. For example, an employee is terminated because of a serious breach of duty. The supervisor of that employee, as well as the employee, knows the situation, but the others who strongly support the employee may not. These supporters become openly hostile toward the supervisor because they perceive the termination to be unjust, yet the supervisor is bound not to convey personal information regarding the termination.

Leaders relying on technological innovations to retrieve, store, or send information must be especially concerned about their information's being captured by others when they send e-mail, use the Internet, make cellular telephone calls, or fax messages. The only way to keep outsiders from obtaining sensitive information from a computer is to not have it connected to the Internet, but this is unrealistic. A realistic option is to buy encryption software that transforms your data into code so others cannot read it. Another option to reduce the likelihood of unintentionally providing sensitive data to the wrong people by using public "proxy servers."

The entire arena of privacy and confidentiality has taken on new significance with the advent of the technology age. The privacy and confidentiality issues inherent in any form of communication—how information is gathered, stored, transmitted, and kept private—are clearly an even bigger issue when they occur electronically. An excellent source of information about electronic privacy is the Electronic Privacy Information Center (http://www.epic.org/privacy/tools.html).

PERSONAL EXPERIENCE: APPLICATION OF THE FRAMEWORK

I have always tried to see the bigger picture, perform at a high level, make a bigger impact, and develop my skills of leadership. I also enjoy relating to other influential people and having access to privileged, special, and even secret information. It is very self-affirming to be taken into the confidence of those in the inner circle. Beyond personal and professional contacts, my gateway to success has often been my ability to gain and use information more effectively than others and my approach to situations in which failure is likely. Regardless of whether I have failed or succeeded, I have used information gained from experience as invaluable in accepting bigger roles and greater responsibilities. What follows are depictions of personal scenarios that illustrate the concepts presented in this chapter.

Finding Good Sources of Information

In any work situation there are workplace politics, but academic institutions have more than their share. One only has to read Jane Smiley's *Moo* (1995) or Richard Russo's *Straight Man* (1997) to get a humorous depiction of the kind and the extent of the politics that operate in our institutions of higher learning. Universities are environments of highly educated, intelligent people competing for limited positions. To penetrate academic administration in a large university is difficult, but as a nurse faculty member, it is nearly impossible. Not unlike other professional situations, if a faculty member climbs through the ranks of tenure and promotion, many of the more senior faculty often persist in perceiving the recently promoted as unprepared to enter a leadership role above their own position.

After receiving tenure and being promoted to associate professor of nursing in 1991, I found myself unable to procure an academic administrative position. I knew I had much to offer as a nurse, as well as much to learn as an academic administrator, but I was competing against people who had achieved tenure earlier than I, many of whom had the rank of professor. One such colleague was elected to the statewide academic senate. She taught me the significance of being one of the university's four representatives to the senate—a policy-making unit composed of elected representatives from the 22 California State University (CSU) campuses at the time. Her participation in local faculty meetings revealed a far greater knowledge of what was happening in the higher education than most faculty members on campus had, knowledge apparently gained from her contacts in the academic senate and her monthly trips to the chancellor's office in Long Beach.

This colleague told me that she would be the newly installed president of a national organization the coming year. Having held a lesser but analogous role in a professional organization myself, I knew she would have to step down from the senator position to fulfill her new role as a president. Successful leadership requires a tremendous amount of energy and commitment, and my colleague's determination to be successful was apparent. I read the bylaws of the academic senate to confirm my suspicion that an ad hoc campuswide election would have to be held to determine her replacement. Using this information, I began preparing for my election as her replacement by campaigning selectively and discreetly. I also knew several people would discount the significance of the election, pretending not to care, in hopes of being "persuaded" to run. By the time my faculty colleague resigned as a statewide academic senator, it was too late for my competition to effectively mount a successful election campaign.

Several of my colleagues were surprised by my election to the senate, as indicated by their interest in how I did it. And, when I honestly shared my reasons and strategies, I gained the trust and confidence of one person who also had aspirations to enter academic administration. She became a wonderful source of information for me in my subsequent role as an associate dean. The election changed the course of my academic career in several ways. It established me as a leader in the academic community beyond nursing. I was able to participate in discussions of the latest issues and to participate in developing strategies for their resolution. Each senate session at the chancellor's office was a policy forum with educational leaders of national stature presenting directly to me as a senate member and agency representative. In summary, I gained access to better information in a more timely fashion and became a much stronger source of information for others.

Asking Questions

When I attended high school in rural Oklahoma, I had a classmate who always asked questions that led to snickers and consternation by most of the class. Her questions always seemed obvious, yet the answers were difficult and often uncomfortable for the teachers. That classmate went on to earn a doctorate from the University of Chicago, became a leading translator for the United Nations, and is quite comfortable in both fiscal and personal affairs. She became a leader.

Growing up, I also witnessed the power of asking questions by listening to my parents make purchases for their businesses. Nether parent accepted the word of vendors at face value; questions were asked that ensured what was purchased was what was really desirable and at the best price. Both my classmate and my parents helped me have the confidence to ask questions. However, it was much later before I learned how to refine my questioning to elicit the best information and to not be perceived as obnoxious for incessant or rude questioning. After all, some questions do not deserve answers.

Once while accompanying a colleague to a meeting with the nursing administration of a medical center, I bluntly asked several questions that embarrassed the administration and subsequently threatened any future collaboration. I had not done my homework or considered the feelings of those present at the meeting. My line of questioning only antagonized others by focusing on what they had not done and what they had not considered in preparing a critical care certification program. Instead of gathering information that would resolve the problems, I created a new problem. Fortunately for me, my approach was refuted in private, which enabled me to grow from the experience.

During graduate school at the University of Texas at Austin, I impulsively took a linguistic philosophy course as a break from my nursing studies. During this course, we read several texts that I still keep on my bookshelves; one of these books was *Challenges to Empiricism* by Morick (1972). This reading exposure reshaped my thinking about questions and proofs that remain with me today. However, I have had to overcome the naiveté that others share my fascination with information and welcome challenging questions or probing.

Serving on the board of directors for a professional nurses' association taught me that refutation of information can be most unpleasant when it identifies weaknesses in the ideas or information people fervently believe in. Refutation is the open expression of disagreement with the information provided (Rieke and Sillars, 1997). During one intense board meeting, I had a nurse request I meet him outside to fist fight. I learned from that experience what refutation can create and now am better prepared for the consequences.

Good questions lead to better information. Good questions led me to better schools than most of my high school classmates attended. My use of information landed me immediate employment and better jobs than many of my classmates in college acquired after graduation. Unfortunately, people may reach a plateau in their professional development that arrests their abilities as leaders. They become comfortable with a particular position and with what they know, so they do not move to new positions or take on new challenges. At times, I also have not taken the challenge.

Frequently, leaders are challenged by germane questions to determine their position on an issue. If asked at the right time and in the right way, these questions can either strengthen the leaders' position or diminish it. Such questions have pushed me out of my comfort zone and made me take up the challenge. I have also used such questioning to push others out of their comfort zones in hopes of creating movement toward a solution to a problem.

A most recent experience points to the expectations of others about questioning. As with any political body, the statewide academic senate that I joined had longstanding members. Some of them seemed to have made an academic career out of serving on the senate but had lost sight of what the real purpose of their office meant to their constituencies. A fellow new senator and I were quickly challenged by a few of these senators who made it clear we were to ask few questions. We were to accept information at its face value.

However, my colleague and I persisted in asking what we considered germane questions, and we carefully analyzed all the information presented, as well as its source. At the completion of our terms, we were commended for our efforts and contributions, and those senators who initially had challenged us had become respected colleagues.

Listening

During my service as academic senator, I participated in a retreat with the university presidents and trustees for the CSU system. I wanted to know who the real decision-makers were. What were their goals? What were their presumptions? I already knew that other persons (e.g., faculty) were trying to become the decision-makers. I purposively sat next to our university president of the time, hoping to distinguish myself as a person of substance to this person who was the leader of over 3000 other faculty and staff. I listened carefully to what my president said and what he did not say. The retreat focused on financial issues facing the CSU system, our academic mission, and where we would need to go in the future. For the first time I understood the president's position because he was not appeasing splinter groups on his home turf but working directly with other presidents and his "bosses."

Before the late 1980s, California was the envy of higher educational systems, but falling state revenues left the state's master plan vulnerable to attack. By understanding how higher education in the CSU system was financed, I easily understood that we were philosophically shifting from a state-supported system to a state-assisted system. I also became aware of battling factions over the state's master plan for higher education in the state and what the state's positions were through debate and policy proposals. I came to see the bigger picture in a much bigger way—this time with better resources, higher levels of expertise, and a new level of commitment. It was during this time that I truly learned to listen to myself and to synthesize my own position beyond what others had said or I had read.

Doing Something With the Information I Acquired

I knew if we were to shift from a state-supported institution to a state-assisted one, the faculty culture would have to change. I needed to learn more about university advancement and raising monies for program support. Subsequently, I linked university advancement, not just nursing advancement, to all my proposals and discussions with upper administration. Using the information I gained as a senator permitted me to begin laying the groundwork for a successful shift to a state-assistance plan for my college. Although many faculty members and a state policy institute were fighting against the philosophical shift to state assistance, I knew the decision to change had been made and was irrevocable.

Opportunities come in remarkable ways. The dean of our college left to become a chancellor of a community college system. Her associate dean became the interim dean, and the college's associate director for development left to become a vice president for advancement at a private institution. I had worked with the associate director for development to fill the gap in my knowledge, and I was the only faculty member perceived to be capable of filling his role until a search for a permanent associate director for development could be completed. All these changes occurred within 2 weeks, and I found myself being relieved of my teaching responsibilities and thrust into academic administration full-time as the college's new associate director for development.

Analogous to my pursuit of the academic senator's position, several of my colleagues did not recognize value in filling the associate director for development role because they were unconvinced that we were truly shifting to a state-assisted academic system. Although I never wanted to be an advancement officer, I knew what the position had to offer. I also knew that the interim dean wanted to be the permanent dean and recognized the importance of the development role. I supported him and worked hard for him. My information was correct, and success in my role as the college's associate director for development established my leadership such that I became a viable candidate for the associate dean position in the largest school in the university.

In 1993, I became the associate dean of a college with more than 5000 majors in 17 degree programs, 12 department chairs and directors, a faculty with 270 members, and a staff of 46. This was a difficult rise to a formal position of leadership considering that I was not a full professor, had been tenured for only 2 years, and had no track record as a department chair or school director within the university. The use of information, coupled with sound political strategies such as timing, placed me in a role that many of my 270 colleagues in the college coveted. Although they had not recognized the power of the other positions I held, I was now acknowledged a part of the college's inner circle.

Based on the information garnered 2 years earlier, I was not surprised in 1994 that the university would experience serious budget cuts, resulting in the elimination of two part-time associate deans and the director of health professions in my college alone. I also rediscovered that leaders don't inflict pain as much as they bear pain. We experienced the loss of the entire tenured faculty in the department of aviation, resulting in no qualified person to assume the chair position for managing a historically outstanding academic unit in the university. Subsequently, I found myself as the sole associate dean and director of health professions for the university's largest college. I also had to serve as interim chair of the aviation department, in which I had no academic preparation or experience other than familiarity with the administrative processes common to all academic units. For the first time in my professional life, I had to develop a strategy for managing information beyond just fulfilling the tasks inherent in my position as a faculty member, family member, and nurse.

My mail in one day would fill a wastebasket, and tracking documents was critical because of the legal implications, in addition to the need to keep the departments and programs operational. I soon discovered what Grove meant when he wrote, "the single most important resource that we allocate from one moment to the next is our own time" (1997, p. 203). It seemed everyone needed or wanted a piece of me.

I also reaffirmed my position that organizational theorists who do not address or consider the intuitive elements of management are making a disastrous error. Although I knew something about human cognition, I was approaching it from a purely rational-logical perspective that did not serve others or myself well. The quote by Herbert Simon (1987) and discussed by Mintzberg (1989) came full force into my thoughts about leadership:

> It is a fallacy to contrast "analytic and "intuitive" styles of management. Intuition and judgment—at least good judgment—are simply *analysis frozen into habit* and into the capacity for rapid response through recognition. Every manager needs to be able to analyze problems systematically . . . Every manager needs also to be able to respond to situations rapidly, a skill that requires cultivation of intuition and judgment over many years of experience and training. The effective manager does not have the luxury of choosing between "analytic" and "intuitive" approaches to problems. Behaving like a manager means having command of the whole range of management skills and applying them as they become appropriate (pp. 61, 63–67).

■ Managing Information and Technology

Up to 1994, I was a fairly conventional user of information, even as a scholar. It was during this time I discovered the real value of e-mail. I also discovered why traditional mail service is referred to as "snail mail." With electronic mail I established mailing lists: one for department chairs and directors, one for the dean's office staff, one for upper administration, and so forth. These lists permitted me to type a message one time, selectively attach documents, and send the message with the appropriate information to everyone at once. It also provided a timed and dated tracking mechanism for all correspondence, as well as a simple tool for reminding people of things with minimal effort. I no longer had to spend hours copying, labeling, and distributing information that frequently seemed to get lost or misplaced.

The best part of electronic mail has been my enhanced ability to communicate frequently with people around the world. I no longer have to wait days or weeks for the coming and going of mail. Beyond the initial investment, and partially because I am in a university setting, the costs have been minimal—no more expensive telephone calls for business conducted during the day.

I have always tried to learn from those around me and make contact with those who can problem solve with me whenever possible. Some of my information sources are perhaps unusual, as I have always been a reader and a closet movie critic. However, what I have gained from the two media forms has been to discover different approaches to common problems and gain exposure to other people's perspectives.

As an associate dean, I learned more about the politics of resource management and greatly expanded my information resources, especially people. I soon recognized the value of a team approach to running a university and the costs of a disjointed administration. My new mentor assigned me to important committees and asked me to chair critical task forces. I went to many regional and national meetings as a representative of the university because he knew I would make contacts there. I was able to get more connected so I could build a network, which enabled me to accept positions that were challenging but highlighted my talents.

■ Becoming Dean

Leaders recognize when it is time for a change, and the change can be a career move. With the support and information provided by others, including my two mentors, I soon recognized it was time for me to seek a dean position. I am fortunate that I did not let distance be a deterrent to my professional relationships. When there was a lull in information sharing, I initiated contact via telephone or sought people when I traveled into their areas. Mutual trust had been built by telling secrets, laying out deficiencies, highlighting weaknesses, identifying fears, and outlining strengths. There were people whom I trusted to tell me how to become a dean.

Recognizing that it was professionally risky for me to apply for administrative positions at other institutions, I needed considerable information from a variety of resources. My application to positions outside the university would indicate that I was either dissatisfied with upper administration or ready to move to another position. Either message would indicate to upper administration that I no longer had the level of commitment to my present role that was expected in a tight administration. Also, I knew there would be a high level of uncertainty, even ambiguity, in my moving from my position as associate dean in an institution where I had spent my last 19 years and now held the rank of tenured professor.

I began by perusing the position announcements in the *Chronicle of Higher Education* and consulting trusted colleagues about dean openings, as well as institutions to avoid. I went on-line to focus my search. I was able to discover much information about the mission, curricula, faculty, organizational structure and governance, and benefits at many institutions via the Internet. The contacts I had made also served as invaluable sources of information on what to do and what not to do. My currency and use of information paid off, as indicated by my success. Although many people are pleased to get one offer in a year, I completed interviews for four separate institutions and was able to choose the one that best fit my leadership goals.

As a dean I have been able to articulate a defining position for my school, as well as my personal goals. To be convincing and clear as the leader, I used the best information available to me from a variety of resources. These resources have included professional and personal contacts and the Internet, as well as written resources. I have taken advantage of having knowledge in areas outside my discipline as well as in nursing. This knowledge has enabled me to see connections and offer solutions that others fail to see.

My development as a dean has not been easy or without failure. Sometimes my lack of information has restricted my position or caused me to make a less-than-desirable decision. In addition to my successes, I have sometimes employed the wrong people, bought the wrong equipment, and even advanced the wrong position, yet I have become increasingly comfortable with the ambiguity of any information, learning much by recognizing what I do not know.

Early on, I knew the power of having information, yet I am continually learning new ways to use information. Being a dean requires me to transform information into action. It's this transformation of information that gives information its real value. I tend to divide information into four types:

1. Information needed for the job at hand
2. Information to be used in the future
3. Information that has interest but no present known value
4. Junk

To determine where any information belongs, I peruse or examine information in the context of assessing cause and effect. Understanding the difference between association and correlation versus cause and effect helps me stay focused on what is most important. I make both quantitative and qualitative comparisons among information sources as much as among the information they provide me. I look for distortions among the sources and the information they provide and ask questions to clarify, validate, and restate information. Although I enjoy novelty, I look at information more for substance than for entertainment, unless entertainment is my wish.

What often compensates for a dean's limitations is choosing good sources, having discipline, and knowing when to let go because it is time to do something else. I gather and use information toward the goal of achieving a vision—it keeps me focused on what I need to know. Most of all, to prevent information overload, I gather and use information until I am tired, not until I am finished. Junk is immediately discarded; information of plausible or actual future value is stored mentally, technologically (e.g., database), or on paper, and the remainder is used at the moment. I continue to put far more energy and time into using information than into storing it. Fortunately, the exponential capacity for information storage by computers and zip drives and the accessibility to databases on-line operate in my favor.

SUMMARY

Being a leader is exciting, exhausting, sometimes nightmarish, but mostly wonderful. My leadership skills have taken me from a small town in Oklahoma to my present deanship in a private university in the state of Washington. I have come to recognize that information technology with the phenomenal growth of the Internet and e-mail applications is redefining health care practices in terms of the leader's required skill set, as well as the health care institution's strategic planning for the future. Certainly, the informational role of the leader is being affected by technology, but what is being redefined pertains more to politics and timing of information—that is, who gets what and when.

Leaders often work with others in a context much bigger than a particular project or discipline. To be successful, it is critical that nursing leaders be aware that compromising autonomy is difficult for people who do not make much money but who are devoted to their work. The issues surrounding nursing to this day pertain to autonomy, accountability, and responsibility. The better information nurses have and the more able they are to transform it into appropriate action, the more comfortable nurses will be in any leadership role.

Nursing leaders increasingly will have to build and connect constituencies. This requires gathering, analyzing, and synthesizing information in new ways. If nurses are unable to gain access to the databases that presently dominate health care decision-making, we will have to create substantial databases that are better and provide key decision-makers with information that has less uncertainty and will reduce the risks while promoting better health care for all. After all, there is great power in information if one knows how to get it and what to do with it.

REFERENCES

Ash, M. K. (1997). The art of listening. In P. Krass (Ed.). *The book of business wisdom* (pp. 137–139). New York: John Wiley.

Baruch, B. M. (1997). My investment philosophy. In P. Krass (Ed.). *The book of business wisdom* (pp. 409–413). New York: John Wiley.

Bryan-Brown, C. W., & Dracup, K. (1998). Thinking outside the box and other resolutions. *American Journal of Critical Care, 7*(1), pp. 1–3.

Burke, J. (Feb. 1998). Government for a world long gone. In D. McKenna (Ed.). *Government technology: Special edition* (pp. 8–15) Sacramento, Calif.: Government Technology.

Dickenson-Hazard, N. (1996). Technology now. *Reflections, 22*(2), 3.

Federwisch, A. (1997). Cybersightings: Patient resources on the Web. *Nurseweek, 10*(23), 7.

Grove, A. S. (1997). Your most precious resource: Your time. In P. Krass (Ed.). *The book of business wisdom* (pp. 203–207). New York: John Wiley.

Henderson, J., & Poulin, M. (1998). Guide to critical thinking about what you see on the web. URL: http://www.ithaca.edu/library/training/hott.html.

Iowa Intervention Project (1997). Proposal to bring nursing into the information age. *Image: Journal of Nursing Scholarship, 29*(3), 275–281.

Jacox, A. (1995). Practice and policy implications of clinical and administrative databases. In N. M. Lang (Ed.). *Nursing data systems: The emerging framework* (pp. 161–165). Washington, DC: American Nurses Association.

Jensen Group. (1997). Changing how we work: The search for a simpler way (http://www.simpler work.com/d/d18.htm).

Jones, L. D. (1997). Building the information infrastructure required for managed care. *Image: Journal of Nursing Scholarship, 29*(4), 377–382.

Kelly, H. H., & Michela, J. L. (1980). Attribution theory and research. *Annual Review of Psychology, 31*, 457–501.

Krass, P. (Ed.). (1997). *The book of business wisdom: Classic writings by the legends of commerce and industry.* New York: John Wiley.

Laudon, K. C., & Laudon, J. P. (1997). *Essentials of management information systems: Organization and technology.* Upper Saddle River, N.J.: Prentice-Hall.

Levinson, H. (1995). Why behemoths fall. In P. M. Williams (Ed.). *Leading transformational change* (pp. 6–14). New York: McGraw-Hill.

Lewis, D. (1996). Dying for information? An investigation into the effects of information overload in the UK and worldwide. Report commissioned by Reuters Business Information.

Mintzberg, H. (1989). *Mintzberg on management: Inside the strange world of organizations.* New York: The Free Press.

Morick, H. (Ed.). (1972). Challenges to empiricism. Belmont, Calif.: Wadsworth.

Rae-Dupree, J. (1997, October 6). Dominating with data. In Business Monday section of the *San Jose Mercury News*, pp. 1E, 4E–5E.

Rieke, R. D., & Sillars, M. O. (1997). *Argumentation and critical decision making.* New York: Longman.

Russo, R. (1997). *Straight man.* New York: Random House.

Sikorsky, I. I. (1997). A mysterious faculty. In P. Krass (Ed.). *The book of business wisdom* (pp. 365–368). New York: John Wiley.

Simon, H. A. (1987). Making management decisions: The role of intuition and emotion. *Academy of Management Executive, 2*, 58–63.

Smiley, J. (1995). *Moo.* New York: Alfred A. Knopf.

Turley, J. P. (1996). Informatics model for nursing. *Image: Journal of Nursing Scholarship, 28*(4), 309–313.

Wells, S. (1998). *Choosing the future: The power of strategic thinking.* Boston: Butterworth-Heinemann.

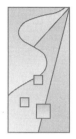

Index

Note: Page numbers in *italics* refer to illustrations.